Managed Behavioral Health Care Handbook

Edited By

E. Clarke Ross, DPA
Chief Executive Officer
Children and Adults with
Attention-Deficit/Hyperactivity Disorder, Inc. (CHADD)
Landover, Maryland

AN ASPEN PUBLICATION®
Aspen Publishers, Inc.
Gaithersburg, Maryland
2001

Library of Congress Cataloging-in-Publication Data

Ross, E. Clarke.
Managed behavioral health care handbook / edited by E. Clarke Ross.
p. cm.
Includes bibliographical references and index.
ISBN 0-8342-1727-9
1. Managed mental health care—United States—Handbooks, manuals, etc. I. Title.
RC480.5.M322 2001
2001021808

Orders: (800) 638-8437
Customer Service: (800) 234-1660

About Aspen Publishers • For more than 40 years, Aspen has been a leading professional
publisher in a variety of disciplines. Aspen's vast information resources are available in both
print and electronic formats. We are committed to providing the highest quality information
available in the most appropriate format for our customers. Visit Aspen's Internet site for
more information resources, directories, articles, and a searchable version of Aspen's full
catalog, including the most recent publications: **www.aspenpublishers.com**
Aspen Publishers, Inc. • The hallmark of quality in publishing
Member of the worldwide Wolters Kluwer group.

Editorial Services: Erin McKindley
Library of Congress Catalog Card Number: 2001021808
ISBN: 0-8342-1727-9

Printed in the United States of America

1 2 3 4 5

This book is dedicated to
Harry Schnibbe and *Elsie Helsel*, my mentors during
early professional life;
Steve Chitwood, for guidance and support during my
doctoral studies;
*Earl Cunerd, Harry Schnibbe, Henry Harbin,
Laurie Flynn*, and the board executive committee
of CHADD for giving me senior management
opportunities;
Each of this book's authors for sharing their
knowledge, insight, and time;
Ron Honberg, a daily role model of personal
commitment and ethics;
Kim Encarnation, for daily quality support and
loyalty; and
Beth Ross for dedicating her life to Andrew.

CONTENTS

CONTRIBUTORS

Neal Adams, MD, MPH
Director
Santa Cruz County Mental Health and Substance Abuse Services
Santa Cruz, California

Christy L. Beaudin, PhD, LCSW, CPHQ
Corporate Director, Quality Improvement
PacifiCare Behavioral Health
Van Nuys, California

Martin D. Cohen, MSW
President/CEO
MetroWest Community Health Care Foundation
Framingham, Massachusetts

Allen S. Daniels, EdD, LISW
CEO, Alliance Behavorial Care
Cincinnati, Ohio
Professor, Clinical Psychiatry
University of Cincinnati, Department of Psychiatry
Cincinnati, Ohio

Stephen L. Day, MSW
Executive Director
Technical Assistance Collaborative, Inc.
Boston, Massachusetts

Veronica V. Goff, MS
Principal
Business Health Network
Washington, DC

Daniel Lieberman, MD
Northeast Regional Medical Director
ValueOptions, Inc.
New York City, New York

David Mee-Lee, MD
Assistant Clinical Professor
University of California at Davis
School of Medicine, Department of Psychiatry
Davis, California

Stephen P. Melek, FSA, MAAA
Principal and Consulting Actuary
Milliman & Robertson, Inc.
Denver, Colorado

John A. Morris, MSW, CHE
Professor and Director
South Carolina Center for Innovation in Public Mental Health
SCDMH/USC School of Medicine
Columbia, South Carolina

Charles G. Ray, MEd
President/CEO
National Council for Community Behavioral Healthcare
Rockville, Maryland

Sara Rosenbaum, JD
Hirsh Professor of Health Law and Policy
The George Washington University School of Public Health
   and Health Services
Department of Health Services Management and Policy
Washington, DC

E. Clarke Ross, DPA
CEO
Children and Adults with Attention-Deficit/Hyperactivity Disorder,
  Inc. (CHADD)
Landover, Maryland

Ian A. Shaffer, MD, MMM
Executive Vice President/COO
University Alliance for Behavioral Care, Inc.
Reno, Nevada

Joel B. Teitelbaum, JD, LLM
Assistant Research Professor
The George Washington University School of Public Health
  and Health Services
Department of Health Services Management and Policy
Washington, DC

Jerome V. Vaccaro, MD
President/CEO
PacifiCare Behavioral Health, Inc.
Van Nuys, California

FOREWORD

The managed behavioral health care movement is certainly among the most important changes in behavioral health care during the last decade. Paralleled only by the introduction of new pharmaceutical agents for the treatment of depression and schizophrenia, managed care has revolutionized the way we conceptualize, organize, finance, deliver, and regulate care.

The movement was driven largely by concerns with rapid cost inflation and a hope that these costs could be contained and quality of service improved through the active management of behavioral health care. In part, the movement also was motivated by a frustration with the effectiveness of process regulation for ensuring quality of care and a hope that, by shifting from a regulatory to an outcome driven scheme, we could control costs and improve the well-being of insured populations. There was even some hope that by better leveraging our public funds through managed care we might be able to expand coverage to parts of the uninsured population.

As is clear from the material included in *Managed Behavioral Health Care Handbook*, these hopes have only been partially realized. Generally, cost containment objectives have been achieved if analysis is restricted to budgeted costs rather than overall social costs. In some instances access to care has also improved as supply side controls have better managed the front door of the treatment system. Knowledge about improvements in quality and outcomes of care under managed care arrangements is still quite limited although there exists little systematic data to indicate that either quality or outcomes have deteriorated substantially. Hopes of abandoning a regulatory model in favor of one that is principally informed by outcomes have not been realized as the adequacy of outcome measures and the ability to link processes of care to outcomes has been disappointing. Purchasers, particularly public purchasers, have also shown a reluctance to abandon process regulations.

What has clearly resulted from efforts to implement and to understand managed behavioral health care, though, is the realization that we continue to confront a series of chronically difficult problems in behavioral health. Determining how to improve clinical and management practices to better conform to our knowledge base is among the most difficult of these problems. The promulgation of treatment protocols—a hallmark of managed care, utilization management techniques, certification and accreditation efforts, performance indicators, and improved market mechanisms do not seem to have solved long-standing problems with improving practice in real world environments. Bringing model technologies to scale in a chaotic treatment and management environment continues to be a challenge.

In light of these persistent questions, the value of *Managed Behavioral Health Care Handbook* is to help identify and reflect upon the strategies that have characterized contemporary efforts at managing behavioral health care. It is only through clearly naming and describing these strategies and understanding their effects in real world settings that we will be able to improve our treatment systems. We must continue this dialogue if we are to operationalize the knowledge from our science base and improve the quality of behavioral health care.

David L. Shern, PhD
Dean and Professor
The Louis de la Parte Florida Mental Health Institute
University of South Florida
Tampa, Florida

PREFACE

Managed behavioral health care is big business. Almost 177 million Americans are enrolled in managed behavioral health care organizations (MBHOs) (Open Minds, 1999). These MBHOs had estimated 1995 revenues of $2.5 billion (Oss & Moghul, 1996). Today, given the significant growth in enrollments, aggregate MBHO revenue may be more than $5 billion. These revenue figures are within the context of total 1997 national mental health and substance abuse treatment expenditures of $85.3 billion (Coffey et al., 2000).

Managed behavioral health care is both a significant economic enterprise and an enterprise undergoing constant change. This book is intended as a guide to the essential elements of managed behavioral health care and the challenges facing this field. It is not a comprehensive reference to managed behavioral health care, but a stimulus about the behavioral health care field offered by management practitioners. It is a practical handbook written by senior-level executives who are, or who have been, facing the realities of managing care within a fixed budget. All are recognized national authorities within the behavioral health care field, and many also have managed care in large, nationally based health care systems. As nationally renowned experts, they grasp academic theory and concept, but what makes them unique is their frontline experience in making managed care *work*.

The practitioners assembled within these covers offer an excellent overview of the issues confronting managed behavioral health care. By reading the material contained in this handbook, readers will understand the core components of managed behavioral health care and appreciate the controversies and public policy issues confronting managed behavioral health care. Essential elements include forms and structures of managing care, payment arrangements, and core operational concepts such as medical necessity. The perspectives of purchasers of care and organized interest groups are offered. Patient rights and consumer advocacy are reviewed, particularly the existing legal protections and existing mechanisms for advocacy. The separation of behavioral and general health care is analyzed. Special populations of the chronically ill—persons with serious mental illness and persons with addictive disorders—are explained. Documented accountability for performance, including the ability of provider-sponsored organizations, is discussed. Professionals in the field—health plan executives, members of boards of directors, current and potential investors, legislators, executive branch governmental agencies, and self-insured employers—will benefit from reading the essential elements contained in this book, as will consumers, families, health plan enrollees, and students of health care administration.

The first chapter presents an overview of managed behavioral health care. It is divided into two sections. The first covers more general topics, such as the forms in which managed behavioral health care is delivered, the carving out of behavioral health care from primary care, the success of managed care in controlling costs, the substitution of outpatient for inpatient care, and the implementation of mental health coverage parity. The second section discusses a range of public policy issues, including the adequacy of behavioral health care services, the role of the concept of medical necessity in restricting care, and the ability of health professionals to manage care directly in provider-sponsored organizations. References to later chapters are included in the discussion of each issue so the readers will know where to look for further information.

The variety of managed care payment arrangements is the subject of Chapter 2. The tendency of these arrangements is to transfer risk to the providers of care, although some of the arrangements do protect providers against excessive losses. The chapter also discusses actuarial models, their use in setting capitation rates, and keys to achieving success in capitation contracts. Providers about to embark on a capitation contract need to know how to manage various kinds of risk, including the risk of underpricing and the risk of large fluctuations in demand for services. The chapter ends with a helpful account of risk-management tools.

Chapter 3 is devoted to the topic of medical necessity. The concept of medical necessity is used in managed care to deny health plan enrollees the provision of some services (those deemed unnecessary) and thereby keep down medical costs. The chapter distinguishes medical necessity from medical appropriateness, discusses one definition of medical necessity, presents two examples showing how the definition might be used to certify or deny services, and examines reasons for variability in behavioral health care treatment, such as differences in training and philosophies of care.

Chapter 4 deals with the ongoing separation between behavioral health care and general health care (primary care) and explores ways of integrating the two. One of the most important ways is to increase communication between health plans and consumers as well as communication among practitioners. Other strategies include enhancing the effectiveness of health screening (so that behavioral health problems are detected early), increasing the accountability of behavioral health care providers (so that other health professionals will have confidence in the efficacy of their efforts), establishing best practices, developing "virtual" systems of care, and improving the education and training of practitioners.

Patients' rights and the regulation of managed care organizations, especially in regard to treatment and coverage decision making, form the core of Chapter 5. The first section provides a historical account of patients' rights, beginning in the fee-for-service era and continuing through the transition to managed care brought about by the passage of the Employee Retirement Income Security Act of 1974. The next section presents key definitions for understanding the issues associated with patients' rights in a managed care environment, including definitions of macro and micro coverage decisions, utilization review, internal and external review of coverage determinations, practice guidelines, and medical necessity. The next section covers legal issues, such as the regulation of utilization review standards, the right to appeal an adverse coverage decision, the right to obtain an external review of a coverage decision, the right to judicial review, the evidentiary standards governing the review process, and penalties for noncompliance with treatment orders. The final section describes the consumer bill of rights and responsibilities that was drafted by the Advisory Commission on Consumer Protection and Quality in the Health Care Industry upon request by President Clinton.

Chapters 6 and 7 discuss purchaser expectations—what purchasers want and expect when seeking to contract with managed care organizations for the provision of behavioral health care coverage. Chapter 6 examines the desires of private purchasers (i.e., employers). Employers are aware that behavioral health problems, especially depression, can seriously impact productivity, and thus they are concerned about treatment effectiveness as well as keeping costs down. In fact, because of the lack of meaningful quality indicators, employers are designing their own, and some employers have found that limiting behavioral health care benefits increases psychiatric disability costs and productivity losses. Public purchasers (state and local governments) are also interested in suppressing costs and improving quality. In particular, they look to managed care as a means to enhance the management and delivery of mental health and substance abuse services, expand the range of such services, and ease the administrative burden of managing public health systems. Chapter 7 ends with two case studies in which government entities contracted with managed care organizations to provide behavioral health care.

Chapter 8 is a critical account of the performance of managed care in serving persons with severe mental disabilities. Whereas employees, as a whole, are basically healthy and usually suffer only short-term and relatively mild mental disabilities, the unemployed, who tend to be covered by Medicaid, often have long-term mental illnesses (which, in some cases, account for their unemployment). Therefore, managed care organizations can offer private purchasers (companies) reasonable capitation rates and provide good care within the limits of their capitation-generated income but yet be unable to adequately treat the seriously ill for the same capitation rates, which puts pressure on them to disenroll such patients or give them insufficient care. Chapter 8 identifies four areas in which public managed care systems have done poorly and describes ways in which they could improve their performance. First, they need to increase the integration of care delivery; second, they need to ensure adequate capitation payments in order to cover the needs of the severely ill; third, they need to increase provider accountability through measuring performance and consumer satisfaction; and fourth, they need to foster meaningful consumer and family participation in operations and decision making.

Chapter 9 discusses how managed care organizations are dealing with another special population, persons with addictive disorders. The first half of the chapter covers the general kinds of treatment that are now in use, including complications-driven treatment; diagnosis, program-driven treatment; individualized, clinically driven treatment; and clinical, outcomes-driven treatment (which, at this time, is more promise than reality, given the current lack of pertinent outcomes data). The second half of the chapter focuses on the needs of persons with addictive disorders and on improving service provision. The chapter explains "where to start in getting there from here," and it covers structural, access, process, and outcomes issues in addiction treatment managed care. Finally, it lists some of the challenges faced by the leaders in this field.

Chapters 10 and 11 both deal with the issue of accountability. Chapter 10 discusses performance measurement, including associated ethical concerns. It outlines the state of the art and highlights one of the major problems in this area: the proliferation of inconsistent performance measurement systems. It goes on to describe attempts by leaders in the behavioral health care field to develop a core set of accepted measures that would allow valid comparisons of different health plans and different providers. Those working toward this goal found they first had to develop a common taxonomy. They then organized the performance measures into three domains: access (the ability of health plan enrollees to receive services), process (the provision of services), and outcomes (the results of the care provided). The chapter notes that the "consensus set" of indicators has some limitations and may not adequately address concerns regarding children and persons with addictive disorders. It also points to other challenges, including the lack of needed performance measurement training among the health care work force, the lack of funds to support performance measurement, and the added technical burden that demands for accountability will place on information management systems.

Chapter 11 addresses the lack of trust that consumers feel toward managed care agents and providers and the importance, for managed care organizations, of measuring consumer satisfaction. The bulk of the chapter consists of a series of case studies of attempts to use consumer satisfaction teams to discover what consumers like and dislike about the care they have been given. It also describes the use of other types of third-party entities for increasing the accountability of managed care organizations, including facility- and program-monitoring teams and ombudsman programs.

Whether provider-sponsored organizations can successfully manage care is the question asked by Chapter 12. This is an interesting issue, because in the old fee-for-service environment (where providers had an incentive to increase the number of billable encounters), "overutilization" of health care resources was among the factors that motivated the transition to managed care. Chapter 12 first provides a brief history of the transition to managed care and offers thoughts about future directions. It then reviews the major stages that a provider-sponsored organization will usually go through on the way to becoming a managed care organization. In the next section, it describes the structure of a typical managed behavioral health care organization, including the main organizational elements and the chief functions, such as utilization management, claims adjudication, contract management, and marketing and business development. It then presents the results of a survey of behavioral health provider-sponsored organizations that indicate that such organizations can indeed manage care successfully. This claim is further defended in the chapter's conclusion, which cites certain characteristics of provider-sponsored organizations that give these organizations an advantage over other managed care organizations.

Chapter 13 deals with the issue of regulation in an environment where interest groups with varying agendas are in competition. It starts with a general analysis of interest group competition and goes on to consider the views of accountability of different interest groups in the health care field. Two foci of conflict are identified: control over finances and control over delivery of care. As part of the battle over these, some groups, especially consumer advocate groups, are calling for the regulation of health plans. Chapter 13 lists some of the recommendations of the Advisory Commission on Consumer Protection and Quality in the Health Care Industry and outlines the provisions of recent federal patients' bill of rights legislation as a way of indicating the core regulatory issues. The chapter ends with a discussion of a public utility model of health care regulation. Using this model, the federal government would establish a health care equivalent to the Securities and Exchange Commission. The mandate of this commission might be to develop measures for comparing plans, develop standardized reporting forms, ensure the disclosure of required information, and generally oversee the health care market.

Chapter 14 consists of a review of the contents of the book and a brief summary of the major conclusions.

This handbook would not be possible without the energy, experience, and willingness of leading managed behavioral health care practitioners to offer their observations and views. Working with these authors over the last several years, I have come to appreciate their honesty, forthrightness, and hard work in preparing their chapters, as well as their commitment to their field. May practitioners, professionals, and students benefit from their efforts.

In addition to the unselfish contributions of the authors, this handbook benefited from the conscientious work of Kim Encarnation, who assembled the fragments of chapters into a coherent whole and facilitated regular communication between the editor and the authors, and Erin McKindley, who took disjoined phrases, sentences, and paragraphs and molded them into clearly phrased and comprehensible statements, while also ensuring that the bibliographic citations were as complete and accurate as possible.

REFERENCES

Coffey, R., Tami, M., King, E., Harwood, H., McKusick, D., Genuardi, J., Dilonardo, J., & Buck, J. (2000, July). *National estimates of expenditures for mental health and substance abuse treatment, 1997*. SMA 00–3499. Rockville, MD: Substance Abuse and Mental Health Services Administration.

Open Minds. (1999). *Open Minds' yearbook of managed behavioral health market share in the United States, 1999–2000*. Gettysburg, PA: Open Minds.

Oss, M. & Moghul, A. (1996). The managed behavioral health care industry: Overview and future prospects. In: *1997 Behavioral managed care sourcebook*. New York: Faulkner and Gray.

CHAPTER 1

An Overview of Managed Behavioral Health Care

E. Clarke Ross

Purpose: This chapter discusses the major issues facing the managed behavioral health care field.

Major Topics: This chapter addresses Forms of Delivery, The Carve-Out Industry, Historical Context, Cost Controls, Service Substitution, The Impact of Parity Mandates, Adequate Services, Coordinated Care, Medical Necessity, Accountability, Enrollee Participation, Conflict and Distrust, Confidentiality, Integrating Behavioral and Primary Care, and Providers as Management Agents.

The introduction of managed care has, without question, caused dramatic changes in our nation's health care system, including changes in the financing and delivery of behavioral health care services. But what is managed care? For purposes of this book, we can use the definition given by Rosenbaum and Teitelbaum in Chapter 5:

> Managed care is any health insuring arrangement in which the corporate entity, either directly or through subcontracts, enters into a formal contractual arrangement with one or more purchasers to both insure a defined group of members and provide the members with care and services delivered through a network of providers selected by the entity and subject to its controls. (p. 94)

Although managed care companies come in many varieties, "the merger of coverage and care into a single corporate structure is what distinguishes managed care from earlier indemnity or service benefit plans that gave physicians and health professionals full discretion over participation and treatment decisions. In managed care, a single entity empowers itself through its control over providers' access to patients to effectively make treatment decisions by virtue of its coverage decisions" (p. 94).

Dyer (1992), relying on Boland (1991), offers a clearer but less legally oriented definition: "Capitated prospective payment to preferred providers based on a performance contracting system: whereby the provider assumes financial risk for the treatment of illness; preferred, whereby providers must demonstrate quality and accessibility; and performance, whereby the provider must earn the reimbursement."

The purpose of introducing managed care is "to control costs through improved efficiency and coordination, to reduce unnecessary or inappropriate utilization, to increase access to preventive care, and to maintain or improve quality of care" (Edmunds et al., 1997, p. 15).

MANAGED BEHAVIORAL HEALTH CARE ISSUES

Managed behavioral health care is currently associated with five major issues:

1. Forms of delivery
2. Carving out of behavioral health care services
3. Ability to control costs
4. Substitution of outpatient behavioral health care for inpatient care
5. Implementation of parity for behavioral health care in health benefit coverage

Forms of Delivery

Although managed behavioral health care is delivered in many ways, managed behavioral health care organizations (MBHOs) dominate the market for such care (Open Minds, 1999). MBHOs deliver services either through (1) direct contracts with payers (known as *carve-outs* because behavioral health care is carved out from other health care) or through (2) subcontracts with managed care organizations (MCOs), which contract directly with the payers.

Other important types of managed care organizations include the full-service health maintenance organization (HMO) and the preferred provider organization (PPO). A full-service HMO provides comprehensive medical care, including behavioral health care, for a fixed annual fee. HMOs come in four varieties: the group model, the individual practice association, the network model, and the staff model.

In a PPO, which is based on a traditional fee-for-service care arrangement, health plan enrollees receive services through a "preferred" network of providers. When an enrollee goes outside of the network (which is allowed), the enrollee is typically required to pay a higher copayment.

A point-of-service (POS) plan is a type of PPO. Primary care physicians are usually the first providers of intervention, and, like in other PPOs, enrollees are charged significant additional copayments when they go outside the network.

Although MBHOs, HMOs, and PPOs deliver the majority of behavioral health care services, the following types of organizations also play a role in the behavioral health care market:

- Administrative services organizations (ASOs) perform administrative services only (e.g., claims processing) and assume no financial risk.
- Employee assistance programs (EAPs) assist employees, family members, and employers in finding solutions to workplace and personal problems.
- Integrated EAPs are assistance programs provided to employees as part of their enrollment in an MCO or MBHO.
- Stand-alone utilization review (UR) or case management organizations clinically review inpatient and/or outpatient services. They also may have case management responsibilities for certain individuals with substantial health challenges. These organizations are usually paid a set fee for each clinical review or each case managed.

Carving Out of Behavioral Health Care Services

The idea behind carving out services of a certain type, such as behavioral health care services, is that it allows the services to be supervised by experts who are especially knowledgeable in the appropriate field and who would seem better able to manage costs. Numerous reasons have been given to explain why so many Americans are enrolled in carve-outs (176.8 million, according to Open Minds [1999]). Among them are the following:

- Many HMOs find the behavioral health benefit too difficult to manage (Surles, 1997).
- Many employees believe MBHOs increase benefit levels and improve the quality of care (Mihalik & Scherer, 1998; Umland, 1997).
- MBHOs deliver more comprehensive behavioral health services than HMOs (Umland, 1997). This belief was confirmed in a Florida comparative study (Shern & Robinson, 1999), which showed that a greater proportion of health plan enrollees and a greater proportion of adults with serious mental illness were served in MBHOs, a greater proportion of schizophrenics received an atypical antipsychotic medication, a greater proportion of persons with major depression received selective serotonin reuptake inhibitor (SSRI) medications, and a greater proportion of individuals discharged from an inpatient facility were seen as outpatients within 30 days of discharge.
- MBHOs are better able to track behavioral health care expenditures (Mihalik & Scherer, 1998; Patterson, 1998).
- MBHOs are better at close tracking of behavioral health care utilization (Patterson, 1998).
- Full-service HMOs and integrated MCOs sometimes do not include a large enough population of behavioral health utilizers to negotiate discounted rates with providers over wide geographic areas (Mihalik & Scherer, 1998).
- MCOs tend to spend most of their money on physical health and offer minimal behavioral health benefits because of the lack of parity between physical health care and behavioral health care in benefit design (Happ, 1998).
- MBHOs use specialized providers and historic community providers and understand how to flex benefits to wrap around consumers (Happ, 1998). The experiences of 180,000 enrollees in United Behavioral Health and Pacific Bell between 1988 and 1995 indicate that MBHOs offer easier access to specialists (Goldman, McCulloch, & Sturm, 1997).
- Historically, mental illness and addiction have been viewed as "fundamentally different" from physical illness (Wiggins, 1997).

Ability To Control Cost

The U.S. Surgeon General (1999) concluded that the

> managed care provision of mental health services emerged partially in response to the overutilization of costly inpatient hospitalization by adolescents in the 1980s. The purpose of managed care has been to control spiraling mental health service costs, mostly by limiting hospital stays and rigorously managing outpatient service usage. . . . Managed care has shortened hospital stays and increased the use of short-term therapy models. Managed care also has lowered reimbursements for services provided by both individual professionals and institutions. This has been accompanied by the construction of provider networks, under which professionals and institutions agree to accept lower than customary fees as a tradeoff for access to patients in the network. (p. 182)

The Surgeon General further observed that

> since 1992, managed care has begun to penetrate the public sector. The prime impetus for this has been an attempt to control the costs of Medicaid, in both the general health and mental health arenas. . . . However, Medicaid populations tend to have a higher prevalence of children with serious emotional disturbance than that seen in privately insured populations. Those children generally need longer-term care. Managed care strategies, which developed in the private sector, are geared toward a relatively low utilization of mental health services by a population whose mental health needs tend to be short term and acute in nature. As a result, the kinds of cost-cutting measures used by managed care organizations, such as reduction of hospital days and encouragement of short-term outpatient therapies, have not worked as well in the public sector with seriously emotionally disturbed children as they have in the private sector. (p. 185)

The Surgeon General went on to describe the phenomenon of cost-shifting and mention the possibility that overall cost savings were not in fact being realized:

Advocates express concern that the restrictions of public managed care on mental health services shift costs of diagnosis and
treatment to other agencies, a process known as cost-shifting.
Under public managed care, hospitalization for mental disorder
is being substantially cut, with youths being discharged from the
hospital before adequate personal and/or community safety plans
can be instituted. Child welfare and juvenile justice agencies
have been compelled to create and pay for services to support
those children who are no longer kept in the hospitals. Thus,
while Medicaid's mental health costs may be decreasing in such
cases, there may be a substantial cost increase to the other
agencies involved, resulting in little if any overall cost saving. (p.
185)

Nonetheless, according to the Institute of Medicine, "Managed care
methods are growing at a faster rate in the behavioral health care sector
than in the rest of the health care system because of their demonstrated
ability to control costs in private health plans and because states are turning
to managed care as a strategy to control Medicaid costs" (Edmunds et al.,
1997, p. 241).

The foremost success of managed behavioral health care is the area of
cost control. Examples include the following:

- "Major corporations such as Dupont, Dow, Federal Express, and
  Xerox have reported cost reductions of 30%–50% over one or two
  years and have increased the flexibility of their mental health benefits
  by eliminating certain coverage limits" (Frank, McGuire, & Newhouse,
  1995, p. 53).
- "Some large employers, such as Xerox, Sterling-Winthrop, Alcan
  Aluminum, and Conoco, have reported overall savings in plan costs
  for mental health/substance abuse care of about 40% over two years
  after the introduction of managed care" (Frank & McGuire, 1995, p.
  108).
- "Mental health services, which once accounted for 17% of employee
  health costs, were cut to 8% of the total after the [Bell South Corpora-
  tion] adopted a managed care program emphasizing alternatives to
  hospitalization" (Pear, 1996).
- Initial results from the Massachusetts Medicaid Mental Health project
  showed that (1) persons using services increased 5%, (2) expenditures

were reduced to 22%, (3) hospital readmissions were reduced, and (4) a more comprehensive array of community-based services were provided (Callahan, Shepard, & Beinecke, 1994).

- The U.S. Department of Health and Human Services Office of Inspector General (DHHS OIG) (2000a) documented that four of seven Medicaid-managed mental health programs saved from $4 million to $12 million the first year, compared with the previous year's fee-for-service expenditures. The other three states limited expenditures to the previous year's expenditures. Four of these states returned "off the top" savings to the state's general fund. The other states used the savings to expand Medicaid to non-Medicaid-eligible persons or to pay for managed care administration.

Substitution of Outpatient Behavioral Health Care for Inpatient Care

The Institute of Medicine (IOM) concluded that "in the late 1980s, the majority (70%) of mental health funds spent by Medicaid and private insurance went for inpatient care, leading many researchers, clinicians, and advocates to question the imbalance and to search for policy changes. Only the introduction of managed care arrangements has led to a significant shift away from costly and often unnecessary inpatient stays to a more appropriate range of outpatient and community-based care" (Edmunds et al., 1997, p. 16).

Study after study (Frank & McGuire, 1995; Frank, McGuire, & Newhouse, 1995) has documented that when managed behavioral health care is introduced, inpatient care declines, psychotherapy declines, and alternative services such as residential treatment, day treatment, psychiatric rehabilitation, and case management increase. Examples include the following:

- In 1993, Value Behavioral Health New York State Employees experienced the following: (1) mental health and substance abuse services increased 20% from the previous year, (2) acute inpatient hospital admissions declined from 6 to 3.8 per 1,000 persons from the previous year, (3) New York State saved $25 million from the previous year, (4) use of outpatient chemical dependency treatment visits rose from 20 to

71.6 per 1,000 persons, and (5) admissions for alternative levels of care increased from 0 to 1.5 per 1,000 persons (Shaffer, 1995).

• From 1986 through 1994 in the Virginia–North Carolina region, FHC (First Hospital Corporation) Options Civilian Health and Medical Program of the Uniformed Services (CHAMPUS) experienced the following: (1) persons enrolled increased from 219,764 to 256,839, (2) persons receiving services increased from 7,600 to 19,180, (3) the average length of hospital stay declined from 58.11 to 7.2 days, (4) the average cost per inpatient admission declined from $18,539 to $2,013, and (5) partial hospitalizations and related day admissions increased from 0 to 3.2 per 1,000 persons (Krupnick, 1995).

Such substitution has resulted in significant tensions between mental health professionals and providers and great hostility toward MCOs, as Exhibit 1–1 shows.

A DHHS OIG report (2000a) documented that seven state Medicaid-managed mental health programs had "dramatic declines" in inpatient costs. One state reduced inpatient costs from 51% of mental health costs to 17% in one year. In two states, there was a reduction of 40% to 50% in available psychiatric hospital beds. In one state, the average length of stay dropped from 30 to 20 days.

Four of these seven states documented increased utilization of services from 1% to 2% after conversion to a managed care system. The seven

---

Exhibit 1–1 Managed Care Networks: Referrals and Reimbursements—Employer Plans, Outpatient Services

1994 Indemnity		1995 MBHO
Referrals		Referrals
85%	Psychiatrists	11%
10%	Psychologists	33%
5%	Social workers	56%
Reimbursements		Reimbursements
$150	Average psychiatrist visit	$90
$100	Average psychologist visit	$75
$85	Average social worker visit	$65

Source: Data from M. Oss and A. Moghul, The Managed Behavioral Health Care Industry: Overview and Future Prospects, in *1997 Behavioral Managed Care Sourcebook*, p. 5, © 1996, Faulkner and Gray, Inc.

states developed new services that previously did not exist—residential services, vocational services, respite care services, in-home programs, clubhouses, day services, and personal services.

In six states, psychiatric hospital readmission rates were higher under managed care, the increases ranging from 4% to 9%. Only one state did not see any "noticeable increase." The DHHS OIG (2000a) concluded that "lower average length of stays and increased readmission rates may indicate that persons with serious mental illnesses are being released from inpatient care too quickly" (p. 1).

In a separate report, the DHHS OIG (2000b) concluded that "reductions of inpatient care for children was greater than that for adults" (p. 2). One state reported that the percentage of children utilizing inpatient care was down 40%, compared with a decrease of 2% for adults during the same period. Another state reported a 30% decrease in psychiatric hospital admissions for children, compared with a decrease of about 6% for adults during the same period.

While outpatient programs expanded in all seven states, "the number of children that access services are still generally below the level of access for adults" (DHHS OIG, 2000b, p. 9). In one state, the rate of adults accessing outpatient mental health services was 123.7 per 1,000 while the child rate was 54.8 per 1,000. In another state, while 6% of adults accessed outpatient services, only 3% of children accessed such services.

Implementation of Parity

Parity is a legislative requirement that mental health insurance benefits be offered in a nondiscriminatory manner (i.e., these benefits must equal the physical health insurance benefits). In 1996, Congress passed a partial mental health parity act. (Although there are three predominant forms of insurance benefit discrimination against mental illness, the Mental Health Parity Act of 1996 only prohibits one of these forms: the use of discriminatory annual and lifetime financial limits. The other two forms are discriminatory day and visit limits and discriminatory out-of-pocket requirements, such as differential copayments.) During the 1990s, 31 states enacted mental health parity laws (National Alliance for the Mentally Ill, 2000b).

A recent trade press headline declared, "Mental Health Benefits Parity Has Been Good for the Bottom Line" (Rudd, 2000, p. 7). The article documents that in states with parity laws, Magellan Behavioral Health experienced new and renewed managed behavioral health care contracts with price increases of 20% to 30% in some cases. Parity is associated with the use of managed care. William M. Mercer Inc. (1998) found that compliance with the federal Mental Health Parity Act of 1996 "is largely an artifact of transitioning to a managed care environment. Specifically, participants reported that the introduction of managed care techniques (e.g., gatekeeping, utilization review, networks, discounts), along with the presence of an EAP . . ., gave [benefits managers], as decision makers, a higher level of comfort with the concept of parity" (p. 3). The study report continued, "Parity was not implemented in a vacuum. Rather, the decision to offer more generous benefits accompanied or followed the decision to introduce or increase the presence of managed care" (p. 3).

Burnam, Escarce, and Escarce (1999) concluded that "recent studies suggest that there is little need for strict benefit limits when care is delivered by a managed care plan" (p. 26). Goldman, McCulloch, Cuffel, and Kozma (1999) similarly concluded that "the findings show the insurability of generous mental health benefits under managed systems of care" (p. 180). There are numerous "recent studies," such as Ma and McGuire (1998); National Institute of Mental Health (1998); Sing, Hill, Smolking, and Heiser (1998); and Sturm (1997).

Goldman et al. (1999) defined the mechanisms of managed care as "prospective and concurrent clinical review, substitution of benefits, individualized treatment planning, provider networks, fixed rates of reimbursement, and use of intermediary levels of care" (p. 180). Their analysis of benefits and costs between 1991 and 1997 indicate that these mechanisms can effectively contain costs "over the long term."

Burnam, Escarce, and Escarce (1999) concluded that "the shift toward managed mental health care makes the parity debate less controversial, because feared cost increases are an unlikely consequence under managed care" (p. 23). In addition, they argued that "managed care also makes benefit parity less relevant to the goals of achieving fairness in the delivery of mental health services" (p. 23).

In analyzing 1996–1998 data from the Robert Wood Johnson Foundation project Health Care for Communities, Sturm and Wells (2000) found that "among individuals with probable mental health disorders, more have lost insurance in those two years than have gained it and more report decreases in health benefits. Individuals with worse mental health consistently report a deterioration of access to care compared to individuals with better mental health" (p. 253).

MANAGED CARE AS PUBLIC POLICY

Historical Background

According to one view, "Managed care is the inevitable consequence of forces that have been building over the past half century. This era is only part of a long process of change" (Schreter, Sharfstien, & Schreter, 1994, p. xiii). In fact, the process arguably began during the time when public mental health services were provided in state-owned and -operated inpatient facilities and continued through the advances in medication and psychotherapy in the 1940s and 1950s, the community mental health center (CMHC) movement in the 1960s and 1970s, and the increased use of state general revenues as a match for federal Medicaid dollars in the 1980s and 1990s. These movements and trends significantly expanded public mental health services, but the "expansions occurred without regard to the cost of the services provided" (Schreter, Sharfstein, & Schreter, 1994, p. xiii).

For example, the share of total state government budgets devoted to Medicaid rose from 8.1% in fiscal year (FY) 1987 to 18.4% in FY 1993. In FY 1993, 39.6% of all federal money coming into the state budgets was used for Medicaid, up from 26% in FY 1987. In 1994, the National Association of State Budget Officers observed that "Medicaid spending is threatening the ability of decision makers to use the budget as a tool for implementing public policy," that Medicaid is now "the single most important cost factor for states," and that "Medicaid has passed higher education as the second largest category of state spending" ("Medicaid," 1994, pp. 15–16). A similar expenditure escalation occurred in private industry, and employee health care costs are now equal to corporate after-tax profits. Thus there is growing emphasis, in both the public and private sectors, on effectiveness and efficiency.

In the mid-1980s, in response to the continuing escalation in behavioral health care expenditures, large private employers began developing EAPs and contracting with organizations that focus exclusively on managing behavioral health benefits. The U.S. Surgeon General's recent report (1999) on mental health characterized the private sector as using "a health insurance model that reimburses for acute medical problems. Under this traditional model, mental health coverage usually entails outpatient counseling, medication treatments, and short-term inpatient hospitalization. Under more generous insurance plans, including some managed care plans, intermediate services such as crisis respite and day hospitalization (also called partial hospitalization or day treatment) are becoming more popular although more traditional insurance plans continue to restrict their use" (p. 182).

The public mental health system, which has a wider-ranging array of mental health services than the private sector, serves as the social safety net for society. Yet "trapped between the private and public sectors is a group of uninsured individuals and families who do not qualify for the public sector programs, cannot afford to pay for services themselves, and have no access to private health insurance" (U.S. Surgeon General, 1999, p. 183). According to the Surgeon General's report, "Managed care represents a confluence [of] several forces shaping the organization and financing of health care. These include the drive to deliver more highly individualized, cost effective care; a more health-promoting and preventive orientation; and a concern with cost containment to address the problem of moral hazard" (pp. 420–421).

Americans receive their mental health care from private insurance primary care providers, private insurance specialty care, and the public mental health system. The IOM observed that "the dynamics of three interrelated sectors—privately funded primary and specialty care and public systems—are complex and also highly idiosyncratic from state to state, community to community, and plan to plan" (Edmunds et al., 1997, p. 3).

While 18.8 million Americans have their behavioral health benefits internally managed through HMO enrollment, 170 million Americans (over 68%) have them managed by MBHOs ("So Much," 2000). Three companies—Magellan Behavioral Health Services, with 69.353 million enrollees; ValueOptions, with 22.154 million enrollees; and United Behavioral Health, with 12.497 million enrollees—represent over 50% of the market (31.51%, 10.07%, and 9.09%, respectively) ("So Much," 2000).

MBHO revenues for 1995 were estimated at $2.6 billion based on the following assumptions (Oss & Moghul, 1996):

- $193.9 million: EAPs (20.2 million enrollees @ $9.60 per year)
- $190 million: integrated programs (9.9 million enrollees @ $19.20 per year)
- $1.6 billion: risk-based network programs (26.6 million enrollees @ $60 per year)

- $404.6 million: non-risk-based network programs (28.1 million enrollees @ $14.40 per year)
- $187.7 million: behavioral health utilization review programs (39.1 million enrollees @ $4.80 per year)

Public Policy Issues

Managed behavioral health care has generated controversy on the following topics:

- Adequacy of services
- Systems of care
- Medical versus clinical versus human necessity
- Public accountability using the performance measures of positive clinical outcomes and consumer satisfaction
- Consumer, family, and enrollee participation
- Distress, distrust, conflict
- Confidentiality
- Integration of behavioral health care and primary care
- Ability of providers to manage care directly

The discussion below highlights the chapters of this book in which these topics are treated in more detail.

Adequacy of Services

While managed care has achieved impressive results in serving the employed, privately insured population, it has been less effective in responding to the needs of populations in which mental illness and addictive disorders are more common, more severe, and of longer duration. Chapter 9 discusses the ways in which health care has historically dealt with addictive disorders and criticizes managed care for focusing on the associated complications of addictive disorders rather than treating the primary addictive disorders themselves.

Systems of Care

Frank and Morlock (1997) observed, "When multiple parties exert partial authority, act according to different rules, and respond to incentives from a variety of financing sources, the result is unlikely to be coordination among complementary community institutions" (p. 3). They concluded that "simple strategies that just manipulate either the organizational or the financial arrangements do not enhance systemic coordination" and therefore proposed the mixed strategies of "blending centralized organizational structure" and of "aggressive management in the form of monitoring, feedback, and education at the provider agency level" (p. 29). Irrespective of the particular expertise of managed care vendors and their degree of social commitment, service will continue to be abysmal if public fiscal and administrative agencies are unable to collaborate on plans of action.

The DHHS OIG (2000c) observed that in seven Medicaid managed mental health programs, "responsibility for care is fragmented with possible cost shifting" (p. 2). It recommended the development of interagency agreements to promote coordination. Chapter 8 describes the lack of coordination that has existed between Medicaid and public mental health programs and presents strategies for increasing the degree of integration in the public mental health system.

Medical Necessity

Managed care uses "medical necessity" protocols in making treatment decisions (Astrachan, Levinson, & Adler, 1975; Bennett, 1996; Ross, 1996). At first blush, the application of medical necessity criteria seems relatively straightforward. Care is medically necessary in any case where a patient has a diagnosable mental illness or addiction disorder, has impaired function, or is clinically unstable. However, professional disagreements over these criteria do occur, and the complex, unique, and sometimes persistent needs of persons with serious mental illness make managed care's reliance on medical necessity protocols problematic in the area of behavioral health care (Hall, Edgar, & Flynn, 1997).

In Chapter 3, Shaffer and Lieberman discuss the evolution of the concept of medical necessity within the managed behavioral health care field. In particular, standardized criteria have been used to govern access. Since the criteria are not universal, however, their use has resulted in "a great deal of confusion and animosity in the provider community toward managed care" (p. 58).

According to Shaffer and Lieberman, in realm of private insurance, treatment is considered medically necessary if it

- is intended to prevent, diagnose, correct, cure, alleviate, or preclude deterioration of a diagnosable condition that is contained in ICD-9 (*International Classification of Diseases*, 9th edition) or DSM-IV (*Diagnostic and Statistical Manual*, 4th edition) or that threatens life, causes pain or suffering, or results in illness or infirmity
- is expected to improve the individual's level of functioning
- provides individualized services that will alleviate the person's symptoms but are not in excess of the person's need
- is based on nationally accepted clinical standards
- is no more intensive or restrictive than necessary to balance safety, effectiveness, and efficiency

Controversy has revolved around the issues of determining when treatment is "not in excess of need," constructing clinical standards (and who should be responsible for their construction), and balancing safety and effectiveness with efficiency.

Professional disagreements abound over the medical nature of many emotional situations, such as marital discord, bereavement, and major life adjustments; over the medical nature of development activities intended to assist persons dissatisfied with themselves or with their interpersonal relations; and over which health professionals working in which treatment settings are most effective. Historically only the more progressive and affluent public mental health systems, greatly aided by Medicaid's rehabilitation option, have paid for psychiatric rehabilitation.

Hollingsworth and Sweeney (1997) documented that in Wisconsin private insurance definitions of medical necessity would cover only 60% of current public-sector treatment of persons with serious and persistent mental illness. Sabin and Daniels (2000) found that all stakeholders in Iowa's Medicaid managed mental health care system agree that "the central source of turmoil" during the initial stages of its implementation "was the clash between private-sector medical necessity criteria and public-sector safety-net functions" (p. 446; also see Hall, Edgar, & Flynn, 1997). The state and its managed care vendor, along with the involvement of consumers, families, and providers, negotiated three changes to the vendor's private insurance model of medical necessity.

First, up to five days of mental health inpatient and one day of substance abuse inpatient court-ordered evaluation are covered under the Iowa Medicaid plan. Second, children may not be discharged from inpatient settings until "a safe living arrangement and a plan for the necessary follow-up for mental health treatment has been arranged" (Sabin & Daniels, 2000, p. 446). As a result, 194 children were retained in inpatient care for an average of 17.6 days each, and for the first time a wide array of alternatives became available. Third, "psychosocial necessity" was added to the operational definition of medical necessity. As a consequence, "environmental factors that inhibit or hamper the effectiveness of treatment" and appropriate rehabilitative and supportive services must be examined (Sabin & Daniels, 2000, p. 446). "Managed care case managers are instructed to specifically consider the potential for services/supports to allow the enrollee to maintain functioning improvement attained through previous treatment" (Sabin & Daniels, 2000, p. 446).

Rosenbaum, Shin, Zakheim, Shaw, and Teitelbaum (1998) documented the tremendous variety in state Medicaid managed behavioral health care structures and contractual obligations. They cited the Iowa contract as a model for the nation. The Iowa contract provides specific guidance on the protocols that are applied in determining the medical necessity of care at various levels and stages of treatment. The contract also establishes an accepted practice standard of coverage for mental illness and addiction treatment.

Chapter 5 provides detailed information on state-specific applications of medical necessity and documents how medical necessity can relate to contractual performance measurement standards.

Public Accountability

In 1997, the IOM found that "the research bases and the development of quality assurance and accreditation standards are far less advanced in behavioral health care than in other areas of health care" and while "quality improvement methods have great potential, [they] are still in preliminary stages for mental health and substance abuse services" (Edmunds et al., 1997, p. 244).

The DHHS OIG (2000a) stated that the "the overall effect on the health of persons with serious mental illnesses" in seven Medicaid managed mental health programs "was not quantified" (p. 2). Further, it stated that none of the states included in its study "had working outcome measures in place before or after they connected to managed care. Even basic utilization data, such as lengths of hospital stays and number of visits, was inconsistently reported by states" (p. 13). The DHHS OIG recommended that the Health Care Financing Administration (HCFA) and the Substance Abuse and Mental Health Services Administration (SAMHSA) collaborate to develop outcome measurement systems.

In some cases, the behavioral health care field has demonstrated leadership and innovation in the development of performance measurement, in particular through the government's Center for Mental Health Services (CMHS); the managed care industry's trade group, the American Managed Behavioral Healthcare Association (AMBHA); the nation's largest family and consumer membership association, the National Alliance for the Mentally Ill (NAMI); and the field's administrative leadership (AMBHA, 1995, 1998; American College of Mental Health Administration, 1997; CMHS, 1996; Ganju & Lutterman, 1998; Hall, Edgar, & Flynn, 1997; Hall, 1998; National Association of State Mental Health Program Directors, 1998; Steinwachs, Flynn, Norquist, & Skinner, 1996). None of the current performance measurement initiatives allows health plan enrollees and their families to compare plan-specific performance, but each has moved forward the concept and practice of performance measurement in managed behavioral health care.

Four states (Colorado, Iowa, Massachusetts, and Washington) studied by the U.S. General Accounting Office (GAO, 1999) require their managed care vendors to collect encounter data, but none of the four systematically uses the data other than to cite penetration rates (i.e., the proportion of an enrolled population actually receiving mental health services). The penetration rates for the managed mental health programs of the four states were as follows: Massachusetts, 25.1%; Iowa, 12.8%; Colorado, 11.9%; and Washington, 7.0%. GAO concluded that data from MBHOs "were untimely, incomplete, or inaccurate" (p. 26). Sturm (1999) stated, "While all companies claim to measure outcome, none are systematically examining key outcomes for people with serious mental health problems" (p. 17).

Clearly, much more needs to be done in the area of public accountability. As Johnston and Romzek (1999) put it, "There is a tendency in privatization efforts, and especially in contracting relationships, to assume that contract management and accountability will take care of themselves or that they can be relatively easily achieved through contract monitoring. The reality is that contract management and accountability do not take care of themselves" (p. 394).

The introduction of managed care represents a paradigm shift (Figure 1–1). The managed care vendor (health plan) is at the core of both decision making and accountability. Under fee-for-service arrangements, providers

Pre–Managed Care

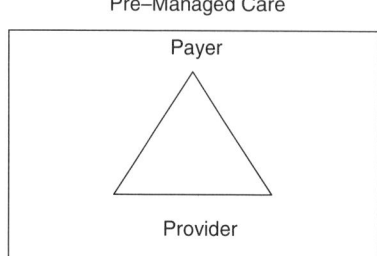

The Management Agent

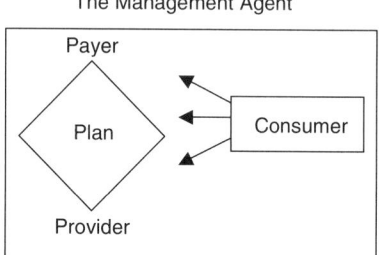

Figure 1–1 Paradigm Shift from Pre–Managed Care to Managed Care

were only responsible for documenting their services in order to receive payment from third-party payers. In the managed care paradigm, two additional parties—the health plan and the consumer—play important roles. The payer, on behalf of the consumer, selects a health plan to manage the health benefits, including making payments to providers. The consumer (the health plan enrollee seeking care and treatment) demands accountability (responsiveness, access, etc.) from the other three entities—the payer, the plan, and the provider.

The collection of data on managed behavioral health care organizations is challenging for two primary reasons:

1. The desire of individual organizations and the legal requirements of federal antitrust mandates to maintain strict ownership and confidentiality related to such data (i.e., the competitive advantage issue)
2. The level of resources (time, money, and personnel) needed to develop the data and put the report results in the requested format

In 1997, IOM concluded, "Overall, the picture is incomplete, inconsistent, and inadequate for making truly informed health care purchasing decisions. To those who are responsible for purchasing care, the absence of consensus on quality measurements is a challenge" (Edmunds et al., 1997, p. 29). This conclusion remains valid today.

Chapter 10 examines a range of issues, including ethical issues and the inconsistency of current performance measures, associated with performance measurement and accountability in managed behavioral health care. Chapter 11 discusses consumer satisfaction and its relationship to other outcome measures, presents case studies of attempts by health care systems to measure consumer satisfaction and use the results to improve their services, and describes other types of programs intended to improve the services provided to managed care enrollees.

Consumer, Family, and Enrollee Participation

Many public purchasers and their management agents fail to meaningfully involve consumers, families, and enrollees in their operations. Consumers lack necessary information. In an October 1998 NAMI (Hall, 1998) survey of its members' experiences with managed care, 55% of the respondents did not know how to file an appeal with their MCO. The respondents were those members who took the initiative to send in a completed survey form, so one would think that they would be among the more involved and knowledgeable of citizens. This finding demonstrates that all parties must make a greater effort to educate citizens about their rights as health plan enrollees.

Pires, Armstrong, and Stroul (1999) studied how MCOs and MBHOs involve families in their operations. By and large, MBHOs involve families significantly more than MCOs. Regarding initial planning and implementation activities, families were significantly involved in 36% of MBHOs, compared with 13% of MCOs. Involvement in current refinements was even more striking: 47% of MBHOs significantly involved families while only 13% of MCOs involved families. And although 77% of MBHOs provided a training and orientation program directed toward families, only 23% of MCOs provided such training.

Sabin and Daniels (1999), advocates of meaningful consumer and family involvement, concluded, "Consumers, families, and the public cannot be expected to trust health care systems that do not hold themselves accountable for demonstrating that their limit-setting policies are reasonable and fair" (p. 883). The DHHS OIG (2000b) recommended that Medicaid managed mental health programs involve beneficiaries and families in the conversion from fee-for-service to managed care and in treatment planning.

Chapter 8 discusses the general lack of meaningful consumer participation in health plan operations, and Chapter 11 describes the role that consumer satisfaction teams and ombudsman and clinical review programs can play in protecting the interests of enrollees.

Distress, Distrust, Conflict

Allies and Adversaries: The Impact of Managed Care on Mental Health Services (Schreter, Sharfstein, & Schreter, 1994) is a leading book on managed behavioral health care written by and for psychiatrists. It describes the clashes that occur between, on the one hand, "clinicians-psychiatrists, psychologists, psychiatric nurses, and social workers—who feel they know what their patients need, especially with regard to quality and quantity" and, on the other hand, "reviewers—an industry whose product is cost savings to those who pay for the care" (pp. xiii–xiv). In this era of limited resources, the clashes have intensified, and to function both clinically and financially, those concerned with mental health policy and services have to understand the forces at work. (Figure 1–2 is a graphic presentation of the organized interests competing for resources and the control of resources.)

Adding to the distress and distrust are the attempts by health plans to reduce the fees charged by health professionals. The lead paragraph of a recent *Boston Globe* article states, "A for-profit company hired by Harvard

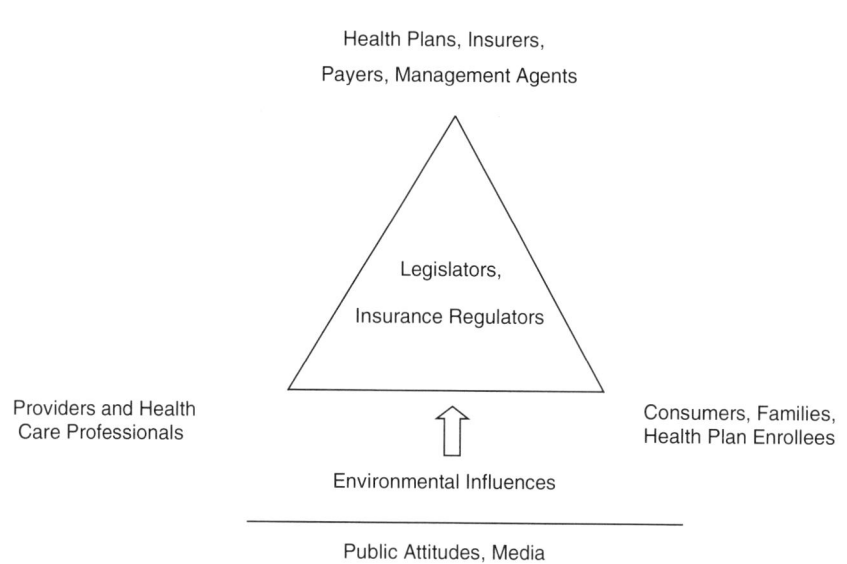

Figure 1–2 Dynamics of the Competition for Resources and Their Control

Pilgrim Health Care to control mental health costs has angered psychologists and psychiatrists by slashing their fees . . ." (Kowalczyk, 2000). Harvard Pilgrim's MBHO subcontractor, ValueOptions, declared that the fee for psychiatrists' 20-minute medication monitoring visits would be reduced from \$57 to \$36 and the fee for their 50-minute psychiatric therapy visits would be reduced from \$78 to \$70. ValueOptions also announced a preference for group therapy and therapy by social workers.

A possible third cause of conflict is the difference between the needs and expectations of basically healthy populations (e.g., workers covered by their employers) and those of populations in which illness is persistent, severe, and disabling. *Stand and Deliver* (Hall, Edgar, & Flynn, 1997), a work published by NAMI, stated that the managed behavioral health care industry "fails in the basic elements of care that people with serious brain disorders need to survive" (p. V).

The imposition of MCO control over providers, however, appears to be lessening over time. For example, between 1996 and 1999 explicit prior authorization requirements declined from 82% to 57% of contracts, and the percentage of contracts requiring a provider to obtain prior authorization from the enrollee's primary care provider declined from 10% to 7% (Rosenbaum, Teitelbaum, Mauery, Zakheim, & Golde, 2000).

Chapter 13 describes the competition among interest groups involved in managed care, the foci of the conflicts between these groups, and alternatives for regulating managed behavioral health care organizations, including the enactment of consumer protections.

Confidentiality

In order to integrate services, avoid one provider's treatment adversely affecting a second provider's treatment, document clinical outcomes and consumer satisfaction, and meet case utilization review responsibilities, MBHOs within a network require the sharing of clinical information. Such sharing has resulted in two types of criticisms: (1) complaints from historically autonomous providers unaccustomed to sharing clinical information with anyone, including consumers and family members, and (2) complaints about the misuse of such information by MCOs. Chapter 4 discusses confidentiality and the potential for confidentiality requirements to obstruct communication between primary care providers and behavioral health care providers.

Integration of Behavioral Health Care and Primary Care

The ongoing failure to integrate mental illness and addictive disorder services is reason to be skeptical that behavioral health care and primary care will be meaningfully integrated in the near term. As Ryglewicz and Pepper (1996) explained, "One of the major problems in treating dual psychiatric and substance abuse disorders has been the routing of mental health and substance abuse clients onto separate trains, sometimes on different tracks—most commonly those of separate agencies" (p. 55).

Three program approaches to serving persons with co-occurring mental illness and addictive disorders are currently in use. Sequential programs treat one disorder, then, after stabilization, treat a second disorder. Parallel programs treat both disorders simultaneously, but two separate agencies, frequently with contradictory philosophies, are involved. Integrated programs treat both disorders simultaneously at the same program site and (ideally) using cross-trained staff. Research by the National Institute of Mental Health and National Institute on Drug Abuse clearly documents that integrated treatment is far "superior" to the "non-integrated" approaches of "parallel and sequential" programs (Camer, 1999; Clark & Drake, 1992; Drake, Mercer-McFadden, Mueser, McHugo, & Bond, 1997; Drake & Mueser, 1996; Mueser, Drake, & Miles, 1997; Pepper, 1998; RachBeisel, Scott, & Dixon, 1999; Ryglewicz & Pepper, 1996).

Despite the evidence-based research, few programs in the nation actually deliver integrated treatment (NAMI, 2000a; National Health Policy Forum, 1998; Ryglewicz & Pepper, 1996). If the behavioral health care field cannot effectively integrate clinical services for persons with co-occurring mental illness and addictive disorders, is the nation ready to integrate behavioral health care and primary care? Chapter 4 is devoted to the issues involved in such integration, including financial issues, the role of treatment guidelines, the use of formularies, and training in best practices.

Ability of Providers To Manage Care Directly

As noted, "the merger of coverage and care into a single corporate structure is what distinguishes managed care from earlier indemnity or service benefit plans that gave physicians and health professionals full discretion over participation and treatment decisions" (quoted from Chapter 5). The single corporate structure might, nonetheless, consist of providers, and one question is whether provider-sponsored organizations can be successful at managing care. This question is dealt with in Chapter 12, which bases its affirmative answer on the results of a study of behavioral health care provider-sponsored organizations done by Dyer and Barkey.

REFERENCES

American College of Mental Health Administration. (1997). *Preserving quality and value in the managed care equation.* Pittsburgh, PA: ACMHA.

American Managed Behavioral Healthcare Association. (1995, August). *PERMS 1.0, performance measures for managed behavioral healthcare programs.* Washington, DC: AMBHA.

American Managed Behavioral Healthcare Association. (1998, July). *PERMS 2.0, performance measures for managed behavioral healthcare programs.* Washington, DC: AMBHA.

Astrachan, M., Levinson, D., & Adler, D. (1976, July). The impact of national health insurance on the tasks and practice of psychiatry. *Archives of General Psychiatry, 33*(7), 785–794.

Bennett, M. (1996, September). Is psychotherapy ever medically necessary? *Psychiatric Services, 47*(9), 966–970.

Boland, P. (1991). *Making managed health work.* New York: McGraw-Hill.

Burnam, M., Escarce, A., & Escarce, J.J. (1999, September–October). Equity in managed care for mental disorders. *Health Affairs, 18*(5), 22–31.

Callahan, J., Shepard, D., & Beinecke, R. (1994, February 16). *Evaluation of the Massachusetts Medicaid mental health/substance abuse program.* Waltham, MA: Brandeis University.

Camer, R. (1999). Retooling dual diagnosis treatment: A consensus is emerging that integrated care and assertive outreach are keys to success. In *1999 Medicaid managed behavioral care sourcebook* (pp. 328–334). New York, NY: Faulkner and Gray.

Center for Mental Health Services. (1996). *The MHSIP consumer-oriented mental health report card: The final report of the mental health statistics improvement program task force on a consumer-oriented mental health report card.* Rockville, MD: CMHS.

Clark, R.E., & Drake, R.E. (1992, Fall). Substance abuse and mental illness: What families need to know. *Innovations and Research*, 3–8.

Drake, R.E., Mercer-McFadden, C., Mueser, K.T., McHugo, G.J., & Bond, G.R. (1998). Review of integrated mental health and substance abuse treatment of patients with dual disorders. *Schizophrenia Bulletin, 24*(4), 589–607.

Drake, R.E., & Mueser, K.T. (Eds.). (1996, Summer). Dual diagnosis of major mental illness and substance abuse disorder. Volume 2: Recent research and clinical implications. *New Directions for Mental Health Services.*

Dyer, R.L. (1992, July 14). The many faces of public managed care in state mental health systems. Paper presented at the summer meeting of the National Association of State Mental Health Program Directors, Arlington, VA.

Edmunds, M., Frank, F., Hogan, M., McCarty, D., Robinson-Beale, R., & Weisner, C. (Eds.). (1997). *Managing managed care: Quality improvement in behavioral health.* Washington, DC: Institute of Medicine, National Academy Press.

Frank, R.G., & McGuire, T.G. (1995, Fall). Estimating costs of mental health and substance abuse coverage. *Health Affairs, 14*(3), 102–115.

Frank, R.G., McGuire, T.G., & Newhouse, J.P. (1995, Fall). Risk contracts in managed mental health care. *Health Affairs, 14*(3), 50–64.

Frank, R., & Morlock, L. (1997). *Managing fragmented public mental health services.* New York, NY: Milbank Memorial Fund.

Ganju, V., & Lutterman, T. (1998). Assessment of performance: The five-state feasibility study: Implementing performance measures across state mental health systems. In *Mental health, United States, 1998* (pp. 45–51). Washington, DC: Department of Health and Human Services.

Goldman, W., McCulloch, J., Cuffel, B., & Kozma, D. (1999, September–October). More evidence for the insurability of managed behavioral health care. *Health Affairs, 18*(5), 172–181.

Goldman, W., McCulloch, J., & Sturm, R. (1997, February). *Costs and utilization of mental health services before and after managed care.* Working paper no. 108. Los Angeles, CA: Research Center on Managed Care for Psychiatric Disorders, UCLA and RAND.

Hall, L.L. (1998, October). Managed care: A survey of NAMI members. Arlington, VA: National Alliance for the Mentally Ill. Internal Report. Not published.

Hall, L.L., Edgar, E., & Flynn, L. (1997, September). *Stand and deliver: Action call to a failing industry—The NAMI managed care report card.* Arlington, VA: National Alliance for the Mentally Ill.

Happ, D. (1998, April). The carve-out: A better alternative. *Behavioral Healthcare Tomorrow, 32,* 37–38.

Hollingsworth, E.J., & Sweeney, J.K. (1997, April). Mental health expenditures for services for people with severe mental illnesses. *Psychiatric Services, 48*(4), 485–490.

Johnston, J., & Romzek, B. (1999, September/October). Contracting and accountability in state Medicaid reform: Rhetoric, theories, and reality. *Public Administration Review,* 383–399.

Kowalczyk, L. (2000, August 18). How to cut psychiatric provider payments; some staff plan to quit Harvard Pilgrim. *Boston Globe.*

Krupnick, R. (1995, November). FHC options. Paper presented to a Global Business Research Conference on Medicaid and Medicare, North Miami Beach, FL.

Ma, C.A., & McGuire, T.G. (1998, March/April). Costs and incentives in a behavioral health carve-out. *Health Affairs, 17*(2), 53–69.

MBHO/EAP enrollment reaches 200 million in 2000. (2000, September). *Open Minds,* 7–8.

Medicaid: The elephant on the budget bus; controlling Medicaid cost: Can states solve the Medicaid problems? (1994, August). *State Policy Reports,* 9–24.

Mihalik, G., & Scherer, M. (1998, Spring). Fundamental mechanisms of managed behavioral health care. *Journal of Health Care Finance, 24*(3), 1–15.

Mueser, K., Drake, R., & Miles, R. (1997). Evolution of integrated treatment. In *Treatment of drug-dependent individuals with comorbid mental disorders*. Bethesda, MD: National Institute on Drug Abuse.

National Alliance for the Mentally Ill. (2000a). *Integrated treatment and blended funding for co-occurring mental and addiction disorders—A where we stand paper*. Arlington, VA: NAMI.

National Alliance for the Mentally Ill. (2000b). *Parity in insurance coverage—A where we stand paper*. Arlington, VA: NAMI.

National Association of State Mental Health Program Directors. (1998). *Five-state feasibility study on state mental health agency performance measures*. Alexandria, VA: NASMHPD.

National Health Policy Forum. (1998, April 14). *Dual diagnosis: The challenge of serving people with concurrent mental illness and substance abuse problems*. Issue brief no. 718. Washington, DC: NHPF, George Washington University.

National Institute of Mental Health. (1998, April). *Parity in financing mental health services: Managed care effect on cost, access, and quality: An interim report to Congress by the National Advisory Mental Health Council*. Bethesda, MD: NIMH.

Open Minds. (1999). Open Minds' *yearbook of managed behavioral health market share in the United States, 1999–2000*. Gettysburg, PA: Open Minds.

Oss, M., & Moghul, A. (1996). The managed behavioral health care industry: Overview and future prospects. In *1997 behavioral managed care sourcebook*. New York, NY: Faulkner and Gray.

Patterson, D. (1998, April). Dealing with the little shop of Medicaid horrors. *Behavioral Healthcare Tomorrow, 7*(2), 32, 35–36.

Pear, R. (1996, May 2). Wider mental health policies seen as feasible requirement. *New York Times*.

Pepper, B. (1998). *Dual disorders: Substance abuse and mental illness—Lecture notes and participant manual*. New City, NY: The Information Exchange, Inc.

Pires, S., Armstrong, M., & Stroul, B. (1999, January). *Health care reform tracking project: Tracking state managed care reforms as they affect children and adolescents with behavioral health disorders and their families*. Tampa, FL: University of South Florida (in collaboration with Human Service Collaborative and Georgetown University Child Development Center).

RachBeisel, J., Scott, J., & Dixon, L. (1999, November). Co-occurring severe mental illness and substance use disorders: A review of recent research. *Psychiatric Services, 50*(11), 1427–1434.

Rosenbaum, S., Shin, P., Zakheim, M., Shaw, K., & Teitelbaum, J. (1998). *Negotiating the new health system: A nationwide study of Medicaid managed care contracts; Special report: Mental illness and addiction disorder treatment and prevention*. Washington, DC: George Washington University, Center for Health Policy Research.

Rosenbaum, S., Teitelbaum, J., Mauery, R., Zakheim, M., & Golde, M. (2000, March). *An evaluation of agreements between managed care organizations and community-based mental illness and addiction disorders treatment and prevention providers*. SAMHSA issue brief no. 9. Washington, DC: George Washington University, Center for Health Services Research and Policy for the Substance Abuse and Mental Health Services Administration.

Ross, E.C. (1996, December 11). The use of medical necessity criteria in managed behavioral healthcare. *BNA's Managed Care Reporter*, 1171–1172.

Rudd, T. (2000, August 17). Mental health benefits parity has been good for the bottom line at Magellan Behavioral Health. *Managed Behavioral Health News*, 7.

Ryglewicz, H., & Pepper, B. (1996). *Lives at risk: Understanding and treating young people with dual disorders*. New York, NY: The Free Press.

Sabin, J.E., & Daniels, N. (1999, July). Public-sector managed behavioral health care III: Meaningful consumer and family participation. *Psychiatric Services, 50*(7), 883–885.

Sabin, J.E., & Daniels, N. (2000, April). Public-sector managed behavioral health care V: Redefining "medical necessity"—The Iowa experience. *Psychiatric Services, 51*(4), 445–446, 459.

Schreter, R., Sharfstein, S., & Schreter, C.S. (1994). *Allies and adversaries: The impact of managed care on mental health services*. Washington, DC: American Psychiatric Press.

Shaffer, I. (1995, May). Value behavioral health. Paper presented to the Center for Mental Health Services Annual Conference on Mental Health Statistics, Washington, DC.

Shern, D.L., & Robinson, P. (1999, April). *Evaluation of Florida's prepaid mental health plan: Year 2 report*. Tampa, FL: University of South Florida, Louis de la Parte Florida Mental Health Institute.

Sing, M., Hill, S., Smolking, S., & Heiser, N. (1998). *The costs and effects of parity for mental health and substance abuse insurance benefits*. SMA98-3205. Rockville, MD: Substance Abuse and Mental Health Services Administration.

So much for integration. (2000, September). *Open Minds,* 1–3.

Steinwachs, D., Flynn, L., Norquist, G., & Skinner, E. (1996, Fall). Editors' notes. New Directions for Mental Health Services. In *Using Client Outcomes Information To Improve Mental Health and Substance Abuse Treatment.* New Directions for Mental Health Services Series. San Francisco, CA: Jossey-Bass Publishers, No. 71, 1–2.

Sturm, R. (1997). How expensive is unlimited mental health care coverage under managed care. *Journal of the American Medical Association, 278*(18), 1533–1537.

Sturm, R. (1999, July). *Tracking changes in behavioral health care: How have carve-outs changed care?* Working paper no. 162. Santa Monica, CA: RAND and UCLA.

Sturm, R., & Wells, K. (2000, April). Health insurance may be improving—but not for individuals with mental illness. *Health Services Research, 35,* 253–261.

Surles, R. (1997, January). *Psychiatric Services.*

Umland, B. (1997, June). Foster Higgins national survey: Trends in behavioral benefits. *Behavioral Healthcare Tomorrow, 6*(3), 57–60.

U.S. Department of Health and Human Services Office of Inspector General. (2000a). *Mandatory managed care: changes in Medicaid mental health services*. OEI-04-97-00340. Washington, DC: DHHS.

U.S. Department of Health and Human Services Office of Inspector General. (2000b). *Mandatory managed care: Early lessons learned by Medicaid mental health programs.* OEI-04-97-00343. Washington, DC: DHHS.

U.S. Department of Health and Human Services Office of Inspector General. (2000c). *Mandatory managed care: Children's access to Medicaid mental health services.* OEI-04-97-00344. Washington, DC: DHHS.

U.S. General Accounting Office. (1999, September). *Medicaid managed care: Four states' experiences with mental health carveout programs.* Washington, DC: GAO.

U.S. Surgeon General. (1999). *Surgeon general's report on mental health.* Washington, DC: DHHS.

Wiggins, J. (1997, January-February). *The National Psychologist.*

William M. Mercer Inc. (1998). *Case studies: A guide to implementing parity for mental illness.* Arlington, VA: William M. Mercer for the National Alliance for the Mentally Ill.

CHAPTER 2

Forms of Payment, Capitation, and Risk Management

Stephen P. Melek

Purpose: This chapter explains how managed care has brought about changes in the forms of payment and describes the various payment techniques used.

Major Topics: This chapter discusses Forms of Payment, Discount Charges, Per Diem Rates, Per Case Rates, Capitation, Risk Pools, Withholds, Actuarial Cost Models, Adequacy of Capitation, Risk Management, Contractual Protection against Adverse Experiences, and System Management Tools.

The evolution of managed behavioral health care has brought about change in the forms of payment for behavioral health care services. Capitation contracts for behavioral health care services are the norm in many health care systems. Moreover, effective risk management has become critical for the ongoing success and survival of behavioral health care systems and providers. This chapter describes provider payment concepts, capitation development and analysis, and risk protection and management issues in managed behavioral health care.

FORMS OF PAYMENT

Until the early 1990s, health maintenance organizations (HMOs), preferred provider organizations (PPOs), insurance carriers, and employers paid health care providers fee-for-service payments based on the provider's

29

billed charges. Typically only a usual, customary, and reasonableness test or discount was applied to the level of billed charges. With no real control over the level of charges or the utilization of health care services, carriers retained the entire risk that health care costs to the insured population would be different from the risk anticipated when setting premium rates. Today, different approaches to provider reimbursement have changed the nature of risk for the carriers and behavioral health care providers. Managed behavioral health care contracts now have provisions that shift risk to providers through guaranteed discounts off billed charges, per diem rates, per case rates, modified case rates, capitation payments, and risk pools and withholds. Various forms of provider incentives also can be structured to influence the way behavioral health care services are provided.

Guaranteed Discounts Off Billed Charges

Discounts from provider billed charge schedules achieve lower behavioral health care costs for carriers but have only a minor impact on the risk to providers. The provider's risk is that the prices paid for the services covered under the discounted arrangement will not cover the provider's costs. However, discounted fee scales can help generate increased volume or market share from additional business. In some cases, providers have been known to "make up in volume" what they gave up via discounts.

Per Diem Rates

Under per diem contracts, hospitals and facilities are reimbursed an agreed-upon dollar amount for each patient bed-day. This can be applied to acute inpatient settings and residential treatment facilities. In addition, day treatment, partial hospital, and intensive outpatient services can be reimbursed under per diem contracts for each "day" of service. These contracts can cover just the facility portion of costs or include the professional charges associated with the facility. This fixed-payment approach shifts the risk that actual costs per day will be more or less than expected from the insurance carrier to the provider. A single per diem rate covering all types of facility stays shifts the most risk to the facility, because the facility is at risk that the patient mix will differ from the prior experience or studies that were used to support the per diem level. Per diem arrangements by service, diagnosis, or diagnosis-related group (DRG) shift less risk to the facility because increased service intensity is reimbursed at higher payment levels.

Per Case Rates

Some payers use a case rate approach to reimbursing behavioral health care providers, making a single payment based on the diagnosis. Case rates can be used for just the facility services, just the professional services, or all services provided to the patient. This approach shifts the risk to the providers not only that the level of charges (intensity of care provided) will be greater than expected, but also that the length of treatment will be longer than expected. This can apply to the length of stay in facilities, the length of psychotherapy treatment by professionals, or the total amount of services consumed by a particular patient when treatment for a condition (e.g., an eating disorder) is reimbursed using a case rate. Unlike the per diem approach that pays more money for a longer length of treatment, the case rate approach yields the same amount of money for a long course of treatment as for a short one.

As with the per diem approach, a single case rate for all types of treatment transfers the most case risk to the providers. Case rates that vary by diagnosis or DRG essentially keep the case-mix risk with the insurance carrier. The risk that the frequency of conditions generating facility or treatment admissions will be more or less than expected also stays with the insurance carrier under case rate approaches.

As acute inpatient utilization for behavioral health care has declined, more acute alternative services are being provided through residential, day treatment, and outpatient programs. In response to this increased use of these acute alternative services, managed behavioral health care organizations have more aggressively contracted on a fixed rate per case for these services.

Modified Case Rates

A newer development in the use of case rates for behavioral health care services involves the use of uncomplicated case rates with an excess day per diem amount. A goal length of treatment is defined for the uncomplicated patient as established by some care path guideline or protocol. Two sets of condition-specific weights are then established—one set reflecting the resource requirements of the uncomplicated patient (patient can be treated within the guideline or care path) and a second set reflecting the resource requirements for extra units of treatment (days, visits, etc.) related to medically necessary complications that cause the patient to "stay longer" than the goal length of treatment.

Two fee multipliers are then established that, in combination with the two sets of weights, produce case-specific reimbursements. The weights are similar to the resource-based relative value scale (RBRVS) while the multipliers are analogous to physician conversion factors that are negotiated between the parties of the contract to set the payment rates. A case rate is paid for each case, and a per diem rate is paid for excess days.

This arrangement was designed to pay the treatment providers fairly for medically necessary services, provide incentives to make patients healthy quickly and cost-effectively, be easy to administer and understand, and be comparable to other provider reimbursement contracts. This type of schedule does not present a strong incentive for providers to reduce lengths of treatment to medically optimal levels. It does, however, avoid some of the concern surrounding "cut corners" and inappropriate care delivery by providers under standard case rate methods.

Capitation Payments

Capitation payments are a budgeted per member per month (PMPM) fee for each member or enrollee in a given health plan. They shift from insurance carriers to providers the risk that:

- The frequency of care will be more than expected
- The level of charges or intensity of services provided will be more than expected
- The case mix will be more severe than expected

Under capitation contracts, the provider essentially underwrites the risk for the scope of services that falls under the contract with the carrier. The issues surrounding capitation arrangements are numerous; they are covered later in this chapter.

Risk Pools and Withholds

Regardless of reimbursement method chosen, there are ways in which the managed care organization and providers can share in the financial risks for behavioral health care services. It is common for physicians to share in the financial risks for facility services because they generally have more influence over the use of such services than do the facilities themselves. The use of risk pools and withholds can accomplish this risk sharing.

The traditional approach to a risk pool is to establish a budget on a PMPM basis for the behavioral services that are being risk-shared. The budget, or expected cost, would be set for a fixed period of time, usually 12 months. The total budgeted dollars would be the budgeted amount PMPM times the number of members enrolled for each month. At the end of the contract period (or at periodic points within it), the total actual expenses would be compared with budgeted amounts. Although enough time should be allowed after the end of the contractual period so that most claims have been paid, it is common for an allowance to be added to the behavioral health care expenses for the expected outstanding unpaid claims.

If the actual expenses are less than the budgeted expenses, there is a surplus that would be distributed to the various parties based on previously established distribution shares. If the actual amount exceeds the budgeted amount, the deficit is shared among the appropriate parties. Typically, the deficit recovery would occur in one of two ways:

1. *Provider payment withhold:* The insurance carrier retains a portion of the amount that otherwise would have been paid to the provider. For example, a 10% withhold would mean that 90% of the agreed on fee schedule would be paid to the provider at the time the claim is processed. The remaining 10% would be "withheld" and returned at the end of the contract or measurement period if there were a surplus. If there were a deficit, the withhold would be used to cover all or part of the deficit.
2. *End-of-year cash settlement:* Providers are required to pay the managed care organization an amount equal to their share of the deficit or the amount that would be withheld from future payments to the providers.

Cash Flow Considerations

Many of these different approaches to provider reimbursement may change the cash flow amounts and timing of receipts that are familiar to the providers. Some of them require additional data to complete the calculation of appropriate payment to the providers. Some may need carefully written terms relating to triggering of payment. Per diem rates need counts of approved inpatient days, case rates need confirmed and accurate diagnosis codes, and capitation rates require accurate counting of covered members under the risk contract—a number that can change on a monthly basis.

In some cases, payments for services can be accelerated, such as case rates that are paid once the diagnosis is confirmed, which could be quicker than the familiar fee-for-service submission process. Capitation rates can result in quicker payments to the providers if member data flow smoothly and accurately. On the other hand, if questions arise as to the accuracy of diagnosis code or membership data, payments could be slowed beyond fee-for-service processing speeds.

In addition, these payment arrangements can result in differences in the steadiness of cash flows. Capitation payments usually result in much steadier cash flows than fee-for-service payments. Case rates and per diem payments can be much less steady, as the payments are triggered by incidence of utilization, much closer to fee-for-service reimbursement cash flow.

CAPITATION

Capitation contracts transfer the entire underwriting risk for the defined scope of services under the contract from the original carrier to the assuming providers of health care. In order to analyze and understand the risks inherent within a capitation proposal, actuarial cost models are typically used.

Developing Actuarial Cost Models

Actuarial cost models present both the probability of an event occurring and the magnitude (cost) of that event. For behavioral health care, an actuarial cost model would include the following data for each type of patient (commercially insured, Medicare, Medicaid, and so on):

- Admit/user rates: These rates are the probabilities of admissions to acute inpatient facilities, residential treatment programs, day treatment programs, intensive outpatient programs, outpatient therapies, and any other type of behavioral health care service provided along the continuum of care.
- Average length of treatment (ALOT) rates: These rates identify the duration of treatment expressed in days, visits, or whatever unit of service is appropriate.
- Service units: The product of the admit/user rates and the ALOT, usually expressed as days/visits/units per 1,000 persons per year.
- Cost per unit of service: The cost per unit could be based on gross charges, net charges, average community charges, marginal cost, total allocated cost, or fixed cost. These unit costs vary by type of behavioral health care service and are usually projected to a specific time period to recognize the impact of inflation.
- Per capita claims cost: The product of the service units and the cost per unit of service divided by 1,000. It often is divided by 12 to attain a monthly cost. Managed behavioral health plans often refer to this value as the PMPM cost.

The items in the model may reflect anticipated statistics (to forecast future results), historical data (for retrospective analysis), or current figures (for operational analysis). Analysis of actual to expected results (variance analysis) based on actuarial models can provide early signs of financial, operational, or clinical practice problems. The model also can establish anticipated utilization and costs to benchmark ongoing experience.

Actuarial cost models are only as good as the data and actuarial judgment used to make them. The following general rules about health system cost models should be kept in mind:

- Rapid changes in behavioral health care cost, managed care efficiency, and delivery systems underscore the need for the most recent data possible.

- A more substantial database (in terms of size and scope) generally will produce more credible results. Utilization rates, in particular, can fluctuate from one time period to another. Inadequate data can lead to inappropriate assumptions, which potentially can lead to disappointing results.
- Data from traditional fee-for-service systems need adjustment for managed care systems. Information about type of service and unit charge or unit cost information can be useful. However, this information is inadequate in terms of the impact of managed care or changes in the degree of health care management.

Sources of data for developing actuarial cost models include:

- Actuarial consulting firms specializing in work with behavioral health care providers and insurance carriers
- State insurance department rate filings made by HMOs, managed behavioral health care organizations (MBHOs), or other health plans
- State-administered databases and surveys
- Publicly available Medicare and Medicaid information
- Health care industry surveys (such as those done by the Health Insurance Association of America [HIAA])
- Behavioral health care industry surveys (such as those done by the American Psychiatric and Psychological Associations and the American Managed Behavioral Healthcare Association [AMBHA])
- Insurance company data

Some caveats should be noted about the data sources described above as follows:

- Actuarial consulting firms specializing in health care risk have meaningful data, but models based on these data should always be reconciled against other known information. A model's users should understand its environment, including significant differences from behavioral health care providers in other regions.
- State insurance department rate filings of HMOs and insurance companies are generally available to the public. Sometimes, rate filings clearly document the assumptions used by HMOs, MBHOs, and Blue

Cross/Blue Shield plans and thus can provide useful figures to compare with a model's assumptions (and filings also may include data on financial performance and volume of business). Unfortunately, there are many ways that a company may categorize its health care costs; therefore, the analyst will need to carefully compare the figures in rate filings to those used in his or her model. In addition, states differ in their auditing of rate filings, with the result that information in rate filings could prove unreliable for comparative purposes.

- State-administered databases can be excellent resources for developing meaningful benchmarks for both unmanaged and managed care situations. States can tabulate acute hospital information by DRG. The more elaborate actuarial cost models present utilization and cost information by DRG.

- Medicare and Medicaid information also can prove useful. In particular, Medicare's data files provide detailed physician information by Current Procedure Terminology (CPT) code. However, because the level and type of services provided to Medicare and Medicaid populations differ from those provided to commercial populations, these data have serious limitations for direct application to commercial situations. However, these files do provide useful geographic information regarding net charges by CPT code.

- Health care industry surveys can examine how costs vary by area and the relative costs of different procedures and categories of care. For example, the HIAA publishes information reported by its members that shows the distribution of physician charges by CPT-4 code and by three-digit zip code. This "prevailing fee" information from the fee-for-service environment can help behavioral health care systems estimate the cost savings a particular discounted fee schedule can produce.

- Claims data repositories, such as health insurer data, provide useful information, if properly analyzed. Because most insurers track the population base that generates claims, an actuary can use insurer data to link health claims to the age, sex, family status, and employment status of the individuals generating a given type of claim. Equally important, insurer databases have information about who does not produce claims. Thus, insurer databases can help develop user rates and costs per 1,000 population.

However, insurer databases have their own flaws, including the likelihood that the data do not reflect managed care operations. Furthermore, the data will reflect an insurer's particular products and approaches to operations, reimbursement, underwriting, and marketing, and they would likely require adjustment for other applications. Last, most insurers guard their information and often will not release the database.

Evaluating the Adequacy of Capitation Rates

The utilization, average costs, and PMPM targets in the actuarial cost model are unique to each contracting situation and are based on a number of key assumptions. These assumptions are as follows:

- Contract period: The period of time during which the behavioral health care risk transfer is effective. It can be a one-year or multiyear period. It also can be months, or even years, beyond the time period when actual experience data are reported and available.
- Geographic area: The state/geozip/county of coverage under the capitated contract. It can range from a small, specific, concentrated area (such as a single county) to a very broad area (such as the service areas covering the employees of a national employer). Area factors or adjustments are used to measure the differences in utilization and average unit costs by type of service. They can vary by state, by geozip, by county, or by other geographic division depending on the data available for measuring such differences.
- Enrollment class (commercial group, Medicare, Medicaid, etc.): Behavioral health care costs vary considerably by enrollment class due primarily to utilization rate differences. Average unit costs also can contribute to the PMPM differences as providers contract at different rate levels across different member groups.
- Degree of behavioral health care management: The use of medical necessity criteria, clinical pathways, and treatment protocols, and the degree of adherence to such standards, results in large differences in utilization patterns and unit costs. Well-managed behavioral health care systems (those that employ comprehensive utilization management techniques with strict adherence) can obtain PMPM costs that are considerably lower (50% or more) than the same costs incurred for the same insured group in loosely managed systems (those that have

very few utilization management techniques, with little or no adherence to standards).

- Patient cost sharing: The deductible, coinsurance, and copayment levels by type of service that are required of the insured members reduce the expected costs to the insuring entities.
- Benefit limits: Calendar year and lifetime limits in inpatient days, outpatient therapy visits, or other behavioral health care benefit reduce the costs under the benefit coverage. The expected cost impact of such limits reduces as the degree of behavioral health care management increases (longer available benefit periods are less utilized in well-managed systems compared with loosely managed systems).
- Provider reimbursement levels: The rates paid for different alternative services available along the continuum of behavioral health care, and the rates paid to the various professionals available within the delivery system, play a critical role in the resulting costs. Increased use of lower cost alternatives to acute inpatient care and increased use of lower cost professionals for certain outpatient services can substantially lower the costs of behavioral health care.
- Definition of capitated services: Understanding the specific behavioral health care services and covered conditions under the contract is vital. Vague descriptions of the services or behavioral conditions that are covered should be avoided.
- Out-of-network services: Many behavioral health care benefits vary based on in-network versus out-of-network provider use by the covered members. The costs for the out-of-network benefits often are still the responsibility of the capitating organization. These out-of-network services are typically more expensive per unit and more difficult to "manage." Use of these services varies based on the degree of difference in benefit coverage between in-network and out-of-network benefits. The volume and skills of the network providers also play a role in out-of-network use.
- Demographic mix of membership: Utilization rates can vary considerably by age and gender. Other characteristics of the covered members also can be key, such as the reasons for eligibility for Medicaid coverage.

These assumptions are unique to each contracting organization and each contracting opportunity. Also, a given contract may include several distinct populations or benefits that should be analyzed separately. Clearly, capitation rates appropriate for one group or situation may not be appropriate for another.

The actuarial cost models in Tables 2–1 and 2–2 represent two different levels of behavioral health care management that have been developed to help Neighborhood Behavioral Healthcare evaluate the capitation proposal made by Quality Health Plan. The utilization targets (expressed as units per 1,000 enrollees) under the loosely managed delivery system (Table 2–1) represent a delivery system with very limited health care management capabilities in Neighborhood's geographical area. The well-managed utilization targets (Table 2–2) represent a "best practice" in the United States and illustrate the improvement potential under a well-managed delivery system. The average costs per unit are based on Neighborhood's target reimbursements, which equal 75% of billed charge levels. They also are expressed as net of insured copayments as defined by the benefit structure. The PMPM figures are a product of units per 1,000 and average costs per unit divided by 1,000 and further divided by 12.

The targets should be based on Quality Health Plan's benefit design and demographic mix. In fact, if the data are available, a cost model should be constructed based on Quality's historical experience.

The utilization rates and PMPM costs in Tables 2–1 and 2–2 are based on inpatient benefits covered at 80% up to 30 days per calendar year (with acute alternative benefits covered from "converting" acute inpatient days) and outpatient benefits covered at 50% for up to 20 visits per calendar year.

Table 2–1 Actuarial Cost Model: Quality Health Plan Capitation Analysis/ Behavioral Healthcare Services—Loosely Managed Delivery System

Service Category	Units per 1,000	Average Net Unit Cost ($)	PMPM Cost ($)
Acute inpatient	40	550	1.83
Residential	0	350	0.00
Day treatment	1	275	0.02
Intensive outpatient	1	125	0.01
Outpatient visits	350	40	1.17
Total benefit costs			3.03
Administrative costs			0.45
Risk margin			0.30
Total			3.78

PMPM, per member per month.

Table 2–2 Actuarial Cost Model: Quality Health Plan Capitation Analysis/ Behavioral Healthcare Services—Well-Managed Delivery System

Service Category	Units per 1,000	Average Unit Cost ($)	PMPM Cost ($)
Acute inpatient	9	550	0.41
Residential	2	350	0.06
Day treatment	4	275	0.09
Intensive outpatient	5	125	0.05
Outpatient visits	225	40	0.75
Total benefit costs			1.36
Administrative costs			0.34
Risk margin			0.20
Total			1.90

PMPM, per member, per month.

They may both be set at higher percentage levels under a well-managed plan. Administrative costs and risk margins are added to the benefit cost targets. Administrative costs will vary depending on the services included under the capitation agreement but could cover claims administration, utilization management, quality assurance, and member service functions. However, it should be noted that although the behavioral health care group will incur administrative costs under a capitation contract, it can be difficult to get the payer to acknowledge the value of the administrative services performed by the group.

The benefit cost targets in the actuarial cost model generally are established at best-estimate levels, which imply that the actual experience will be higher than the targets 50% of the time and lower than the targets 50% of the time. A risk margin should be added to the best-estimate benefit cost targets to increase the probability that the capitation will exceed actual costs.

The Quality Health Plan capitation proposal can be evaluated by comparing the proposed capitation with the loosely managed and the well-managed targets. A proposed capitation of $2.50 PMPM is equal to 66% of the loosely managed target. With minimal behavioral health care management, the capitation would equate to only 66% of Neighborhood's fee targets, or 50% of billed charges (66% × 75%). However, if Neighborhood could become optimally managed, the Quality capitation would yield 132% of its target or nearly 100% of billed charges (132% × 75%). This analysis also indicates that Neighborhood would have to perform about

34% ($2.65/$3.78 = 66%) better than a local unmanaged system to achieve its fee targets.

The actuarial cost models also can provide standards against which to compare actual experience after the capitated contract is signed. Variances in actual experience from the targets can be used to identify areas where improvement in efficiency or opportunities for savings could occur. More detailed versions of the actuarial cost model can further identify problem areas or opportunities. For example, the actuarial cost model could include targets by DRG, CPT code, or type of facility or professional.

Neighborhood Behavioral Health Care will need to address a number of issues in addition to the above development of actuarial cost models and capitation adequacy, including the following:

- The behavioral health care system's ability to educate and work with its professional staff and network to manage the use of various behavioral health care services efficiently
- The presence or creation of a professional incentive program to support its management objectives (In particular, can Neighborhood develop incentives for the professionals that will produce appropriate lengths of treatment?)
- The cost and risk of covering services at other facilities and by other out-of-network providers (These services could be negotiated out of the capitation contract, but this could be difficult.)
- Stop loss coverage could be obtained to protect against large claims under the capitation contract (The payer or other stop loss provider charges Neighborhood for this stop loss coverage, which should be evaluated for reasonableness by obtaining an actuarial review or by comparing the charges among various insurance carriers.)
- The capitation could be structured to vary by member age and gender to better protect Neighborhood against the risk of changes in Quality Health Plan's membership

Keys to Success under Capitated Contracts

Capitation requires a significant change from traditional fee-for-service reimbursement and may continue to become a much more prevalent form of behavioral contracting in the future. Some keys to success under capitation contracts include the following:

- New vision and mind-set. Capitation contracting requires a change in strategic vision and operations. The strategy will make the transition from filling beds, programs, and professional offices to managing the behavioral health care needs of a fixed population. All departments within the delivery system will now become cost centers. One of the keys is to share a common vision and incentives with the providers within the system.
- Professional incentive programs and buy-in. Physicians and behavioral health care clinicians control the use of acute hospital, other facility services, and various professional treatment alternatives, and they must be appropriately incented and involved in planning for success under capitation. The various facilities and professionals should have the same incentive to manage the use of behavioral health care resources appropriately. One approach is to invest in provider education programs. Some portion of existing provider education programs could be refocused on medical efficiency and the appropriate use of behavioral health care resources.
- Medical management. Another key to capitation success is the need to develop guidelines for the appropriate use of behavioral health care resources. Providers must participate in, and buy into, this guideline-setting process.
- Cost accounting and other reporting systems. A good cost accounting system is needed to identify fully how and when costs and resources are used. It should be noted that the system must account for lines of business and buyer groups as well as traditional health care accounting items. Managed behavioral care information systems will be needed to measure costs, support management of care, and evaluate required behavioral health care outcomes. These systems will need to support measurement of actual costs against the targets in the actuarial cost model for each contract. In addition, the delivery system should have a professional profiling system that supports analysis of professional performance related to facility-based and outpatient care, both for individuals and groups of behavioral professionals.
- Administrative services. It will be important to identify who is responsible for what services. The behavioral health care group will need to

negotiate with the plan for part of the plan's administrative fee. However, this may be difficult because the plan is not likely to give the behavioral group much credit for its administrative service contribution.

- Need for subcontractors. The behavioral group may be capitated for a wide range of behavioral health care services, some of which could be subcontracted to other providers. This could transfer the risks for certain services or conditions to certain behavioral health care specialists (such as substance abuse or eating disorders). This relationship with subcontracted providers also has a risk and should be as carefully evaluated as that with a managed care organization or health plan.

RISK MANAGEMENT

Like other businesses, behavioral health care providers face many kinds of risks; often these risks are interrelated. In addition, the risks faced by behavioral health care providers today contain new elements. For purposes of this chapter, these new elements of provider risk fall into three categories:

1. *Underpricing:* Expenses are greater than revenues because the prices charged are too low. Underpricing is not a new risk, but today's environment requires new approaches to forecasting and managing revenues and expenses.
2. *Fluctuation:* This refers to random, "unlucky," or infrequent events such as a run of high-cost, low-frequency behavioral health care conditions requiring extensive acute inpatient treatment. In medical settings, a run of premature infants or transplants would describe this risk. Many organizations associate this kind of risk with Lloyds of London. Health care executives may be particularly concerned about fluctuation, especially if they also are worried about underpricing.
3. *Business:* New kinds of business risk arise from the risk-sharing arrangement, including managing and distributing capitation payments, collecting required copayments, and assessing the financial stability of potential partners.

Although behavioral providers face other new risks, such as regulators constraining the kinds of business that a provider can enter, this chapter concentrates on the basic issues.

Underpricing Risk

How much should a behavioral health care provider charge for a particular service? How much should it charge for all the services that 100,000 people will need in one month? *Underpricing risk* is the danger that the provider will charge too little. Similarly, overpricing can mean the provider will become uncompetitive.

The common-sense idea that a company will get into trouble if revenues are less than expenses is made more complex by new risk arrangements. For example, a behavioral health care facility may agree to an HMO's per diem reimbursement because it believes that the per diem will generate sufficient revenue. However, if the HMO's physicians reduce length of stay (LOS), reimbursement may decrease more than the facility's expenses and the facility could lose money on this particular group of patients. This will happen unless the facility becomes more efficient, because the days that are not eliminated—the first days of the stay—are likely the most expensive for the facility.

Underpricing risk also occurs when facilities and other providers charge HMOs marginal rates. Such rates may cover the cost of providing services to an additional volume of patients, given the total current patient volume, but may not cover the average cost of all patients. Expenses include fixed and variable components; marginal pricing may cover all or a major part of the variable portion but little or none of the fixed portion. This practice can lead to a downward pricing spiral as follows:

- The HMO's lower marginal cost may give it a significant cost advantage.
- This cost advantage allows the HMO to sell its products at lower premium rates, attracting more members.
- Larger enrollment and volume of business give the HMO leverage to demand larger discounts from providers.
- The HMO has an even greater cost advantage, and the cycle continues.

If the provider's own costs do not decrease, the cycle may cause the provider to lose money under the HMO contract. Underpricing risk clearly causes more complexity for the provider. No longer can expenses be grossly identified and a simple margin added to develop fees for services.

Fluctuation Risk

Some people call fluctuation risks "insurance risks" because these are the kinds of risk that they associate with insurance companies (e.g., a homeowner's insurance protection against the unlikely occurrence of a fire). *Random risk* ("bad things happen") occurs on both a large scale (such as epidemics) and a small scale (such as an unusually high number of heart transplants). Aside from these examples, fluctuation risk also includes situations where a normally simple case or procedure goes awry and expensive complications set in. Examples of fluctuation risks are as follows:

- *Epidemics:* Death rates soared during the 1918 influenza epidemic. If such an epidemic were to occur again, the health care costs could be enormous. Would insurers, HMOs, or capitated providers become insolvent?
- *Coincidence:* In 1993, there were two heart transplants among the 2,000 people covered by the author's firm's health benefits program, which was about 20 times the national average rate of 5 per 100,000 people for the under-65 population. Was this coincidence, or is the group a bad risk? Who bore the loss?
- *Severity:* Cholecystectomies are fairly routine operations, with an average LOS of somewhat more than three days. However, in rare instances something goes wrong and the patient stays for a month. If the patient were a Medicare DRG patient, his or her LOS would cause the hospital to lose a lot of money. Are events like this random, or are they associated with improvable physician practices?

Fluctuation risks become much more dangerous financially if the provider has underpriced services or faces unusual business risks.

Business and Administrative Risk

Business risk is not new, but in the changing environment, there are many new forms and health system management has new responsibilities. A few examples of this risk follow:

- *Capitation management:* Providers are paid per covered member and must carefully track enrollment to ensure payment for all patients who might receive care. Capitation distribution also must be fair and auditable to ensure that facilities, professional providers, and others receive appropriate portions of revenue and profit.

- *Copay collection:* Suppose an HMO contracts with a facility for a $500 mental health per diem, but the facility must collect a $500 per admission copayment. The $500 per diem charge may be adequate, but if the facility does not develop the administrative systems to bill and collect the patient-pay portion, the contract could lead to large losses.

Financial Stability and Legitimacy of Partners

Like other businesses, managed care organizations and insurers can become insolvent. Payer financial and system problems can lead to delayed and uncertain payments. In many cases, system problems result from (or are related to) financial problems. Furthermore, most HMO contracts with providers contain hold-harmless provisions that prevent the provider from collecting bills from patients in the event of HMO insolvency.

Entrepreneurs and existing organizations are creating new kinds of provider, marketing, risk-taking, and payer ventures. Sponsors of these ventures may include: (1) health care providers such as physician group practices, medical societies, and hospitals or facilities; (2) insurance agents or brokers; (3) third-party administrators; (4) insurance companies; (5) HMOs or PPOs; and (6) venture capitalists. These entrepreneurs and organizations may bring important pieces of the health care market and important skills to health care networks. Nevertheless, management should ask these difficult questions before entering into a contractual relationship:

- Does the venture have sufficient capital to cover start-up costs? What is the level of sufficient capital?
- Can the venture actually deliver the promised volume of patients and revenue?
- Can the venture actuarially demonstrate that promised cost advantages are likely to materialize?
- Does the venture have all necessary regulatory approvals or a plan to obtain such approvals? What is the impact of a regulatory decision that the venture is really an insurance company or HMO and must be licensed?

- What do the partners bring in terms of skills, market and political connections, capital, and so on? What makes their proposal better than competing proposals—or the status quo?
- Does the proposed arrangement enhance the delivery of high-quality, efficient services?

Tools That Providers Can Use To Control Risk

The tools to manage risk under a reimbursement contract with a managed care organization fall into three general categories:

1. *Contractual tools:* These tools relate to modifications that would be made in the reimbursement contract to control or limit the extent to which risk is transferred.
2. *Health care delivery management tools:* These tools relate to the methods that the providers use in carrying out their main line of business, which is the actual delivery of behavioral health care services.
3. *Business tools:* These tools relate to general management techniques that can be used to manage any type of business risk.

Contractual Tools

The following section describes approaches to contractual protections against adverse experience.

Stop-Loss Insurance.   A common contract provision establishes that the carrier must make additional payments to the provider on catastrophic claims. For example, a catastrophic claim might be defined as one in which the provider's billed charges exceed $50,000 on an individual patient. The $50,000 threshold operates as a deductible. When the threshold is exceeded, the stop-loss insurance carrier would assume liability for, perhaps, 90% of all charges in excess of $50,000. The providers might obtain this stop-loss insurance through their contract with the managed care organization, or they could purchase it from a company specializing in such insurance.

Outlier Payments.   Outlier payments are made by the managed care organization on cases in which the contractual reimbursement to the provider varied significantly from the billed charges incurred by the patient. Theoretically, the outlier provisions of a contract could either increase the reimbursement to a provider or decrease it on a particular case.

For example, an outlier provision under a case rate reimbursement approach might provide that whenever the case rate is less than 50% of actual billed charges, the managed care organization will make a supplemental payment to the provider to bring the total reimbursement for that case up to the level of 50% of billed charges. It also could provide that whenever the case rate is greater than 80% of billed charge on a particular patient, the case rate will be reduced for that patient so that the provider does not receive more than 80% of billed charges in total reimbursement.

Risk-Sharing Provisions.   There are contractual provisions that can allow providers and the managed care organization to share the risk of adverse claims experience. Methods for sharing this risk could include a combination of the following:

- *An experience refund provision:* In this method, if capitation payments exceed actual billed charges by some predetermined amount, the excess amounts (or percentage thereof) will be refunded to the managed care organization.
- *A supplemental capitation provision:* In this method, if the actual billed charges exceed the capitation payments by some predetermined amount over the course of the year for the entire enrollment group, the managed care organization will supplement its reimbursement to the providers with additional capitation payments.

Both of these techniques are common provisions in insurance carrier contracts with large self-funded employers. They are becoming more common in provider reimbursement contracts.

Risk-Adjusted Capitation Rates.   The capitation payments made by the managed care organization can be adjusted to reflect key indicators of the future health costs of the individual enrollees. The most common key indicators (risk characteristics) are the enrollee's age and sex, but certain health status indicators also might be used. This type of risk classification for determining premium rates is a long-standing practice of insurance companies. Indicators of health costs should be easily determinable, the cost differences should be measurable and material, and the indicators should be practical to implement.

Subcapitation to Other Providers. Primary acceptors of capitation rate payments, who are responsible for providing all contractual behavioral health care services to the covered members, may choose to carve out some of these services or covered conditions and capitate them to a second provider under a separate contract. For example, services for eating disorders could represent a good subcapitation prospect if the primary provider group does not provide these specialized services. The primary group thus has limited its risk for the costs of providing these services by passing it on to another organization. The goal of the primary capitated group is to retain the risk only on those services over which it has some control. Care should be exercised when subcapitating specific conditions that may be complicated by comorbidities. Both parties must understand their risk division for patients who have conditions that may bridge between the two provider groups.

Escalator Clauses in Multiyear Contracts. Multiyear contracts commonly have an escalator clause that increases the rate of reimbursement for each 12-month period. This approach is superior to having a flat rate for the entire period. The most common inflation escalator clauses are based on the consumer price index (CPI), using the all-items CPI or the medical care CPI. In each case, it is likely that the CPI understates the true increase in provider costs. As an alternative to using the national CPI, the escalator could be based on the CPI for the metropolitan area in which the providers are located or for the nearest metropolitan area for which the CPI is calculated. Another alternative would be simply to have a fixed-percentage increase included in the contract (e.g., 5% per year).

Health Care Delivery System Management Tools

Behavioral delivery system management tools include any methods or approaches leading to the more efficient delivery of behavioral health care services. Meeting or beating the targets implied in the reimbursement contract with respect to length of treatment, intensity of service provided, number of admissions, and so on depends on greater efficiency. The providers need to develop medical management strategies and work with the individual professionals to develop clinical guidelines, protocols, and treatment paths. Other activities might include the following:

- Recruitment and training of medical directors experienced in managed care
- Recruitment and training of nurses with managed care experience
- Development of utilization management guidelines for clinical care
- Development of case management guidelines

Analysis of the utilization of services will be a key component in measuring and modifying the efficiency of delivering behavioral health care services. For example, comparing actual experience with clinically developed target LOS by DRG is an effective approximation of the current level of acute behavioral health care management. Medical chart audits that examine the level of efficiency and severity of cases at facilities also help improve the efficiency of health care delivery.

Resource planning is yet another tool to be used to help achieve the necessary levels of efficiency. Examination of historical utilization experience for closed population groups supports reasonable estimates about the resources needed as the capitation population grows. Resources such as the number of acute inpatient beds, residential treatment facility beds, day treatment program "slots," and so on are dependent on the level of behavioral health care management in the system and on the characteristics of the population base (such as age and sex). Resource planning supports efficient use of resources and discourages overutilization of services for which the providers are at risk. It also helps plan for the required number of providers as capitation contracts and populations are added.

General Business Tools for Managing Risk

Beyond seeking contractual protections and building systems to ensure optimal efficiency in behavioral health care delivery, health care executives should formulate a systematic approach to reviewing the operating assumptions of their managed care business. The following sections detail the key elements that should be a part of this ongoing review.

Risk Selection and Underwriting. Behavioral health care providers will want to take all necessary steps, whether contractual, through observation, or through periodic auditing, to make sure the insurance carrier or HMO is following sound risk selection and underwriting guidelines. Risk selection and underwriting (to the extent allowed by state insurance departments) are important in any insurance product line. As providers accept risk transfer, they must evaluate the methods of risk selection and underwriting employed by the managed care organization. The provider reimbursement rates in the contract are based on certain assumptions as to the health status of the insured population. It is important that the risk selection and underwriting techniques employed by the managed care organization be consistent with those assumed in the pricing of the insurance product and in the reimbursement rates for the facilities and other behavioral health care providers.

Market Assessment.   Many "markets" may supply patients to behavioral health care providers, and each one has its own expected behavioral health care costs. Each of these markets also may require different levels of needed resources and different approaches to utilization management. Typical health insurance markets include the following:

- Large employer groups (typically with self-funded health benefit plans)
- Mid-size employer groups (typically insured with insurance companies, Blue Cross/Blue Shield plans, or HMOs)
- Small employer groups (fewer than 15 employees who make insurance purchasing decisions based primarily on price and, perhaps, on the specific health care needs of individual employees)
- Individuals (who purchase their own health insurance based on perceived need)
- Medicare (mostly the elderly who, because of their age, have a variety of health care needs and often purchase insurance to fill the gaps in their Medicare coverage)
- Medicaid (the low-income population, who often have more health problems than the employee-related population and no family physician)

Each of these markets should be evaluated separately to capture the different cost and utilization expectations. For purposes of rating, projecting financial results, and analyzing financial experience, each market should be treated as a separate line of business. The analysis of financial results and the decisions about adjusting rates should be done for each market independent of the others.

Management Reporting. Good management reporting should be thorough, timely, and accurate. Management reports should give management the information to test all the assumptions that have been made in the product pricing. Management should track assumptions made in pricing with respect to utilization of services and the average charge per service for each type of behavioral health care modality along the continuum of available services. This should include acute inpatient, residential, day treatment, intensive outpatient, psychological testing, individual and group therapy, and medication management. Separate analysis of mental health and chemical dependency conditions should be completed. Separate use of different types of professional providers should be analyzed. Last, out-of-network use and cost levels must be analyzed carefully if the provider group is at risk for these services. These assumptions should be tested separately for each market or line of business.

For per diem contracts, management reports should match each service reimbursement category. For example, the contract may have a per diem for mental health DRGs, substance abuse DRGs, residential days, and so on. For each service category, the group should track admissions per 1,000, average length of stay (ALOS), cost per day, allocated cost per day, and revenue per day. The contractual per diems should be compared with the average charge per day and average cost per day to see if the underlying discount is reasonable or if the contract needs renegotiating.

Under a capitation contract, the providers should capture encounter data and the associated billed charges. They should then compare the actual billed charges and allocated costs for all services provided under the capitation contract with the capitation rate plus any copayments received, coordination of benefits and subrogation revenue, and any incentive risk pool payments. This comparison will reveal the effective discount in the capitation rate.

Additional management reporting should include tracking provider liability for any incentive pool payments to be made to other participants in the contract. In addition, reporting should include claims incurred but not reported for services performed by other providers for which the behavioral group is liable (such as specialists to whom the patients have been referred).

Financial Projections.   Financial projections of revenues and expenses should be developed as part of any feasibility study for a new venture. These projections then can be used as a test against the realities of the marketplace to see if the new venture and products are feasible. In addition, the projections act as a budget once the new venture is operational. A two-year financial projection is probably adequate in the health care insurance market (although regulatory agencies may require longer projections); projections beyond 24 months are less reliable due to changes in health cost trends. Projections should be detailed by type of service, including specific budgeted line items for acute inpatient services, residential services, day treatment, intensive outpatient, additional lines for professional services, and so on, and they should be updated frequently (perhaps quarterly, but at least semiannually) using actual data from experience monitoring reports.

Monitoring Reports.   Frequent monitoring of actual experience is essential if management is to make timely and informed repricing decisions. Experience monitoring warns of revenue shortfalls and any need to revise rates. Monitoring should include actual versus budgeted utilization, average charges per service, and dollars of expense by type of service in detail. Trends in utilization and costs also should be monitored to anticipate needed capitation revisions.

Periodic Price Adjustments.   Monitoring experience and comparing it with budgeted costs allows adjustment of prices with managed care organizations. For example, if effective LOS declines, the behavioral organization can attempt to increase its market share by agreeing to lower per case rates. However, a shorter LOS may mean that the providers will need to increase per diem rates under its per diem contracts to recognize the more intensive services provided on a daily basis for the shorter LOS. If the facility's operating costs increase, a price increase in its per diem and case rates will be necessary to increase its margins.

The providers should monitor the markets to see what price adjustments the market will allow and to charge accordingly. There is a tradition in health insurance of annual price adjustments to keep pace with inflation and other trends and to correct for past estimates of health care costs. Managed care organizations and employers should anticipate that their providers will request annual price adjustments under their contracts.

Cost Structure.   It is fundamental to successful financial management to know what it costs to bring a product or deliver a service to the market.

Providers should know their fixed and variable costs for delivering services under their contracts with managed care organizations. These costs are important to recognize for their impact on case rates if patient LOS or length of treatment (LOT) drops. Many providers do not have adequate cost accounting systems, which means, among other things, that there is no cost history on which to base their pricing decisions. Until that history can be compiled, providers have to estimate their costs when developing prices under their managed care contracts.

CONCLUSION

Provider reimbursement arrangements have changed the nature and degree of risk for both carriers and providers of behavioral health care services. Managed behavioral health care contracts often are shifting different types of "unaccustomed" risk to the providers and also adding new incentives for care delivery. Providers must learn to understand the nature of the various risks that they acquire before embarking on new contractual arrangements. Capitation rates should be analyzed and evaluated for adequacy. Provider health care delivery habits may need to change to manage utilization targets that are developed to manage risk contracts successfully. Moreover, risk management actions should be undertaken to enable organizations to protect their long-term viability as well as short-term cash flow. Providers that take the time to evaluate, analyze, understand, and manage the various payment patterns and risk characteristics of their managed behavioral health care contracts will more likely be winners as the industry continues to change in the years ahead.

CHAPTER 3

Clinical Delivery
and Medical Necessity

Ian A. Shaffer and Daniel Lieberman

Purpose: This chapter explains the evolution, significance, and controversy surrounding the concept of medical necessity.

Major Topics: This chapter discusses medical necessity's relationship to the evolution and goals of managed care, medical appropriateness, and clinical evidence. The examples of obsessive-compulsive disorder and personality disorder are presented. Variability, in both diagnosis and treatment, is identified.

INTRODUCTION

Medical necessity is a term that has been closely associated with managed care, and one that has created a great deal of controversy. It is a concept that has held a variety of meanings, but in general has not been understood well. This chapter discusses the concept of medical necessity in the development of managed care. It uses one definition of medical necessity and presents case examples to demonstrate its interpretation. Special focus is placed on some of the conflicts associated with this concept. The discussion concludes with a presentation on some of the future goals for managed care in relation to medical necessity and clinical delivery.

EVOLUTION OF MANAGED CARE

Managed behavioral health care began in the early 1980s. While managed care organizations had been present prior to that time, there was little emphasis on behavioral health. Frequently, managed care organizations offered a limited benefit for behavioral health treatment; even when the benefit was present, access was highly restricted. The limitation of benefit, accompanied by fears of stigma, yielded little use of behavioral health treatment.

Due to the perceived stigma, individuals suffering from behavioral illnesses tended not to speak up. They were a silent, underserved population. At that time, the limitation of treatment in this population did not raise sufficient concern to make any changes. Specifically, the limitation of benefits supplanted the need for medical necessity determinations in many cases.

On the other hand, in companies with indemnity insurance or those that were self-insured, rapidly escalating behavioral health care costs, increasing in excess of 20% per year, were present. Companies found these increases difficult to accept for a number of reasons. First, when companies looked at some of the information they received, it appeared that patients received highly variable treatment that was not explained. Moreover, they had no method to measure the value of the treatment that was being received by their beneficiaries. Last, the reasons for stopping treatment did not seem to be based on a clinical status, but on consumer choice.

The advent of managed behavioral health care and the concept of medical necessity began to address these concerns. Practicing clinicians were asked specific questions about the nature of the disorder, the treatment plan, and endpoint goals for each person they saw. Within this new evolving model, specific treatment plans were expected for specific clinical conditions. Clinical criteria for each level of care and evidence of medical necessity became the watchwords for authorizing the treatment that would be reimbursable under the health plan. During the initial stages of managed behavioral health care, the definition of medical necessity and the criteria for certifying care were viewed as proprietary and not released to the provider community. There was a great deal of confusion and animosity in the provider community toward managed care. Providers did not clearly understand what was expected of them, and, as a result, many of their requests for authorization were denied.

Over time, the definition of medical necessity and level-of-care criteria were made public. Nonetheless, confusion continued regarding the application of the definition of medical necessity in managed care. Much of the confusion centered on providers assuming that medical necessity determinations were disguised cost-cutting strategies. The managed care companies, on the other hand, viewed medical necessity as an approach to objectify clinical decision making and thereby as an essential element in the development of evidence-based medicine. Cost-efficient care is a natural outgrowth of this approach.

GOALS OF MANAGED CARE

Many people who became involved in managed care almost 20 years ago describe a sense of idealism. They wanted a more objective approach to the assessment and treatment of those suffering from behavioral illnesses. They believed a more standardized approach would yield cost efficiencies that would allow the reinstatement of broader benefits. In fact, managed care, in part, led to the passage of the initial federal act providing parity for mental health benefits. A recent study done for Congress by the National Advisory Mental Health Council (1998) demonstrated that in a managed care environment the cost of parity is less than 1% of the total health care cost. On this basis, a number of leading employers moved to parity for behavioral health care.

This new system demanded an increase in accountability through clarity of treatment plans and goals. This has paved the way for increased benefits. A significant portion of the responsibility for this accountability fell on providers. They are now being asked to provide comprehensive assessments, develop diagnoses, and create treatment plans for each individual they see. A significant complicating factor is that many providers' training did not follow this model. In fact, many followed a psychoanalytic or social approach in which nondirected therapy was provided with the goal of unearthing issues underlying the consumer's difficulties. In managed behavioral health care, providers must be much more specific about the problems that are being treated, the methods of treatment that are being utilized, the specific measurements of improvement that are being used throughout treatment, and what level of improvement results in an end of treatment. Medical necessity definitions in many cases are built on this paradigm. In exchange for receiving this specificity, payers are asked to provide enhanced benefits and improve overall access to treatment.

This dichotomy between specific targeted treatment and open-ended therapy has led to mixed reactions from consumers. Those with long-term illnesses are hopeful that managed behavioral health care, through increased benefits, will open the door to greater access to treatment and provide benefits that will allow for the long-term care they require. Those with acute illnesses look forward to a specific diagnosis, clear treatment plans, and a defined endpoint. At the same time, those individuals who look to therapy to improve their self-understanding and ability to relate to others react negatively to limitations placed on those therapies by managed care.

Another goal of managed care has been to contain and decrease the escalating costs of behavioral health care. The most significant component of this expense related directly to the high utilization of inpatient programs. Managed care, through encouraging the development and use of alternatives to inpatient approaches, has been instrumental in increasing the utilization of partial hospitalization and intensive outpatient programs. Many individuals who had previously been admitted to hospitals are effectively treated in these alternative levels of care. Moreover, they are able to remain at home receiving the support and encouragement of their family members and friends.

The second area of cost impact is the more focused approach to outpatient treatment. This meant that individuals who were receiving therapy must have specific functional deficits and a diagnosis to explain the treatment being received. Individuals receiving long-term treatment over many years on a weekly basis and who were clearly stable would no longer receive reimbursement. Further, people in treatment with no stated goal of treatment were no longer eligible for reimbursement for that care. On the other hand, those with long-term illness were able to receive the long-term maintenance treatment they needed at a level that was affordable for them.

The overall impact of managed care was a significant decrease in cost. In the late 1980s and early 1990s, many self-insured, large corporations moved to managed behavioral carve-out programs for their mental health and substance abuse treatment benefits. In many of these cases, companies experienced 20% to 30% decreases in cost over the first several years, while there was a 15% increase in the number of individuals accessing care.

MEDICAL NECESSITY

In order to look at medical necessity, it is necessary to first consider medical appropriateness. There are treatments that are appropriate for a condition, but not necessary. The confusion about these two concepts accounts for a good deal of the tension between manager and provider. Intensive treatment and hospitalization might be appropriate for an adolescent with a significant conduct disorder but not necessary. Treatment at a lower level of intensity may be equally effective. The use of psychoanalysis and other dynamic psychotherapies can be appropriate for goals of increasing awareness and overall growth. However, in that context they would not be seen as medically necessary. It is important to keep in mind that while a treatment may not be medically necessary, it can be medically appropriate and have a value to the individual receiving it. The difference has to do with whether a treatment is reimbursable under a benefit plan.

There is a separate group of treatments that are not appropriate. Schuster, McGlynn, and Brook (1998) state that approximately 30% of health care treatments provided to people are inappropriate. While there is some tension between clinicians and managers on inappropriate or highly questionable treatment, the issue when a medically appropriate treatment is not necessary is a much more significant issue.

In order to discuss medical necessity more fully, the definition from the *ValueOptions Provider Manual* (1999) is used for reference. ValueOptions is a managed behavioral health care organization. While each organization's manual may be different, the concept is consistent across most managed behavioral health care organizations. The definition will be discussed in a generic format; examples of the use of the definition in both acute care and long-term characterologic illness will be reviewed.

ValueOptions, as stated in its provider manual, defines medically necessary services as those services that are:

- Intended to prevent, diagnose, correct, cure, alleviate, or preclude deterioration of a diagnosable condition (*International Classification of Diseases*, 9th edition [ICD-9] or *Diagnostic and Statistical Manual*, 4th edition [DSM-IV]) that threatens life, causes pain or suffering, or results in illness or infirmity
- Expected to improve an individual's condition or level of functioning
- Individualized, specific, and consistent with symptoms and diagnosis and not in excess of patient's need
- Essential and consistent with nationally accepted standard clinical evidence generally recognized by mental health or substance abuse care professionals or publications
- Reflective of a level of service that is safe, where no equally effective, more conservative, and less costly treatment is available

- Not primarily intended for the convenience of the recipient, caretaker, or provider
- No more intensive or restrictive than necessary to balance safety, effectiveness, and efficiency
- Not a substitute for non-treatment services addressing environmental factors

In reviewing this definition, it becomes clear that the first element of medically necessary services is the presence of a diagnosable condition. Medically necessary services are utilized to diagnose and treat a condition or for maintenance care in those with a long-term illness. Services are used to maintain the individual's level of functioning and minimize the risk of relapse. Note that a goal is to improve an individual's condition or level of functioning. This specifically addresses the treatment issue where improvement is expected. Maintenance of functioning in those with long-term illnesses such as schizophrenia is an equally valid reason for providing services. One of the issues that will arise later is the level of intensity to which maintenance treatments are needed.

The third component of the medical necessity definition requires that a specific treatment plan be generated to address the patient's symptoms and diagnosis, including severity. A single diagnosis such as depression may have medically necessary inpatient care in some cases and monthly medication management follow-up in others. The managed care model requires that those admitted to higher levels of care not only have the symptoms and diagnosis of a significant illness, but also that the severity of their symptomatology requires the intensity of service being provided.

It is extremely important to keep abreast of the clinical evidence for the treatment of various illnesses. Treatment should be consistent with that evidence. It is interesting to note that behavioral health is one specialty in health care where a provider's orientation and philosophy can drive treatment as much as the clinical evidence. While there may be multiple approaches depending on the orientation of the provider, all these orientations should come from the body of knowledge about the specific illness being treated. Over the past decade, many evidence-based practice guidelines have been published. While a number of organizations have published guidelines on the same topics, most of these guidelines have many similarities that should be taken into consideration. There continues to be significant resistance to guidelines, which adds to the tension between practitioners and managed care organizations.

The fifth point states that the services must be safe. In health care, ensuring the safety of the individuals under practitioners' care must be paramount. Because all treatments have both risks and benefits, clinicians must consider both when deciding on treatment. One should not be placed in a treatment program where the potential risk outweighs the potential benefits. Just as one would not provide surgery for someone who could be treated for ulcer disease with medication, one should not provide inpatient care for someone suffering from mild depression. Moreover, given that resources for health care are finite, we must consider efficiency as well; when two equally valid treatments are available, it is prudent to select the one that is more cost-efficient.

Services provided must be based on the assessment, diagnosis, and treatment plan. Services should not be for the convenience of the consumer, family, or provider. That is not to say that there are not situations where a higher level of service is provided given an individual's particular situation. For example, in rural areas one might have to travel several hundred miles to a partial hospitalization program. In that situation, an individual is likely to be admitted to an inpatient program because the partial hospitalization program is impractical. Impracticality is different from convenience. A provider a number of years ago suggested that he did not like to discharge people on a day when the weather was inclement because it was more difficult for family members to pick up the individual. Except in highly unusual circumstances, the presence of inclement weather should not be a reason for an individual to remain in an inpatient facility.

Treatment should be provided when potential benefits outweigh potential risks. Risks and benefits are measured at a personal, family, clinical, and overall program level. One must ensure that the individual is safe and that the treatment being prescribed is safe and can be utilized based on the potential benefit one hopes to achieve. Further, treatment must be based on its potential to be effective. Consider the individual with a long-term disability who is receiving ongoing treatment with the eventual goal of returning to work. That individual should not be in treatment to return to work if there is no evidence that returning to work is possible. In those situations, the individual should receive appropriate long-term maintenance treatment to maintain progress made with the necessity of such maintenance being based on maintaining gains to date and an understanding of the risk of relapse. Last, treatment services cannot be utilized to substitute for other services that might be needed. Where an individual's living situation is impractical, it is unreasonable to request inpatient care in lieu of having that individual change his or her current living situation. For example, a substance-abusing individual should not be in an inpatient program solely to keep him or her away from an area where drugs are readily available. The environmental issues must be addressed in order to obtain success in substance abuse treatment for such an individual but they do not justify a specific level of care.

OBSESSIVE-COMPULSIVE DISORDER

Obsessive-compulsive disorder (OCD) provides an example of the use of the medical necessity definition in the certification of medically necessary services. An individual presenting with obsessional thinking or compulsive behavior must be assessed; with the diagnosis of OCD made and the deficits in an individual's functioning outlined, the first component of the medically necessary definition has been met. A number of treatments for OCD are known, and the selection of any of these would be an appropriate initial course of action. One, for example, might choose the use of behavioral therapy or specific medications and supportive therapy as the initial treatment program. Both of these can be expected to improve the condition and are reasonable selections. Given that the treatment is addressing the patient's diagnosis and is selected based on a body of evidence suggesting the possibility that these services will be helpful, the third and fourth components of the medical necessity definition are met. These services are known to be effective. Thus, the fifth component is met, as is the sixth as treatment is being designed to address a disorder. The final two components of the definition also are met.

It is clear that this disorder has a body of evidence that supports the treatment being requested. One might put forward that there is a need for family therapy given the impact of this disorder on the family's life and the impact of changes. One such example involves a 42-year-old woman who was successfully treated for OCD with medication. She had been engaging in compulsive behavior related to cleanliness, wherein she washed all of her family's clothes every night and was not available to spend time with her family. This continued over 10 years while her children, who are now 14 and 16, were growing up. Once the compulsive behavior diminished to almost zero, she was interested in engaging in activities with her family. Her husband and children reacted negatively, stating that they had developed a life to work around the patient's disorder and that they were not prepared to change what they were doing to meet her new state. It became clear that it was important to work through many of the issues the family had toward this individual in order to allow her to reengage with her family system. Here again, this is a focused treatment approach with a clear goal.

One final note is in order in working with acute illness. In OCD, one could start therapy with medication or behavioral therapy. Either of these choices would be appropriate, but regardless of which is chosen first it is not necessarily going to be effective. It is very important for the clinician to monitor the impact of the therapy. If progress is not being made within a reasonable period of time, the clinician should consider an alternative approach. While there are complaints that some general medical providers do not allow sufficient time for behavioral health treatment to be effective, behavioral health clinicians have a tendency to stay with an ineffective treatment for an excessive period of time. Progress must be measured carefully by the treating clinician and decisions made as to what is effective and how long one is going to allow the individual to experience the disorder without moving to a second, potentially more effective, alternative approach. The medical necessity definition would be reviewed here as treatment is expected to improve the individual's condition. One major area of tension between managers and clinicians revolves around how long to stay with a particular treatment. Clinicians see managers as focusing on cost. Managers see clinicians as being overly attached to a treatment model. Ultimately outcome data will help define future direction.

PERSONALITY DISORDER

Personality disorders have been particularly problematic within managed care. The individuals suffering from these disorders generally do not see themselves as having a problem and may not give evidence of functional deficits that would allow for the certification of medically necessarily services. The conflict between the managed care organizations and providers arises when the provider believes that change within the individual can be effective in the long term and the managed care organization does not see definable symptoms, diagnosis, or functional deficits. Thus, treatment of the character component of that individual may not be certified as medically necessary. On the other hand, other clinical issues of the individual may require treatment that would be certified as medically necessary.

One such example is that of the schizoid withdrawn individual. A person may be isolated and not involved in any long-term interpersonal relationship. Providers may believe that the provision of psychotherapy will assist this individual by improving his or her ability to relate to others. However, if that individual were working in an environment where interaction with others at his or her employment was minimal and he or she was comfortable living alone, then the provider will have difficulty meeting the definition and intent of the medical necessity definition.

While a personality disorder diagnosis is required in the first part of the medical necessity definition, it would be difficult to show how the situation threatens life, causes pain and suffering, or results in some form of infirmity. While the therapist takes the position that there is pain in isolation, the individual may not experience it; the lack of the functional deficits based on this individual's lifestyle raises significant doubt about medical necessity. There always has been controversy over whether such psychotherapy would improve the individual's level of functioning and how individualized and specific the treatment needs to be. It is difficult in these situations for a therapist to present specific treatment goals and how progress toward these goals will be measured. While there may be standards of care for people with character disorders, and the service may be safe, the first three components of the definition must be met. Often the acute components of illness are certified as medically necessary, but long-term treatment for characterologic change is more difficult to justify. It is likely that such treatment will meet the sixth component of the definition, as services are not for the convenience of the individual. Again the issue of intensive therapy is raised in the seventh component. While safety may not be an issue, effectiveness and efficiency become vague if treatment goals are unspecified and a mechanism to measure progress is not included, making it difficult to state how one would know treatment was effective. In fact, the task of the therapist is to develop with the patient specific treatment goals and a way to mutually monitor progress toward those goals. The eighth component is not a concern here.

In many situations the character component of an individual may not meet the medical necessity requirement; however, other issues may be present that lead to the certification of care. For example, an individual with a personality disorder who is significantly depressed with suicidal ideation should receive medically necessary services for the treatment of the suicidal ideation and depression. Once the depression and suicidal ideation resolve, it is likely that the personality disorder will not be certified for treatment absent the presence of definable functional deficits.

It is no doubt clear from the definition and from this discussion that it is extremely important that a comprehensive assessment takes place. Such a comprehensive assessment should address the clinical signs and symptoms and the individual's level of functioning within himself or herself, within his or her interpersonal sphere, and in his or her occupational or educational life. A specific diagnosis should be made. The presence of the diagnosis provides us with a natural history of the illness, as well as an understanding of which treatments the literature suggests might be effective. A specific treatment then can be chosen, and measurable goals can be defined. In the presence of that specificity, it is relatively straightforward for an individual to receive certification for services being requested.

VARIABILITY IN BEHAVIORAL HEALTH CARE TREATMENT

This section discusses some of the issues that this approach has surfaced for practitioners and some of the struggles that it raises within managed behavioral health care.

Diagnostic Variability

Geographic Variability (Philosophical Differences in Training)

For clinicians who have had the responsibility or opportunity to engage in peer review or otherwise have reviewed numerous clinical cases, one can hardly ignore the variation in both diagnoses and subsequent treatment approaches for the same or similarly diagnosed patients. Consequently, one is left to ponder the causes of these variabilities. Is the diagnosis accurate? Do clinicians diagnose disorders differently depending on their geographic location, where they were trained, or according to their mentor's or supervisor's proclivities for making a particular diagnosis (provider preferences)? Second, once diagnostic differences are analyzed, then what is the basis for choosing a particular treatment strategy?

The literature is replete with examples of practice variability associated with provider preferences and philosophies based on particular training institutes. Anecdotally, psychiatrists have been prone to favor choosing a particular Axis I diagnosis based on what was emphasized at their training program. So, for example, in the same urban center, a patient could be diagnosed as suffering from schizoaffective disorder or bipolar disorder depending on the particular training of the clinicians in the emergency department where the patient presented. While the presence of a definition for medical necessity does not resolve these issues, it adds to the continuing search for greater specificity of diagnosis and concordance of diagnosis, functional deficits, treatment plan, and overall treatment goals.

Moreover, with this specificity and after treatment, in the event of a relapse, that same person might present to a different emergency department affiliated with a different training program. It would be possible for the individual to receive a different diagnosis with similar presenting symptomatology. Another work-up would ensue, and the treatment plan would change, as would the course of subsequent treatment decisions for this individual. As Pomerantz (1999b) comments, "The fact is, we don't practice on the basis of evidence: witness the wide variations in practice styles or in outcomes for essentially any problem in any specialty. We practice according to the way we were trained—according to our experiences, our prejudices, our habits and our hopes. The available information changes, but our practice styles don't necessarily keep pace."

On a positive note, psychiatrists have begun to make great strides in diagnosing illness accurately and reliably. Bowden (1996), in his article on depression and bipolar illness, reported that "Axis I psychiatric diagnoses are made with a high rate of reliability, generally around 0.7, which is greater than the reliability of reading an exercise electrocardiogram for heart disease (0.3). The diagnostic reliability for bipolar disorder is particularly high (around 0.8), mostly because a manic episode is only recognized as such if symptoms occur that are uncharacteristic of almost any other medical disorder, thus improving the certainty of the diagnosis." Nonetheless, diagnostic variability continues in a number of categories such as personality disorders. Many payers have questioned the variability of diagnosis and treatment in apparently similar cases. They see the medical necessity definition as moving us toward greater specificity. Practitioners, on the other hand, feel that diagnosis is overemphasized and, as a result, see medical necessity definitions as missing the mark.

Belief Systems

Do a clinician's individual belief systems impact the use of the diagnostic manual? On how many occasions has one heard a behavioral health care clinician comment he or she did not want to label a person with a particular diagnosis because of its severity and the spoken or unspoken stigma attached to a mental or substance abuse disorder? Is the lexicon of our diagnostic manual itself the culprit? Is the diagnostic manual an adequate tool for cataloging diagnoses?

For example, take the case of schizophrenia in a 16-year-old patient whose symptoms have been evolving over the past year. The treating clinician is biased against making the diagnosis, not wanting to label such a young person with such a serious diagnosis. Imagine the scenario. The patient is out of town. He or she begins to experience an acute exacerbation of symptoms. "My doctor told me I have an adjustment disorder," he tells the emergency department physician, who may initiate a treatment that will be inappropriate, not knowing the patient. Can you imagine a cardiologist telling a cardiac patient that it was heartburn, not angina secondary to cardiac disease, that he or she was experiencing, not wanting to worry or label someone? Behavioral health care clinicians are somewhat more disposed to vagueness in diagnostic clarity partly because of the time-held concerns in society regarding the stigmatization of having a mental illness diagnosis. Many clinicians will not even call the person they are treating, "a patient." They use the term "client." Cardiac patients are patients. Why are persons suffering from a mental illness or substance abuse disorder different? Are behavioral health care professionals adding to the continued stigmatization associated with the field? More recently, the term "consumer" has evolved. It implies collaboration between those providing care and those receiving it. Irrespective of the term, we must endeavor to eradicate the stigma and demystify the illnesses. Correct descriptions of illnesses are key. Misdiagnosis leads to ineffective treatments and an inability to identify disorders and track treatment-associated outcomes systematically.

The variability in diagnosis that occurs as a result of clinician belief further complicates the determination of medical necessity and therefore the tension between practitioner and manager. As the managed care clinician reviews the clinical case used in this section, there is a disconnect between the presenting picture and the diagnosis. Quality-of-care concerns are raised by the managed care organization and anger at being questioned rises in the provider. What we may have is an information disconnect with the result that there is difficulty receiving certification for care. At the same time more complete clinical reporting may have met the requirements for medically necessary care and the receipt of certification.

Treatment Variability

Standardization in the delivery of behavioral health care is greatly complicated by the issues outlined in regard to diagnostic validity and reliability. The task then turns to an analysis of provider practice patterns once particular diagnoses and functional impairments have been identified. The medical literature documents wide variations in provider practices and treatment. Geyman (1998) reports

> During the last 15 years, many studies have reflected the extreme practice variations from one part of the country to another, and even within a given state. Wennberg found, for example, 20-fold differences in utilization rates for carotid endarterectomy in 16 large communities in 4 states. Within single states, he found the odds of tonsillectomy during childhood ranging from 8 percent in one Vermont community to 70 percent in another, while in Maine the range for hysterectomy varied from 20 percent to over 70 percent. A study of procedure rates for Medicare patients in 13 large metropolitan areas of the country showed variations of more than 300 percent for more than one half of the procedures. Recently another study found a fourfold variation in adjusted odds ratios for the likelihood of warfarin (an anticoagulant) use for people with atrial fibrillation in the South compared with the Midwest. All of these examples stretch the bounds of clinical credibility way beyond any reasonable variations that might be defended based upon clinical, demographic, or other geographic differences. These large practice variations call into question scientific truth in each instance; shifting to a more evidence-based style of practice would have to narrow these variations.

Moore (1997), adding to the argument, comments: "The differences in patterns of care could not be explained away by case mix, inadequacies in data or methods of analysis, or any other confounding factors."

These issues are equally cogent in behavioral health care. All too frequently, when a person arrives for an evaluation with a behavioral health care provider, multiple treatment choices are possible. For example, a depressed individual might be offered one of a variety of psychotherapies, one of a number of antidepressant medications, an herbal remedy, a holistic approach, music, art, humor, or even pet therapy. The problem is not that any of these treatments is necessarily inappropriate, but rather how to identify the most effective. The determinants of the type of treatment embarked upon and where the care will be delivered are not often data driven, but more a function of the following factors:

- Provider's technical training: Behavioral health care clinicians frequently offer treatment in which that particular clinician has expertise, regardless of the existence of an evidence-based outcome matching the treatment to the disorder.
- Provider's physical location: Providers tend to treat people where they themselves practice and are comfortable; inpatient clinicians will tend to recommend inpatient care despite availability of clinically appropriate alternative levels of care.
- Institutional training: Training institutes frequently are attached to a particular philosophy of care in which they excel; trainees tend to limit their scope of expertise to that specific modality.
- Availability of true expertise in a specialty modality of treatment: An area of concern is the dearth of formally trained short-term and cognitive behavioral therapists. Cognitive behavioral therapy and other short-term therapies require rigorous and formal training. There are few training institutes in these specialties; therefore, there are few formally trained clinicians.
- Individual variations in skill level of delivering treatment.

There are particular concerns regarding treatment variability in outpatient therapy, based on what appears to be a paucity of expertise in modalities other than long-term dynamic psychotherapy. Recent literature clearly suggests that focused psychotherapies may be as or more effective than medications for the treatment of depression (Pomerantz, 1999a).

Here, again, the component of medical necessity that focuses on specific treatments shown to be effective for specific illnesses comes to the fore. While there are a number of equally valid treatment regimens for several disorders, managed care still requires specificity of goals and progress milestones based on the particular treatment program selected. A number of treatment approaches are nonspecific and nondirected. Here, again, the differences between managed care and the practitioner community add to the tension and frustration.

FUTURE GOALS

As discussed throughout this chapter, medical necessity criteria have been developed as a response to the rising cost of health care delivery, an attempt to be more specific in providing treatment, and an effort to decrease inappropriate variations in the quality of care delivered. A key goal in developing specific treatment guidelines is an attempt to decrease unexplained variation within treatments for individuals suffering from the same disorder on the one hand and clearly defend the variables in treatment for others. In order for this to evolve, providers and managers must share a more unified vision recognizing the need for development and implementation of evidence-based clinical practice guidelines. By definition, these guidelines are "systematically developed statements to assist practitioner and consumer decisions about the appropriate health care for specific clinical circumstances" (Moore, 1997). Treatment chosen will then be based on a combination of those that are known to be effective and the consumer's current situation. From within those choices, one will be agreed upon between the provider and the consumer of care. While it is not the goal of managed care to provide cookbook-like treatment guidelines, it is managed care's intention to raise questions on the issues that went into a provider's decision to recommend a form of treatment. These forms of treatments would be suggested by the nature of the illness and the information known about treatment, and not by a provider's philosophy or belief structure. At the same time, there is significant variability within treatments. For example, cognitive behavior therapy is done a number of different ways by different therapists. It is not possible for, nor is it managed care's intent, to begin to separate these elements within treatment. However, managed care is in a position to continue to encourage measurement of progress toward stated goals and encourage providers to reassess treatments they are providing if improvement is not taking place in a reasonable timeframe.

As mentioned at the outset, many providers have not been trained in this model of assessment, diagnosis, and treatment. Often providers enter into managed care contracts and must retrain themselves in order to function within the managed care environment. While some providers will solve this problem by moving away to areas where there is little or no managed care penetration, others do wish to be in communities where managed care is highly penetrated. They, therefore, will work with managed care companies to receive the training that moves them closer to a model that conceptualizes cases with the development of a treatment plan supported by the data and evidence-based treatment information. Providers are frequently being asked by managed behavioral health care companies to show evidence that critical thinking went into the development of a specific treatment approach and that the treatment approach selected is by individual need. There are, unfortunately, still practices where all those who enter a particular therapist's office receive the same form of treatment, most frequently once-a-week psychodynamic psychotherapy. Individual needs for therapy are not regimented to a once-a-week model. We must work with academic centers to train providers to think through the intensity of treatment that is required and the justification. At some points in time, individuals will need less frequent care. For example, an individual with a long-term illness such as bipolar disorder who is stable may need to be seen only once every one to three months. However, if that same individual suffers a relapse, he or she may need to be seen several times a week during that acute episode and, once improved, return to a less frequent maintenance program.

To be successful, managed behavioral health care organizations, providers, and academic institutions must come together to develop a model that highlights the critical thinking that is necessary in developing a meaningful treatment program. This would be very effective in diminishing the current tensions that exist between the consumer, provider, and manager in determining which services will be seen as medically necessary.

In the end, provider training that emphasizes conceptualizing a problem and utilizes a treatment plan derived from evidenced-based data will eventually remove from managed care the necessity to oversee medical necessity criteria and will move us to the study of outcome information. That information, which will demonstrate the result of the treatment both clinically and functionally, will allow us to gain further treatment specificity and a demonstrable improvement in outcomes in the ongoing evolution of best practices.

REFERENCES

Bowden, C.L. (1996). Depression and bipolar disorder: Implications for medical care in an era of managed health care. *Medscape Mental Health, 1*(11).

Geyman, J.P. (1998). Evidence-based medicine in primary care: An overview. *Journal of the American Board of Family Practice, 11*(1), 46–56.

Moore, K.G. (1997). Evidence-based clinical practice guidelines. *Drug Benefit Trends, 9*(4), 37–45.

National Advisory Mental Health Council. (1998). *Parity in financing mental health services: Managed care effects on cost, access & quality. An interim report to Congress.* Bethesda, MD: National Institute of Mental Health.

Pomerantz, J.M. (1999a). Focused psychotherapy as an alternative to long-term medication. *Drug Benefit Trends*, *11*(7), 2, 5.

Pomerantz, J.M. (1999b). Behavioral health matters: Clinical practice guidelines. *Drug Benefit Trends*, *11*(4), 2–BH.

Schuster, M.A., McGlynn, E.A., & Brook, R.H. (1998). How good is quality of healthcare in the United States? *The Milbank Quarterly, 76*(4), 517–563.

ValueOptions Provider Manual. (1999). Fairfax, VA: ValueOptions.

CHAPTER 4

Integrating Behavioral Health and Primary Care: Finding New Solutions to Long-Standing Problems

Jerome V. Vaccaro and Christy L. Beaudin

Purpose: This chapter discusses the goal and status of integrating behavioral and primary health care.

Major Topics: This chapter discusses Definitions, Core Concepts, Prevalence, Detection, Diagnosis, and Psychiatric Liaison. It also explains the controversies of Confidentiality, Organized Delivery Systems, Financing, Treatment Guidelines, Formularies, Communications, Best Practices, and Turf Wars. In response to these controversies, solutions based on existing practices are identified.

INTRODUCTION

Integrating behavioral health and general health care is a topic ready to occupy center stage. Volumes are devoted to it, accreditation and regulatory agencies cite and promote its importance, and yet no one can define or offer strategies for effective operations that satisfy everyone. Furthermore, forces are aligned to resist integration from many quarters, as it challenges old ways, traditions, and institutions, and it will lead to significant role changes among providers and management agents. Its rise in importance is occasioned by the accountability for outcomes and costs that was ushered in by managed care: Purchasers and other stakeholders demand that managed care organizations and health care delivery systems look for ways to provide affordable, effective care that considers the comprehensive needs of the consumer.

In no other area of health care has there been such a significant and well-developed specialty sector as exists for behavioral health. The reasons for this are many including underlying beliefs about the mind/body dichotomy, the early development of the state hospital system, and initiatives such as the community mental health movement of the 1960s and 1970s. This high degree of specialization, while furthering the development of care and financing models, also has marginalized behavioral health within the health care system.

The attention to integration forces managed care to examine the status quo and find new solutions to long-standing problems. How well we do this will depend on a clear understanding of the challenges we face, a vision of what the possibilities are, and our creativity in finding solutions that are manageable. Thus, integration carries with it the requirement that we change our roles and processes in dramatic ways. In this chapter, we will attempt to move beyond the lofty reasons for integration and suggest a framework for accomplishing some of its core elements, highlighting terms and concepts, addressing areas of controversy, pointing out what has worked in the past, and suggesting directions for the future. Last, this description may fall short in the reader's view in terms of what actually works to improve the coordination of behavioral and primary care. Effectiveness research is not yet readily available about existing programs that are considered the state of the art.

DEFINITIONS AND CORE CONCEPTS

Integration/Coordination

From its earliest days, medicine has struggled with the concept of integration—first at the level of the individual patient, then in considering the assignment of roles among health care professionals, and last in the design of systems of care. The concept of integration is attractive largely due to presumed benefits to the individual through a comprehensive approach to care. Intuitively, this is quite attractive; yet, for many reasons it has not been achieved in most settings.

For our purposes, *integration* is the alignment of goals, incentives, and systems such that consumers are provided with well-coordinated, comprehensive, and efficient care with individual offerings that are synergistic rather than conflictual. This definition raises a series of questions, perhaps the most hotly debated being the role of the two primary approaches to managing behavioral health care delivery: carve-in and carve-out models. There are those who decry the use of managed behavioral health care organizations (MBHOs), saying that they promote fragmented and uncoordinated care. Indeed, this is a potential pitfall of any arrangement where multiple entities work toward managing the process of care. Equally persuasive, though, is the argument that a dedicated focus on behavioral health care is beneficial or even necessary, and that the potential downside is offset when organizations develop interdependencies, "permeable boundaries," and aligned incentives (Feldman, 1996). Further, it is the authors' opinion that one size does not fit all. There is no one approach (carve-out or carve-in model) that suits all environments; it is best for stakeholders such as purchasers and consumers to debate the merits of these models and arrive at informed choices best suited to their own needs.

Prevalence, Detection, and Diagnosis of Mental Disorders

It is estimated that 17% of the general population has a diagnosable behavioral health disorder (Regier et al., 1993). There is disagreement about what proportion of these individuals requires the attention of behavioral health care specialists. However, it is clear that less than one third of such individuals actually receive services from behavioral health specialists in most settings. Among primary care patients who have other medical conditions, comorbidity of behavioral health disorders ranges from 20% to 40%, depending on the health condition involved (Wells et al., 2000). In all, then, behavioral health disorders are highly prevalent both in the general population and among persons seen in primary care settings. Relatively few of these individuals receive care targeted to these disorders.

Vast underdetection of mental disorders in primary care populations compounds effective integration of behavioral health with primary care. While nonpsychiatric physicians prescribe more than two thirds of psychotropic medications, fewer than half of patients with depression are recognized as such by their primary care doctors (Depression Guideline Panel, 1993). The picture is even bleaker with chemical dependency, where the majority of persons with substance use disorders go with the condition unrecognized (National Institute on Alcohol Abuse and Alcoholism, 1993).

Finally, while detection programs may help remedy these problems in detection, not all primary care practitioners have the time, skill, or inclination to diagnose, let alone treat, behavioral health disorders accurately.

Whether the high prevalence of persons presenting with mental disorders in primary care settings is seen as a result of the way our systems are designed or due to consumer choice, there is a clear imperative to address behavioral health problems in these settings.

Prevention

Talk of prevention in behavioral health generates considerable emotion and relative inaction. Until accrediting agencies turned their attention to this area, few systems of care outside of community mental health agencies and employee assistance programs (EAPs) paid it much heed. The National Committee for Quality Assurance (NCQA) launched its MBHO accreditation program in 1996 to provide employers and the 140 million Americans enrolled in MBHOs at that time information about the quality of those organizations (NCQA, undated). It was at this time that MBHOs began developing such programs in earnest. Indeed, many health maintenance organizations (HMOs) began devoting attention to this important area as a result of their own accountability for prevention programs.

How to implement prevention programs effectively in a managed care environment also has become central to government agencies. For example, the Center for Substance Abuse Prevention (CSAP) and the Substance Abuse and Mental Health Services Administration (SAMHSA) sponsored the "CSAP Prevention Benchmarks and Managed Care Working Group" held in San Francisco, California, in September 1999. The purpose of the work group was to identify benchmarks for substance abuse and mental health prevention programs that would be included in benefits for managed care plans. One of the topic areas addressed was the development of realistic goals and how to promote a shift from tertiary prevention models toward a primary prevention model. Related issues such as practice guidelines, integration with primary care, accreditation standards, contracting language, quality improvement, performance measures and indicators, outcomes, and the potential for realistic prevention benchmarks were discussed. These forums likely will increase the focus on prevention in managed care organizations (MCOs) and raise the performance bar.

Consultation/Liaison Psychiatry

This subspecialty field (albeit not recognized by way of certification) has seen its popularity wax and wane over time. At its core, it is an approach that is devoted to the integration of care at the consumer level by providing consultation services (seeing patients or rendering advice to medical colleagues) in medical settings and developing ongoing liaison with medical colleagues in the form of educational offerings and system linkages. Its main goal is the provision of integrated care through a collaborative effort among health and behavioral health care providers. Oftentimes, it is interpreted as being devoted to specific sets of disorders (e.g., somatization disorder), medical-psychiatric interfaces (e.g., identifying whether a condition has an underlying "medical" versus "psychiatric" cause; addressing medical-psychiatric comorbidity), types of patients (e.g., the "difficult patient" in the medical setting), or enhancing the care of persons with chronic diseases (e.g., health improvement and disease management).

CONTROVERSIES

The literature is replete with suggestions about how the care of persons with behavioral health disorders can be managed. For example, David Mechanic (1997) offered six models for integrating behavioral health with primary care: mainstreaming, psychiatric/collaboration, new practitioner, independent carve-outs, functionally integrated carve-outs, and extended care models. However, models aside, there are numerous barriers to realizing truly integrated care. They range from systems deficits through problems posed by role confusion, individual skill deficits, and bias.

Confidentiality: Real Concern or Shield from Accountability?

Early efforts to facilitate communication between behavioral health and health care providers were stymied by concerns over confidentiality. Psychotherapists expressed apprehension that sharing details of their treatment would hamper the therapy they were providing. Primary care practitioners, in fact, did not and do not want reports about intimate details provided during psychotherapy. Instead, they seek information relevant to their own work with their patients, namely medications prescribed; the fact that a patient is getting treatment for an identified behavioral health concern; or suggestions about ways to address treatment, disease management, or compliance problems.

The consumer also may be a source of concern for the sharing of clinical information among his or her treating practitioners. There is both reluctance and misunderstanding about the "what" and "with whom" that serve as barriers to sharing information to advance a treatment plan. The misunderstanding over the desired information has been a powerful driver for the special protections sought for behavioral health records in legislative and regulatory patient confidentiality initiatives. In response to these concerns, MBHOs and MCOs have developed clear protocols (some outlined below) for sharing of information, so that only essential data are shared. When these protocols are implemented, and patients are made aware of the reasons for sharing specific information, care is improved and all stakeholders (providers, consumers, and MBHOs/MCOs) meet their responsibilities and needs.

Organized Systems of Care versus Organized Delivery Systems

Conversations about integration reach a feverish pitch when it comes to defining specific solutions. Battle lines are drawn between advocates of closed, organizationally/physically integrated systems and those who argue for the maintenance of separate entities such as MBHOs. Doherty, McDaniel, and Baird (1996) defined levels of collaboration or integration along a continuum from level I (minimal collaboration) through level V (close collaboration) in a fully integrated system.

These levels can be interpreted to mean that the desired state is one in which a system is organizationally, physically, and financially integrated; this is, in fact, the flash point for many debates about integration. Whether this interpretation is correct seems not to be the point. In today's highly sophisticated technology environment, it becomes feasible to speak about fully integrated systems that are aligned through clinical, organizational, and financial agreements and supported by information systems that become the glue in a new "virtual system of care." Most citizens and payers have chosen to maintain the unique American system of non-staff models of care, and so it appears incumbent on health system administrators to design and run these virtual systems.

Financing

Opinions are like certain anatomic parts: everyone has them. Nowhere is this more apparent, and nowhere are opinions more firmly held, than in the area of health care financing. For every stakeholder who believes that provider risk sharing is worthy or essential, there is an opponent of such arrangements. The waxing and waning in popularity of capitation, case rating, and other approaches make for great drama and confusing strategy. The argument in favor of risk sharing is that it aligns providers' and health plans' incentives. Early systems, in which safeguards were less well developed, generated concern that access to care might be blocked with provider risk sharing. Accrediting bodies such as NCQA and state regulatory bodies have developed robust oversight requirements to establish and maintain patient protections.

A mid-course redirection in these arrangements involves the use of financial rewards for improvements in quality. Generally speaking, these involve rewarding providers for improvements in certain aspects of care, based on both process and outcome measures. While these have been used in a limited manner thus far, and not very extensively to spur integration, this approach represents promise for improving best practices for care integration.

A final note about financing should include discussion of the perceived inadequacy of behavioral health funding. Over the past decade, behavioral health funding has not kept pace with health care; in fact, some believe that behavioral health resources have actually declined by as much as 40% to 50%. Some have argued that this may be redressed through the redirection of health care dollars through demonstration of "cost offsets," or through decreased resource consumption by persons who receive additional or adequate behavioral health treatment. While attractive in theory, this has not been implemented, nor is the notion of cost offsetting widely accepted as fact in real-world settings.

Treatment Guidelines

Fascination with treatment guidelines rose and fell like a rocket. The early enthusiasm with the idea that promulgating "best practices" guidelines would alter treatment practices has been replaced by the sober awareness that changing practice patterns is a laborious, difficult, and costly process. Today, the average health or behavioral health practitioner works with four to six MCOs, all of whom develop and disseminate treatment guidelines in response to accrediting bodies' mandates to do so, or the desire to keep up with industry competitors, or simply wanting to incorporate evidence-based practices into care delivery. It is no wonder, then, that the impact of publishing guidelines is limited. Efforts to make guidelines "live" and be used in real time are now the focus.

Throughout health care, data show that the incorporation of research findings into clinical practice is slow and irregular. Whether examining the usage rates of efficacious medications in cardiovascular disease or tracking compliance with a full course of antidepressant medication among depressed patients, success rates rarely exceed 40% in unmanaged, real-world settings. Success stories in actual practice settings come only with an almost obsessive focus on improving quality. Common success factors include distilling treatment guidelines into one- or two-item practices and then repetitively communicating the importance of the particular treatment element. Wells and associates (2000) developed and tested evidence-based intervention materials (training guides, slides, brochures, and videos) designed for clinicians, nurse specialists, psychotherapists, and patients by incorporating them into a quality improvement program that was a resource tool kit for primary care practices. The program did not require any services beyond those that already were covered by the health plan. The study found that patients with both severe and mild forms of depression improved their outcomes under the program, and that the program was similarly effective whether it provided extra resources for medication management or for psychotherapy.

Formulary

Rising pharmacy costs and the use of formularies are the lightning rods of current managed care debates. The use of restricted formularies is becoming increasingly popular while also being judged as wrong-minded. Especially in behavioral health circles, where the consumer and advocate communities are better developed than in many areas of health care, controlling access to drug therapies is a highly charged issue.

Wherever the debate ends, it is important for behavioral health specialists to join with our health care colleagues in dialogue. We must contribute to the debate in policy-making forums within health care organizations, and we must help advance the understanding of the total costs of care by linking MBHO data sets with those of pharmacy benefits management (PBM) companies and MCOs. It also is critical that we involve other stakeholders in this debate, including pharmaceutical manufacturers, payers, and consumers.

Training for Best Practices

Related to discussions about poor penetration of best practices is the inadequacy of providers' skills. The U.S. Department of Health and Human Services report (1999) titled *Mental Health: A Report of the Surgeon General* highlights the historical tendency of training programs not to equip new professionals with the knowledge and skill needed to deliver effective treatments. Nowhere in health care is this better illustrated than in the case of psychotherapy. For example, while cognitive behavior therapy (CBT) has been demonstrated to be effective for the treatment of depression, few professionals are able to deliver this specific intervention with any reliability (Wells et al., 2000). Furthermore, few professionals are trained in the collaborative models of care that are required for success in the integrated treatment environment of the future. Last, few programs prepare graduates for practice in managed care settings (Di Lorenzo & Williamson, 1997).

What is required is extensive retooling of our educational and training institutions and programs so that they offer didactic and practical work in these areas. This may include some competency measurement of practitioners in preprofessional and postgraduate academic training programs that would permit graduates to have immediate entry into managed care panels and would indicate competency to work in public sector systems in higher levels of responsibility without additional training. To achieve this proficiency, both intellectual and experiential content would need to be taught using a multidisciplinary approach (involving both traditional faculty along with consumers and family members as faculty) that would incorporate the values and standards of contemporary behavioral health care (American College of Mental Health Administration, 2000). Topics may include developing the ability to integrate or work with primary/ specialty care practitioners and deliver prevention and health education. While this is easily stated, and has actually been highlighted for years, academic institutions remain sluggish at best as they contemplate such shifts in focus and attention.

Turf Wars

Health care turf wars are perhaps at their worst at the interface between health and behavioral health care. Battles may become pitched over where a patient is best served or, conversely, where not served. However, the adequacy of mental health services is confounded by variation in service availability and variation in practice. This includes diagnosis by setting, patient groups, and diagnostic criteria; the management of mental health needs in the primary care setting beyond depression; competing tasks and demands; and, finally, the organization of services and incentives (deGruy, 1997). Concerns over payment in our now highly specialized and fragmented field tend to make these battles seem fiercer. Rather than place blame or add to a frenzied and often irrational debate, we are served better by identifying and addressing the needs of the "big three"—the consumer, the provider, and the purchaser.

Considering the nascent behavioral health/health care alignment, consumers are best served by beginning with systematic application of rational clinical protocols. These should be processes that use scientific approaches to identify clinical needs, then articulate the focus of care (what is to be delivered), and finally decide on the appropriate locus of care (where it is best to be delivered). Once decided in this manner, the appropriately credentialed, licensed, and privileged providers may be deployed to meet a consumer's needs. These components of our system are necessary, but certainly not sufficient, in the endeavor to deliver effective, efficient care.

The administrative apparatus that supports appropriate care is the glue in this system. Too frequently, qualified and well-intentioned providers offer the right care at the right time, only to find that they failed to consider some administrative rule in their environment. It is incumbent on the architects of these systems to work out, in advance, who pays for what under what circumstances and according to what rules.

SOLUTIONS/MODELS

Concern remains high with the lack of penetration of best practices throughout our systems of care. This section frames the main areas of focus for quality improvement and then illustrates these with workable solutions or model programs. In each case, an attempt is made to define the critical success factors so that the reader may use these solutions in varied practice settings, highlighting mechanisms that incorporate clinical utility, reduced administrative burden, and reliability. Without a supportive, efficient system that facilitates integration, none of the individual efforts of providers are likely to impact outcomes or succeed in meeting the expectations of consumers, purchasers, and accreditation organizations.

Screening/Detection/Diagnosis

One of the most vexing clinical problems at the interface between behavioral health and health care is the recognition of behavioral health disorders in their most common locale, the primary care office. The sobering realization that the vast majority of behavioral health problems first present here and remain undetected has led many organizations to galvanize their efforts around improving detection through the use of validated screening instruments in numerous formats. Following closely on the heels of detection difficulties is the problem of accurate and reliable diagnosis. This dilemma is difficult enough to solve in behavioral health settings, but it is made more challenging in health care settings where focus, time, and expertise are more limited.

Harvard Pilgrim Health Care established a program for the early detection and treatment of depression in a primary care setting. Using these principles in planning—focus, simplification, minimization of practice interference, and starting small—enabled the mixed-model HMO to implement a successful program with its primary care providers. The program components included depression screening (three item "yes" or "no"), education (learning modules), mental health consultation during working hours, patient and physician supports (videos and treatment summary cards), and outcomes evaluation. Finally, a key financial incentive was built into the basic capitation to encourage the ongoing success of the program (Stelovich, 1997). The initial results suggested that undetected depression was being uncovered but the true program effects had not yet been analyzed.

Consumer Communication

Seeking any and all avenues of communication with members has been a focus of MCOs/MBHOs. To fulfill standards for prevention and quality improvement under NCQA, communication that is targeted to member need is one critical pathway to successful accreditation. Different purchasers have different expectations, and the rates paid to MCOs/MBHOs may not be commensurate. So, focused and well-planned member services activities consume both development time and committee time in every organization.

Raytheon serves as an exemplar of a purchaser working with its health plan, Blue Cross and Blue Shield of Massachusetts (BCBSM), in a partnership to improve the delivery of both the behavioral and medical aspects of delivery (Langman-Dowart, Gatti, & Duval, 1997). To improve communication, Raytheon and BCBSM tackled key problem areas with respect to transition of care by sending letters emphasizing the importance of primary care and distributing a monthly newsletter. A health information line, Infodial for Health, was made available that uses a modified Zung tool to screen members confidentially and offer referral information. Finally, Blue Care Line provided 24-hour access to members who needed immediate assistance or advice. About 6.3% of the Blue Care Line calls are Raytheon members. At the end of the partnership's first year, a measure of success was that approximately 50 cases were co-managed with medical and behavioral health triage (Langman-Dowart, Gatti, & Duval, 1997).

Several of Magellan Behavioral Health's Regional Service Centers have implemented primary care physician (PCP)–related medical integration activities. These can be divided into five key areas:

1. PCP educational activities
2. PCP 800 help lines
3. Prevention activities/programs that actively involved PCPs
4. Member educational materials/activities designed for PCP offices
5. Integration of behavioral health screening, assessment, and referral into chronic medical disease management

Magellan is in the process of developing several different systems that will utilize interactive voice technology to improve the collaboration and coordination of care between medical and behavioral health practitioners. The first of these systems to become operational is the centralized version of the postpartum depression (PPD) prevention program that become operational in late October 1999 and is serviced 24 hours per day, 7 days per week by medical nurses trained in mental health through the Magellan Specialty Health nurseline. The goals of the PPD program include the early identification, appropriate referral, and treatment of depressive disorders in new mothers. One of the goals is the education of members and health care providers including PCPs and obstetricians as to the signs and symptoms of postpartum depression. Early identification and treatment of PPD also may affect the link drawn between maternal postpartum depression and child functioning.

A PCP depression/anxiety testing system also is being developed that will be piloted with a teaching hospital in San Francisco. Ultimately interactive voice technology systems may be developed that would link PCPs, pharmacy benefit managers, health plans, and MBHOs. These systems could provide valuable profiling information back to MCOs regarding PCP's psychotropic prescribing patterns and behaviors, with the ultimate goal of improving appropriate prescriptive patterns and decreasing inappropriate patterns. With these systems, Magellan will be able to offer solutions to health plans that are searching for ways to meet the NCQA MCO Standard Quality Improvement 9 that looks to the MCO to provide evidence of ensuring the continuity and coordination of care that members receive.

Practitioner Communication

Practitioners sometimes see the process of coordinating care as time consuming; in addition, it has not become part of the fabric of delivering care in many settings. For these reasons, PacifiCare Behavioral Health (PBH) developed a system of easy-to-use forms, decision support tools, and targeted reminders to improve primary care integration efforts. Enhancing communication with provider partners is central to this effort. First, a simple, one-page document, the Health Care Coordination Form (HCCF), is required of practitioners for all patients seen; this form is sent to the PCP. The HCCF contains the following two sections:

1. Section 1 obtains the member's signature for permission to share information about current behavioral health treatment
2. Section 2 provides a summary of relevant clinical data from the behavioral health practitioner

In addition, reminder letters are sent to practitioners when members meet criteria for coordination of care based on an analysis of the Provider Assessment Report (the treatment plan). It reminds them of the importance of coordinating care with other practitioners. In its first year of operation, this program improved performance significantly.

Formulary Strategy

Pharmacology is a critical component of treatment for behavioral health disorders. MCOs and MBHOs seek innovative solutions to the management of pharmacy benefits. ValueOptions uses an integrated approach to care management—Rx Innovations (RxI), which is an affiliate of its parent company FHC (First Hospital Corporation) Health Systems. Data warehousing technology is key to facilitating the linkage of pharmacy services and medical outcomes. RxI provides analytical and disease management services and pharmacy management services. Moreover, RxI's PBM services can be integrated with behavioral health programs to manage care and pharmacy through performance-based contracting and full-risk capitation through an integrated behavioral health services program. Through these programs, ValueOptions helps its providers understand which drugs have the best rates of consumer adherence and clinical outcomes, promoting evidence-based formulary decisions. Finally, provider and consumer medication utilization profiles present opportunities to target educational initiatives.

Outcomes Management

Studies show that clinical results vary considerably from one provider or system of care to the next. Without the accountability introduced by managed care, systems have no incentive to focus on outcomes measurement, let alone improve clinical outcomes. Throughout health care, this area has become integral to the success of health plans and practitioners alike. Within behavioral health care, the measurement of indicators of clinical outcome has lagged behind the rest of health care. As a result, primary care practitioners often view behavioral health efforts with skepticism. In recent years, managed behavioral health care organizations have taken this problem to heart and begun to address it.

MBHOs have adopted existing instruments, such as the SF-12/20 and BASIS-32, or developed their own to provide some measure of success for treatment effectiveness. For example, the ALERT (ALgorithms for Effective Reporting and Treatment) system is an outcomes management program developed by PBH that includes consumer self-report data for both adults and youth. This system, designed to promote outcomes management rather than simple outcomes measurement, permits meaningful comparisons to be made at larger system levels. The program begins with instruments that are sensitive to detecting real change by analyzing change based on self-report items in combination with provider-reported data. Reports are then generated that are used in case management, network management, resource allocation, and outcomes evaluation as follows:

- The ALERT system connects the patient, the provider, and PBH in an information loop that provides timely reports on critical risk factors and changing levels of distress for the consumer.
- ALERT captures data and generates reports with high efficiency and low burden on consumers and providers. These reports then guide modifications in the treatment plan to help ensure better clinical outcomes.
- Aggregate level reports demonstrate clinical outcomes for entire systems of care and for specific provider groups.

Regardless of the setting or the funding source for behavioral health care services, the value of services must be demonstrable to all stakeholders. While it is important to measure variables such as client satisfaction, service quality, and essential clinical processes, it is vitally important to demonstrate positive clinical outcomes as well. Overall, behavioral health services are quite beneficial for those in need of care, and programs such as ALERT give clients the empirical evidence to prove this to payers and consumers.

THE FUTURE

What, then, does the future hold? We predict increased attention will be paid to the integration of behavioral health and health care, as demonstrated by the many efforts of all stakeholders: payers, consumers, accrediting bodies, regulatory agencies, and managed care organizations. This attention will lead to the extension of those efforts outlined in this chapter and development in the areas noted below.

Best Practices

We live in a society in which consumers expect demonstrated value in their purchases. In no industry but health care has the prevailing lack of accountability for consistent delivery of high-quality services been tolerated. This situation will end. Stakeholders will demand that systems of care demonstrate continued advancement in best practices, including consistent delivery of care, reduction or elimination of medical errors, and better clinical outcomes. This will place greater emphasis on MBHOs' and practitioners' initiatives to measure what they do and take responsibility for processes and outcomes of care. We must find ways to advance the science of our field, thus tangibly improving outcomes, while at the same time providing superior service.

Development of Virtual Systems of Care

As the Internet and related technologies become more firmly ensconced in our lives, we will see these facilitators bind our current disjointed systems. Primary care and behavioral health practitioners will be in immediate contact with one another and will influence one another's treatment decisions, allowing for true synergies in care to develop. This will move the dialogue away from the frivolous debates about "carve-in" versus "carve-out" to more productive debates about demonstrable quality improvement.

Pay for Value: Quality Performance Management

As in other fields, consumers will leave systems of care that do not deliver expected value. Especially as end-users/consumers become increasingly responsible for health care costs through greater cost sharing and other means, they will "vote with their feet" and leave plans and providers who do not measure, demonstrate, and report better outcomes. In recent years, the use of financial and other incentives for delivering truly better outcomes has become more prevalent. We expect this trend to continue. Simultaneously, health plans will gravitate from intrusive utilization management programs toward quality improvement–based management of providers. Thus, through greater consumer informed choice and health plan/MBHO selection and direction to high-quality providers, those who deliver truly integrated care will thrive.

Training and Education

In our increasingly inter-linked health care systems, training programs are less immune to true accountability. Previously unrestricted funding streams that were tied to questionable reimbursement practices are largely a thing of the past. Institutions must now demonstrate to a wide audience of stakeholders that they produce value. They will be forced to demonstrate that they are training professionals for practice in today's environment. Their survival will depend on their ability to promote best practices in care delivery: They must equip their trainees with scientifically valid therapeutic skills, and their trainees must be taught to use them in newly integrated, accountable systems of care. Training of primary care practitioners needs to include curriculum and experience that will help them deal with psychological issues encountered in the primary care setting. This might include familiarity with screening tools for depression and other behavioral health disorders, facilitating disclosure of symptoms by patients that will lead to definitive diagnoses and treatment plans, and an increased understanding of psychotropic medications (Mechanic, 1997).

In all, we live in turbulent times; change and uncertainty are disconcerting, but they present new opportunities to improve care, particularly at the interface between behavioral health and the rest of health care. We should seize the opportunities and chart new paths to high-quality, outcome-driven, error-free, and fully integrated care.

REFERENCES

American College of Mental Health Administration. (2000, March 15–19). Changing the actions, strategies, and behaviors of clinicians, consumers, families and organizations: The critical role of education and training. Paper presented at the Santa Fe Summit, Sante Fe, New Mexico.

deGruy, F.V. (1997). Mental healthcare in the primary care setting. *Families, Systems & Health, 15*(1), 3–26.

Depression Guideline Panel. (1993, April). *Depression in primary care: Volume 2. Treatment of major depression. Clinical practice guideline, number 5.* AHCPR publication no. 93-0551. Rockville, MD: U.S. Department of Health and Human Services, Public Health Service, Agency for Health Care Policy and Research.

Di Lorenzo, T.M., & Williamson, H.A. (1997). Training for interdisciplinary practice: Trends in clinical psychology and family medicine. In J.D. Haber & G.E. Mitchell (Eds.), *Primary care meets mental health*. Tiburon, CA: Centralink Publications.

Doherty, W.J., McDaniel, S.H., & Baird, M.A. (1996). Five levels of primary care/ behavioral healthcare collaboration. *Behavioral Healthcare Tomorrow, 5*, 25–27.

Feldman, S. (1996). A marriage unconsummated. *Behavioral Healthcare Tomorrow, 3*, 47–48.

Langman-Dowart, N., Gatti, E., & Duval, D. (1997). Building partnerships of lasting value in health care: The Blue Cross and Blue Shield/Raytheon collaboration. In J.D. Haber & G.E. Mitchell (Eds.), *Primary care meets mental health*. Tiburon, CA: Centralink Publications.

Mechanic, D. (1997). Approaches for coordinating primary and specialty care for persons with mental illness. *General Hospital Psychiatry, 19*, 395–402.

National Committee for Quality Assurance. (Undated). MBHO accreditation. http://www.ncqa.org/pages/policy/accreditation/mbho/mbhotext.htm.

National Institute on Alcohol Abuse and Alcoholism. (1993). *Alcohol and health: Eight special reports to the U.S. Congress from the Secretary of Health and Human Services.* NIH publication no. 94-3699. Rockville, MD: U.S. Department of Health and Human Services, National Institutes of Health.

Regier, D.A., Narrow, W.E., Rae, D.S., Manderscheid, R.W., Locke, B.Z., & Goodwin, F.K. (1993). The de facto U.S. mental and addictive disorders service system. Epidemiologic catchment area prospective 1-year prevalence rates of disorders and services. *Archives of General Psychiatry, 50*(2), 85–94.

Stelovich, S. (1997). Depression and its management in primary care: The Harvard Pilgrim Health Care experience. In J.D. Haber & G.E. Mitchell (Eds.), *Primary care meets mental health*. Tiburon, CA: Centralink Publications.

U.S. Department of Health and Human Services. (1999). *Mental health: A report of the Surgeon General.* Rockville, MD: U.S. Department of Health and Human Services, Substance Abuse and Mental Health Services, National Institutes of Health, National Institute of Mental Health.

Wells, K.B., Sherbourne, C., Schoenbaum, M., Duan, N., Meredith, L., Unutzer, J., Miranda, J., Carney, M.F., & Rubenstein, L.V. (2000). Impact of disseminating quality improvement programs for depression in managed primary care: A randomized controlled trial. *Journal of the American Medical Association, 283*(2), 212–220.

Treatment and Coverage Decision Making in Managed Care: Patients' Rights under Publicly and Privately Sponsored Managed Care Arrangements

Sara Rosenbaum and Joel B. Teitelbaum

Purpose: This chapter examines the complex issues associated with patients' rights and treatment and coverage decisions in the context of managed care.

Major Topics: This chapter discusses public policy and legal provisions governing patients' rights and insurance coverage under the Employee Retirement Income Security Act (ERISA), Medicaid, and Medicare. Provisions discussed include Coverage Determinations, Utilization Review, Internal and External Review and Appeals, Practice Guidelines, Medical Necessity, and the legal concepts of Burden of Proof and Minimum Evidentiary Standards. Two appendices present examples of medical necessity clauses in employer-sponsored health insurance and in Medicaid managed care programs.

INTRODUCTION

This chapter examines the complex issues that arise in any analysis of patients' rights in the context of managed care treatment and coverage decision making. The subject of patients' rights in matters of health insurance coverage is a long-standing one that has its roots in the earliest efforts by public and private insurers to curb health care spending. The advent of managed care, however, made matters more complicated. From both a practical and legal standpoint, managed care represents a merger of both the treatment and coverage decision-making process, thereby raising a host of substantive and procedural problems that earlier forms of health coverage essentially avoided. Furthermore, available data on the downward effects of managed care on health care spending suggest that no group of insured individuals may be more likely to encounter these problems than persons with mental illness–related health needs. In the space of a single decade, spending on mental health–related services has declined significantly, underscoring the apparently powerful effects of managed care on access to and utilization of care (Goldman, McCulloch, Cuffel, & Kozma, 1999). Based on existing data, it is not possible to know the implications of these changes in spending patterns for the quality of care.

For purposes of this chapter, *managed care* is any health insuring arrangement in which the corporate entity, either directly or through subcontracts, enters into a formal contractual arrangement with one or more purchasers to both insure a defined group of members and provide members with the care and services that it insured through a network of providers selected by the entity and subject to its controls. Managed care companies can take many forms, ranging from nonprofit companies to investor-owned insurance companies. A single company may offer many different types of managed care products, ranging from products that are loosely configured to those that are tightly managed, with greater or lesser discretion given to members and providers alike to make decisions regarding the consumption of health care resources. Regardless of the type of product, however, the merger of coverage and care into a single corporate structure is what distinguishes managed care from earlier indemnity or service benefit plans that gave physicians and other health professionals full discretion over participation and treatment decisions. In managed care, a single entity empowers itself through its control over providers' access to patients to effectively make treatment decisions by virtue of its coverage decisions.

This chapter begins with a brief history of insurance coverage decision making that considers the issues that arose under pre–managed care arrangements. This section also discusses the transformation to managed care and the organizational and structural hallmarks of the new system and introduces key concepts and terms. The chapter then presents a typology of the legal issues that arise in any discussion of treatment and coverage decision making. This section is followed by one that outlines the current areas of debate in both publicly and privately sponsored managed care arrangements including, in the case of employer-sponsored health plans, the questions of who should have the power to decide if health care is medically necessary and therefore covered, what types of coverage disputes should be subject to an impartial review process, and whether individuals who claim to be injured as a result of a managed care organization's negligent treatment and coverage decisions should have the right to sue for damages. The chapter closes with a discussion of likely future directions on these matters, particularly the question of how medical necessity cases are decided in employee benefit plans and what remedies are available to persons who are injured as a result of negligent coverage decisions.

No single chapter can give full treatment to the rights of patients in a managed care treatment and coverage decision-making context. This is true for two basic reasons. First, at least as of the time of this writing, there was no uniform federal law defining patient protections in managed care treatment decision making. The American health care system tends to set separate standards for different forms of coverage, with patient protections highly dependent on whether an individual is insured through Medicare, Medicaid, an employer covered by federal employment law, or some other form. By the end of the first term of the 106th Congress, both the House (H.R. 2990) and the Senate (S. 1344) had completed debate on patients' rights legislation that would, for the first time, establish at least some form of basic statutory framework governing some or most managed care products. However, final action on these bills did not take place before the end of the 106th Congress. Second, the nature of the American legal system itself makes discussion of patients' rights very difficult. Depending on the form of coverage, an individual's legal rights under the system may be governed by a host of federal and state statutory, regulatory, and constitutional laws. This welter of laws also means that managed care companies must operate in an extremely complicated legal environment in which the level of protections they afford to their members depends on which entity—an employer covered by federal law, one who is not, Medicare, or Medicaid—is paying for the membership.

Because the law surrounding patients' rights in managed care is so multidimensional and currently in a state of ferment, this is a particularly challenging time to study this topic. We live in a period of shifting private expectations and public policies, and it may be years (if ever) before a clear picture of patients' rights in managed care emerges. However, while the legal framework for managed care may be in a state of flux, the issues raised by this chapter are enduring and can be expected to occupy center stage in the ongoing debate over managed care coverage decision making. Even if managed care companies were to dramatically reduce their day-to-day management of health professionals' treatment decisions, their overall control of the environment in which health resources are amassed and allocated would be sufficient to cause these issues to remain central in the ongoing debate.

BACKGROUND AND OVERVIEW

Patients' Rights against Insurers in the Pre–Modern Managed Care Era

There was a time, in the early years of health insurance, when the topic of patients' rights was virtually nonexistent. This was because physicians, hospitals, and other health care providers designed the earliest forms of insurance and, until relatively recently, insurers paid providers the amount they charged for the services they considered necessary (Rosenblatt, Law, & Rosenbaum, 1999/2000). In other words, insurers were essentially passive financing companies formed by the health care industry itself to help individuals finance the cost of health care.

Both public and private insurance operated along these lines, at least at the beginning. Employer-sponsored health insurance coverage in the United States, which began in the early 1930s and reached its apex by the latter half of the 1970s (Gabel, 1999), paid providers what they sought for the treatment they elected to furnish, although coverage was far narrower in the early decades of the system. Similarly, the Medicare program, which was designed to parallel the private insurance scheme of the time with respect to coverage and provider compensation, contained virtually no checks on provider treatment discretion (Rosenblatt, Law, & Rosenbaum, 1997). Medicaid, which is a means-tested welfare program and not insurance in the legal sense, extended significant discretion to states to structure their coverage and compensation policies (Congressional Research Service, 1993).

Within several years of Medicaid's enactment in 1965, however, the U.S. Supreme Court, in a series of landmark decisions, extended constitutional protections to welfare assistance (*Goldberg v. Kelly*, 1970). By extension, these decisions were held to apply to Medicaid as well (*Wilder v. Virginia Hospital Association*, 1990). These constitutional protections not only established procedural protections in the case of "adverse decisions" (e.g., timely and adequate notice, an evidentiary hearing before an impartial examiner), but also prohibited states from instituting actions against persons who made a timely request for a hearing (i.e., before the date on which the intended action was scheduled to take effect) until the hearing was conducted and a decision rendered (*Goldberg v. Kelly*, 1970). These constitutional protections ultimately were codified in federal regulations (42 C.F.R. §431.210) and have had the effect of significantly constraining state conduct in the area of benefits. Medicare beneficiaries enjoy similar constitutional protections with respect to notice and hearing rights before an impartial administrative body (*Mathews v. Eldridge,* 1976); however, the question whether coverage must be continued at pre-reduction levels is a matter that is currently under debate, as discussed further below.

Thus, as of the beginning of the 1970s, public and private insurance, which covered fewer services than are found in typical policies today, also paid for the services that it covered in accordance with the individual decisions of providers and on a compensation basis that met providers' expectations. Medicaid covered more but paid at lower rates, and constitutional requirements prohibited states from arbitrarily reducing or denying coverage. Even in the present period, when Medicaid payment rates in many cases have fallen dramatically below those available under other forms of coverage, Medicaid agencies appear to make coverage decisions in accordance with professional opinion more frequently than do private insurers (Finkelstein, Silvers, Marrero, Neuhauser, & Cuttler, 1998).

By the early 1970s, the consequences of public and private insurance design choices on health care costs were becoming increasingly evident. Medical care inflation rose at twice the general rate even as the concept of insurance was expanded to include both primary and preventive services, and coverage increased for greater levels of costly treatment. In the face of this, price controls remained nonexistent (Bovbjerg, 1975), even as both employers and Congress (in the case of Medicare) demanded control over the cost of coverage, and insurers began to experiment with both "macro" (i.e., memberwide program design issues) and "micro" (individual enrollee) controls over spending. Macro controls in the public arena took the form of rate setting, fee schedules, and across-the-board limits (e.g., visit and day limits) on coverage (Rosenblatt, Law, & Rosenbaum, 1997). Micro controls in both the public and private sectors involved the development and application of utilization review techniques designed to curb spending on individual enrollees (Rosenblatt, Law, & Rosenbaum, 1997).

These original spending controls were applied retrospectively after treatment had been rendered (Rosenblatt, Law, & Rosenbaum, 1997). In the case of private insurance, these efforts to control costs resulted in legal challenges to insurer practices in court by individuals alleging a breach of contract (*Van Vactor v. Blue Cross Association,* 1977). Ultimately, however, insurers began to apply utilization controls on a prospective or concurrent basis, attempting to make coverage decisions either in advance of or concurrent with care. As efforts to control costs prospectively grew, their impact on access to care rapidly became evident. By the mid-1970s, courts had begun to apply common law tort principles to insurance coverage decision making in order to fashion remedies for injuries flowing from physical and psychological injury, pain, and suffering sustained as a result of negligent or bad faith denials (*Gruenberg v. Aetna Insurance Co.,* 1973; Henderson, 1992; *Sarchett v. Blue Shield of California,* 1987). Damages also could be recovered under these tort theories for punitive purposes (Rosenblatt, Law, & Rosenbaum, 1997). In the case of Medicare and Medicaid, persons injured as a result of negligent coverage decisions could seek compensation for damages against state and federal officials under federal law, although damage awards would be subject to limits (Federal Tort Claims Act, 28 U.S.C.S. §§1346 et seq., and the Civil Rights Act of 1964, 42 U.S.C. §1983; note that injured persons cannot recover damages against state officials for past financial injuries [*Edelman v. Jordan,* 1974]).

In sum, by the 1970s, state law controlled the rights of individuals against private health insurers. Lawsuits were relatively rare, since few insurers made adverse decisions and those that did tended to make decisions on a retrospective basis, after care already had been rendered. While lengthy and costly disputes over coverage could and did arise as insurers became more aggressive in their use of micro-control techniques, these battles typically occurred after the fact. For the most part, state insurance departments, unlike the Medicare and Medicaid programs, did not provide for a system of review of insurer decisions by impartial administrative officials. Persons who were aggrieved by their insurer's decision could sue in court under various legal theories, including breach of contract, insurance and general consumer fraud, and, in cases where injuries occurred, tortious conduct.

The Transformation to Managed Care

The enactment of the Employee Retirement Income Security Act of 1974 (ERISA) altered the debate over the rights of privately insured persons in a treatment and coverage context. Enacted as a comprehensive remedial statute, the purpose of which was to protect pension rights, ERISA transformed the American health system, as well as patients' rights within the system. By releasing employers from the traditional structure of provider-sponsored health insurance plans, ERISA served as the basis for the modern managed care structure; by insulating employers from the effects of most state laws without substituting federal standards in their place, ERISA permitted employers to achieve this transformation in a wholly unregulated environment (Rosenblatt, Law, & Rosenbaum, 1997).

ERISA preempts most state laws that apply to employee benefit plans, including employee health benefit plans. Courts have ruled that the law provides for both "conflict preemption," which merely states a federal defense but does not provide a basis for federal jurisdiction or removal, and "field preemption," that is, a preemption of the entire "field" of state regulatory law as it applies to employee benefit plans, even where federal standards are lacking and therefore no conflict exists (*Shaw v. Delta Airlines,* 1983).

According to legal experts in the field, this unusual level of preemption was the result of overriding congressional concern for the standardized application of uniform legal principles to employee benefits in a national economy (Langbein & Wolk, 1995). Most observers assumed that content standards would follow the enactment of the law. In the area of pension benefits, it occurred; in the case of health benefits, however, national reform never took place. Thus, no content standards ever were developed (Rosenblatt, Law, & Rosenbaum, 1997). ERISA's field preemption is therefore often referred to as the ERISA "vacuum," since preemption of state laws (including state consumer protection laws) can occur regardless of whether there are substantive requirements to take their place (Rosenblatt, Law, & Rosenbaum, 1997).

ERISA's broad preemption provisions did make one exception to the normal rule, "saving" from preemption state laws that "regulate insurance"

(ERISA §514 (b)(2)(A); 29 U.S.C. §1144(b)(2)(A)). However, whether a state law is one that regulates insurance is considered by courts to be a matter of federal law (*American Medical,* 1997; *Metropolitan Life,* 1985; *Union Labor,* 1982; *Unum Life,* 1999), and many types of state laws that apply to insurers nonetheless are not considered to be laws that "regulate insurance." Thus, state laws that protect against consumer fraud and create a legal right to sue for damages suffered as a result of injuries sustained as a result of the misconduct of an insurer (*Pilot Life,* 1987), or that create administrative rights and external review hearing systems for persons who wish to contest an insurer's decisions (*Corporate Health,* 1998), are not considered to be laws that regulate insurers. Furthermore, where an employer self-insures (i.e., insures its own health plan while contracting with an insurer or managed care company simply to administer the plan), even state laws that regulate insurance would not apply, since under ERISA self-insured plans are not considered to be insurance companies. Since the overwhelming majority of privately insured Americans (as of 1999, approximately 50 million privately insured Americans were enrolled in self-insured plans) (Rosenblatt, Law, & Rosenbaum, 1999/2000, p. 115) derive their health care coverage through employers, the effect of ERISA was to wipe out many state legal protections that either existed at the time of passage or that states have attempted to institute as the health care system has undergone its managed care transformation.

Not only did ERISA preempt most state laws protecting individuals against the wrongful conduct of insurers, but also ultimately drove the transformation to managed care. At the time of ERISA's enactment in 1974, a very small number of Americans were members of prepaid group practice health plans such as Kaiser Permanente and Group Health, the conceptual and structural precursors of the modern managed care corporation (Rosenblatt, Law, & Rosenbaum, 1997). Twenty-five years later, nearly 90% of all employer-insured persons were enrolled in some form of managed care (Employee Benefit Research Institute, 1999). By preempting even state insurance laws in the case of self-insured plans, ERISA effectively freed employers from the strictures of provider-fashioned health insurance schemes and allowed them to create health benefit plans that contracted selectively with providers and that demanded deep financial concessions and agreement to a wide variety of practice constraints as the price of participation (Rosenblatt, Law, & Rosenbaum, 1997). Providers that sought to resist these demands faced exclusion from networks; when they attempted collective action against purchasers, they were charged with violation of state and federal antitrust laws that, until the mid-1970s, exempted the "learned professions" from their reach. (In *Goldfarb*, 1975, the Supreme Court struck down the learned profession exemption and allowed lawyers for the first time to competitively advertise their services. This decision was followed by *Arizona*, 1982, which stripped physicians of the learned profession exemption as well as effectively ceased the practice of provider-set fee schedules that had dominated the insurance industry ever since the creation of the first Blue Cross plans.)

Thus, even as ERISA swept away most state law applicable to employee health benefits, it failed to establish federal standards in its place. The assumption on the part of leading members of Congress at the time of ERISA's enactment was that the preemption of all state law was part of a general national health reform effort; however, that reform effort never took place. As a result, employers that elect to self-insure have nearly complete discretion over the structure and design of their benefit plans (*Jones*, 1999; Rosenblatt, Law, & Rosenbaum, 1997). Furthermore, all employers, self-insured and otherwise, are insulated against state laws that establish consumer protections outside of the insurance regulation arena, such as an external review process to which individuals can appeal denials of care on medical necessity grounds.

Federal law does create certain procedural protections for participants and beneficiaries in employee benefit plans. ERISA plans are based on the law of trusts and must be overseen by a "fiduciary" who is obligated to manage plan assets for the welfare of its participants. (Interestingly, this "welfare" standard does not prohibit per se an insurer from acting as a plan fiduciary, even though the conflict of interest would appear to be obvious.) Fiduciaries found to have breached this trust standard may be held liable for such a breach, although the extent of the liability and the remedies available are not clear, at least in the health arena (*Shea v. Esensten*, 1997).

Individuals who are dissatisfied with an ERISA plan administrator's decision regarding benefits (such as the denial of health benefits on medical necessity grounds) have a right to a "full and fair hearing" through a process established by an employer that meets certain basic federal regulatory standards (ERISA §503; 29 U.S.C. §1133). Furthermore, courts have the power to hear cases involving "claims for benefits" that arise under ERISA plans (ERISA §502; 29 U.S.C. §1132). In the event that a claimant prevails, a court may award him or her the value of the benefit as well as attorneys' fees and certain "extra-contractual" remedies. Thus, for example, persons who are denied benefits on the ground that their care is not considered to be "medically necessary" may obtain a "full and fair hearing" of the decision. Existing ERISA fair hearing regulations do not provide for expedited procedures in the event that a hearing concerns an urgent need for medical care and lack other procedural safeguards that would be important in a medical hearing, such as provisions regarding the inspection of medical evidence used by the health plan. As with the Medicare appeals process, which similarly has been challenged as providing insufficient legal protections to patients in a managed care context (*Grijalva*, 1998), the full and fair hearing process may not suffice in emergency and urgent care medical situations.

While federal law does extend procedural protections aimed at helping individuals enforce their benefits under their ERISA plans, at the same time federal law is limited in the remedies it provides for persons who suffer injury because their benefits were wrongfully withheld. The rationale for this limitation is the fact that the ERISA statute was grounded in the law of trusts, which has as its basic underpinning protection of trust assets from depletion (such as from massive liability awards). Enacted in a pre–managed care era and conceived as a law that regulates retirement income, not health insurance, ERISA is designed to protect pension benefits, not to address issues of medical care liability. Even as its preemption provisions were extended to state laws that permit injured persons to recover against insurers for wrongful conduct, there was no evidence that Congress intended to remove such basic rights from insured Americans, simply because their insurance was derived from an employer-sponsored plan (Rosenblatt, Law, & Rosenbaum, 1997). Moreover, ERISA's sponsors did not conceive of the potential for managed care to merge health care and health benefits or create a situation in which the denial of care by an insurer ultimately could cost an individual his or her life in the absence of a rapid system for review.

Courts ultimately softened the potential reach of ERISA by drawing a distinction between claims for benefits that result in a preemption of state-created rights and remedies and claims that challenge the quality of the care itself (*Dukes,* 1995; *Pegram,* 2000). In the first case, an individual is limited to his or her ERISA remedies (i.e., the value of the benefit and attorneys' fees). In the latter, the individual has full access to state-created remedies, because the lawsuit is treated not as a "claim for benefits" but as a complaint about the quality of care, which is an issue not reached by ERISA. As a quality claim, a case may raise a variety of allowable state law theories regarding the company's liability, including theories of "corporate negligence" (e.g., the selection of an incompetent provider network; *Shannon*, 1998) or "vicarious liability" (i.e., liability for the negligence of the company's provider-agents; *Boyd*, 1998). While this quantity/quality distinction has helped preserve state law remedies for injuries caused by poor quality care, recent court decisions (*Andrews-Clarke*, 1997; *Moscovitch*, 1998) also point to the difficulty in distinguishing when a lawsuit involves claims of quantity as opposed to quality. Furthermore, the viability of the lawsuit may come down to the creativity of a plaintiff's lawyer in crafting the pleadings in the case to be understood as a quality—not a quantity—case. By blurring the distinction between coverage and care, managed care has produced a plethora of court rulings that often produce inconsistent results, sometimes casting plan conduct as coverage, sometimes as quality.

KEY CONCEPTS AND DEFINITIONS

With this overview of current law, it is now possible to consider the issues raised in a discussion of patients' rights in a managed care era. There are many concepts and definitions relevant to an understanding of enrollee rights in managed care generally and of medical necessity determinations specifically. A number have been discussed as part of the brief history set forth above. The others are outlined below.

Macro versus Micro Coverage Determinations

As noted, insurers and health plans make two types of decisions: macro and micro. Historically, insurance companies made macro coverage determinations as a matter of marketing, since insurers tailored their benefit packages to meet the needs and desires of their customers. Understandably, then, traditional health insurance generally covered hospitalization and surgery for acute health problems, since these were the most expensive services private employees—insurers' core market—were likely to encounter. A macro decision goes to the design of the plan and answers the question whether a particular service (e.g., mental health benefits, hospitalization, pharmaceuticals) is covered for *any plan member* (Rosenblatt, Law, & Rosenbaum, 1997). A micro matter concerns whether a particular benefit enumerated in the plan is covered for *an individual*.

Legal disputes that emanate from health care coverage determinations can be either macro or micro. For example, coverage for mental health benefits may be available except where the condition was preexisting. Depending on whether the condition at issue was preexisting, coverage may fall within or outside the limits of the contract. Often the issues boil down to a legal interpretation of the document by a court, but this type of dispute can involve significant debates over the facts of an individual's case as well.

A medical necessity decision represents a classic example of a micro decision. In a medical necessity case, the insurer or health plan does not dispute whether the service is covered *at all*; instead, the dispute concerns whether, *for a particular individual*, the covered service is medically necessary as defined by the insurance contract or other applicable law. An example of such a dispute would be a decision to terminate a patient's inpatient mental health care on the grounds that the care is no longer medically necessary (*Andrews-Clarke,* 1997). Experimental treatment decisions are sometimes discussed as micro issues, but they are really macro issues: Once a procedure is labeled experimental, it is not covered for anyone under virtually all insurance plans, no matter how necessary or worthwhile.

In sum, both macro and micro decisions can raise factual questions as well as questions of law. Deciding either type of case can call for both legal expertise (e.g., construing the meaning of certain contract terms), as well as extensive testimony by health professionals designed to elicit the essential characteristics of the conditions and medical procedures against which the law will be applied. For example, were an insurer to deny a certain form of mental health therapy as "experimental," issues of both fact and law could arise. A judge or hearing officer with legal expertise would have to examine the documents to determine whether the term "experimental" is defined at all and, if so, how. The judge or hearing officer would then need to hear the factual testimony of experts who could testify as to whether the procedure in question fell within or outside the definition. Thus, if a contract defines experimental treatment as treatment that has not yet been become part of the standard practice of medicine in the relevant field, experts on psychiatric care might be brought in to testify whether a certain psychiatric treatment should be considered accepted practice for a given condition.

Utilization Review

Utilization review (also termed utilization management) is the process by which health care providers evaluate the appropriateness and cost-effectiveness of proposed health care services. Utilization review is the process that leads to medical necessity determinations; reviewers of health care service utilization undertake to determine the medical necessity of, for example, a patient's hospitalization generally and the length of the patient's stay specifically. While utilization review techniques are in some respects related to the quality of care (Snoe, 1998), the main thrust of the review may be to contain costs by denying payment for unnecessary health care and related services (Rosenblatt, Law, & Rosenbaum, 1997).

There are several utilization review techniques that generally involve the reviewing organization's approval or denial of full or partial payment for health services (Snoe, 1998). When the review takes place, who performs it, and how it is conducted, all are issues that frequently are discussed in the patients' rights debate. Insurance companies may employ their own in-house program or may contract with companies that specialize in utilization review services (*Corcoran,* 1992). Alternatively, an insurer might market its utilization services to employers and other organizations either as a stand-alone service or as part of a third-party administrator (TPA) service contract through which the TPA provides all administrative support for the employers' health plan. Some utilization review companies limit themselves to specialized areas such as mental illnesses and drug and alcohol addictions. Because health maintenance organizations (HMOs), independent practice associations (IPAs), and other alternative delivery systems are prepaid for health care, most operate their own review programs (Snoe, 1998).

The Coverage Determination Process

The coverage determination process is composed of a series of distinct steps. Pursuant to the terms of an insurance contract or employee benefit plan, certain procedures may have to be referred to a utilization management program. The utilization management entity then, at least in theory, examines the facts of the patient's case and compares those facts with the entity's treatment standards. (In theory because cases involving challenges to denials of care frequently reveal utilization processes in which the reviewer failed to consider anything about the individual patient at all and instead simply denied the care as inconsistent with the company's practice guidelines [*Bedrick,* 1996; *Wickline,* 1987].) The process would take a defined time period, with results communicated back to the patient and/or provider. Most utilization review is done prospectively or concurrently, meaning that it is performed either before or at the time of treatment. The process for determining coverage prior to care also is known as prior authorization.

Retrospective utilization review (i.e., reviews performed after care has been rendered) is probably most typical in cases involving emergency care, where treatment has been rendered and a decision regarding payment must be made. In the case of Medicare and Medicaid managed care, utilization review regarding emergency care can take place only after treatment has been rendered, and the standard for reviewing such claims is whether a prudent layperson (not a medical expert) would have considered the condition to be an emergency. Employer-sponsored plans that self-insure are free to decide for themselves whether to permit or prohibit prior authorization in the case of emergency care and are free to adopt or reject the prudent layperson standard. Employers that purchase insurance may be subject to state insurance regulation on this matter, although the standards may vary from state to state. As of 1999, more than 30 states had adopted a prudent layperson standard for emergency care. (According to the National Conference of State Legislatures [1999], in March 1999, 31 state laws specified automatic coverage for emergency medical conditions "of sufficient severity, including severe pain, that a prudent layperson, who possesses an average knowledge of health and medicine, could reasonably expect the absence of medical attention to result in placing the person's health in jeopardy." The number of states with special standards governing mental illness–related emergencies is unknown.

In theory, personnel who have qualifications and expertise in the areas under review conduct utilization review. In practice, the review may or may not be conducted at the initial stage by such personnel; experts may be brought in (if at all) only at the internal appeals stage.

Internal and External Review of Coverage Determinations

As noted above, the procedures for reviewing coverage determinations made during the utilization review process vary depending on the applicable law. In the case of ERISA-covered health plans (basically all employer-sponsored plans other than those offered by public employers), the process of internal and external review is governed by ERISA. Public employees have whatever process is created under state law and their own employee benefit contracts. Members of Medicare managed care plans have the right to a process that is set forth in federal regulations. The Balanced Budget Act of 1997 considerably overhauled this process, establishing a new expedited internal and external appeals process for persons whose medical needs necessitate rapid appeals.

As with so many aspects of health policy, Medicaid rules governing the review of coverage determinations are the most complex of all. Federal law (Section 1932(b)(4) of the Social Security Act) requires managed care organizations (MCOs) to maintain an internal grievance process. Where the MCO's decision amounts to a denial, reduction, or termination of coverage, the beneficiary also has the right to a fair hearing directly from a state, since the MCO is considered to be an agent of the state. If the hearing is requested in a timely fashion, then the MCO must continue to furnish care to the beneficiary while the decision is pending.

Practice Guidelines

Put simply, practice guidelines (also known as "practice parameters" or "practice protocols") are concisely formatted information that prompts physicians and other health care practitioners on how to act in a given medical situation (Brook, 1989). The National Guideline Clearinghouse, a public resource for evidence-based clinical practice guidelines sponsored by the Agency for Healthcare Research and Quality (formerly the Agency for Health Care Policy and Research) in partnership with the American Medical Association and the American Association of Health Plans, adopted the following definition: "Clinical practice guidelines are systematically developed statements to assist practitioner and patient decisions about appropriate health care for specific clinical circumstances" (Field & Lohr, 1990, p. 39).

The National Guideline Clearinghouse (2000) explains that the practice protocols it provides are

> not fixed protocols that must be followed, but are intended for health care professionals and providers to consider. While they identify and describe generally recommended courses of intervention, they are not presented as a substitute for the advice of a physician or other knowledgeable health care professional or provider. Individual patients may require different treatments

from those specified in a given guideline. Guidelines are not entirely inclusive or exclusive of all methods of reasonable care that can obtain/produce the same results. While guidelines can be written that take into account variations in clinical settings, resources, or common patient characteristics, they cannot address the unique needs of each patient nor the combination of resources available to a particular community or health care professional or provider. Deviations from clinical practice guidelines may be justified by individual circumstances. Thus, guidelines must be applied based on individual patient needs using professional judgment.

The use of practice guidelines has flourished under managed care since, like prospective utilization review techniques, they can be used to control physicians' use of resources. The U.S. General Accounting Office (1996) estimated that by 1996, about 75 separate organizations had developed over 2,000 guidelines in a sweeping range of areas. By 1995, approximately three quarters of all HMOs and one quarter of preferred provider organizations (PPOs) were using written practice guidelines as one means of measuring provider performance (Gold, Hurley, Lake, Ensor, & Berenson, 1995).

Medical Necessity

As noted at the beginning of this chapter, prior to the 1970s, traditional notions of physician autonomy generally permitted physicians' medical opinions to carry the day with respect to insurance coverage. Physicians' medical determinations largely dictated coverage, and private and public insurers rarely challenged such decisions. Commercial insurers, on the one hand, were traditionally providers of indemnity insurance and chose to restrict coverage in ways that shied away from involvement with providers. Medicare and Medicaid, on the other hand, were required by statute beginning in 1965 to limit payments to medically necessary care, but the early years of both programs were generally marked by an inclination to follow the lead of private payers in not challenging physicians' judgments. Blue Cross and Blue Shield, still heavily under the influence of the hospital industry and medical profession until the late 1970s, were not inclined to question providers' coverage determinations (Rosenblatt, Law, & Rosenbaum, 1997).

However, several factors during the 1970s combined to end this extraordinary level of physician autonomy and led to the rise of the medically necessary coverage standard. Chief among these factors was the increasing cost of health care that began in the mid-1960s and the subsequent pressure on employers and government to hold down these spiraling costs. Two other factors included the continued development of expensive and potentially dangerous medical technologies that were thought by some to be of limited efficacy in certain circumstances, and medical research that found disturbing geographic differences in the rates at which physicians used certain treatments. Both of these factors thus called into question treating physicians' judgments (Rosenblatt, Law, & Rosenbaum, 1997).

Insurers now routinely make treatment decisions as part of the coverage determination process and thus independently determine what goods and services are medically necessary and therefore insured. This blurring of the line between medical care and coverage decision making is particularly pronounced in managed care, since control over health care access and utilization lies at the heart of most managed care arrangements. Insurers' power to determine coverage thus potentially gives them the power to dictate professional standards of practice for all but the wealthiest Americans who can afford to pay out-of-pocket for care not covered by their plans.

Insurance contracts typically contain definitions of medical necessity. In the case of Medicaid contracts, these definitions may or may not mirror the definitional language related to medical necessity that exists within the federal statute and regulations (Rosenbaum, Sonosky, Shaw, Zakheim, Shin, & Repasch, 1999). Employer plans and private insurers are free to construct their own definitions. Examples of medical necessity definitions taken from litigation involving employer-sponsored care can be found in Appendix 5–A, while definitions taken from Medicaid managed care contracts can be found in Appendix 5–B.

One last point regarding medical necessity is in order—its relationship to performance measurement. An essential component of any health care contract is an explanation of how performance on a particular specification will be measured and the information that the purchaser requires of the contractor (i.e., the health plan). Performance measurement standards are particularly important in public contracts because due process considerations require clarity in compliance measurement. Performance measurement—including both internal quality performance assessment and external review—regarding medical necessity determinations requires a combination of structure, process, and outcomes measures. Examples are as follows:

- Structure Measures: All written materials furnished to network providers regarding coverage, applicable limitations, and exclusions; an explanation of how medical necessity determinations will be made; and identification of services and procedures that require prior authorization.
- Process Measures: Explanation of how medical necessity determinations are carried out (e.g., timelines for determinations, qualifications of personnel making determinations, and descriptions of evidence considered and the protocols used), description of the prior authorization program, copies of all practice guidelines used, forms for submission of evidence, and sample forms used to explain coverage decisions.
- Outcomes Measures: The results of reviews of individual medical necessity determinations for selected services chosen by the purchaser, with ratios of approvals and denials to requests for prior authorization (Rosenbaum & Teitelbaum, 1998).

TYPOLOGY OF LEGAL ISSUES REGARDING PATIENTS' RIGHTS IN THE AREA OF TREATMENT AND COVERAGE DECISION MAKING

Whether the population whose rights are at issue are individuals whose membership is sponsored by an employer, Medicare, or Medicaid, or totally financed from personal funds, the issue of managed care protections raises the same set of questions. However, depending on the source of financing (i.e., public or private), constitutional due process considerations may cause the resolution of these issues to vary somewhat, particularly with respect to the procedural protections related to the external review process as well as to the discretion of the company, as the agent of the state, to reduce or terminate care pending the outcome of the hearing process.

Questions on managed care patients' rights can be both substantive and procedural. Furthermore, while certain patient protection issues are unique to managed care because of its merging of treatment decision making and coverage decision making, other issues are common to all forms of health insurance.

Concern over managed care has triggered action at all levels of government to consider patient protections. Most states now have passed some form of managed care regulation that, to a greater or lesser degree, focuses on at least some of the issues discussed in this section. Medicare and Medicaid managed care reform legislation enacted by Congress in 1997 includes a number of patient protections of the type discussed here (Schneider, 1997). At the congressional level, the Consumer Bill of Rights issued by the President's Advisory Commission on Consumer Protection and Quality in the Health Care Industry led to several years of congressional debate about the protection of managed care members. In 1999, during the first session of the 106th Congress, both the House and Senate enacted bills that, while similar in certain superficial respects (Borzi & Rosenbaum, 1999), differ profoundly on a number of matters, the most far-reaching of which is the extent and depth of rights that patients in ERISA and other types of health plans would have to contest adverse treatment and coverage decisions. Whether this legislation is ultimately enacted into law remains to be seen.

The major managed care patient protection issues among Medicare, Medicaid, and ERISA are presented in Table 5–1 and discussed in more depth below. The issues are complex, and their resolution will determine the extent to which Americans' expectations regarding their health coverage can be enforced. The issues range from the degree to which plans' internal workings will be regulated to the degree to which plans will be held accountable through external review procedures for the consequences of their decisions.

The Regulation of Internal Utilization Review Procedures and Standards

The starting point of the patient protection debate is arguably the plans' own internal review process: Should a managed care company's internal utilization review process be regulated? If so, to what extent?

The issues that arise in debates over the regulation of utilization review frequently are procedural in nature. They include the qualifications of utilization review personnel, the timing of the utilization review proce-

Table 5–1 Managed Care Patient Protection Issues

Patient Protection Issue	Medicare	Medicaid	ERISA
Regulation of internal utilization review procedures	Establishes prior authorization timelines and prohibits the use of prior authorization in the case of emergency care.	Prohibits the use of prior authorization in the case of emergency care.	No similar provision.
Internal appeals	Requires managed care organizations to provide internal appeals procedures to review any determination "on the health care services an enrollee is entitled to receive, or any amounts the enrollee must pay for services."	Requires managed care organizations to provide internal appeals procedures to "challenge the denial of coverage . . . or payment [of medical] assistance."	Provides all beneficiaries and participants with full and fair hearing rights before a plan fiduciary.
External review	Beneficiaries have the right to external administrative review of health plan decisions. Medicare's external review system is federally administered and is subject to minimum federal standards.	Beneficiaries have the right to external administrative review of health plan decisions. Medicaid's fair hearing requirement effectively acts as an external review mechanism for all health plan conduct involving benefits, since health plans are considered to be agents of the state.	Provides no external review process other than permitting a direct appeal to court of any claim for benefits.

continues

Table 5–1 continued

Patient Protection Issue	Medicare	Medicaid	ERISA
Judicial review of external decisions	Beneficiaries are entitled as a matter of federal law to judicial review of any decision affecting benefits.	Beneficiaries are entitled as a matter of federal law to judicial review of any decision affecting benefits.	Provides access to judicial review of claims denials.
Burdens of proof in the review process	Beneficiaries receive an external review that effectively shifts the burden of justification to the plan. Information used by the plan is submitted to the external reviewer, which places the burden on the plan to submit sufficient evidence to justify its decision.	Similar to Medicare, in that in the case of a denial of coverage by a Medicaid agency or its health plan agent, a court or fair hearing officer would effectively be determining whether the agency's decision was justified by the facts it presents.	Burden falls to claimants to prove coverage at all levels, including during the full and fair hearing and during judicial review.
Evidentiary standards governing reviews	Federal due process principles effectively require adherence to rules of good evidence.	Federal due process principles effectively require adherence to rules of good evidence.	No standards provided for internal review.
Power to define coverage terms	Coverage terms and definitions generally are governed by federal law, thereby binding federal agencies and their health plan contractors.	Coverage terms and definitions generally are governed by federal law, thereby binding federal and state agencies and their health plan contractors.	Provides limited content standards for health plans (e.g., the Mental Health Parity Act, COBRA, HIPAA).

continues

Table 5–1 continued

Patient Protection Issue	Medicare	Medicaid	ERISA
Penalties for non-compliance with treatment orders	Health plans that fail to comply with treatment orders can be subject to enforcement orders in court. Also, if available under state law, beneficiaries have the right to sue their plans for injuries suffered as a result of damaging treatment decisions.	Health plans that fail to comply with treatment orders can be subject to enforcement orders in court. Also, if available under state law, beneficiaries have the right to sue their plans for injuries suffered as a result of damaging treatment decisions.	Health plans that fail to comply with treatment orders can be subject to enforcement orders in court. Also, enrollees have the right to recover damages for injuries in health care *quality* cases; claims for injuries resulting from coverage decisions are preempted.
Regulation of plan/professional relationships	Prohibits physician incentive arrangements that specifically reward health professionals for withholding medically necessary care.	Prohibits physician incentive arrangements that specifically reward health professionals for withholding medically necessary care.	No prohibition on physician incentive arrangements that specifically reward health professionals for withholding medically necessary care.

ERISA, Employee Retirement Income Security Act; COBRA, Consolidated Omnibus Budget Reconciliation Act; HIPAA, Health Insurance Portability and Accountability Act of 1996.

---

dures (e.g., 72-hour, rapid prior authorization procedures for urgent health care needs), and a prohibition against the use of prior authorization techniques in certain circumstances. Both the federal Medicare managed care statute and regulations (42 U.S.C. §1395w-22(d) and 42 C.F.R. §422.122), as well as legislation enacted during the first session of the 106th Congress (Borzi & Rosenbaum, 1999), establish prior authorization timelines and prohibit the use of prior authorization techniques in the case of emergency care.

More significant utilization review regulatory proposals have surfaced in recent years. These proposals are substantive in nature and would reach the content of the practice guidelines permissible for use by utilization review personnel, as well as the definitions of coverage that they are allowed to employ. In the congressional debate over managed care quality in 1998 and 1999, managed care companies rejected these proposals as unduly intrusive and an attempt to codify into federal utilization review law the "professional standard" of practice. This practice standard, which has governed Anglo-American medical liability law for some 250 years, relies on expert testimony to establish the prevailing practice by knowledgeable professionals in the relevant medical or health field (i.e., professional custom) to determine both medical necessity and the quality of health care (*Slater,* 1767). Industry-developed practice guidelines that are contrary to professional custom would not be considered to meet a professional standard of practice. Industry leaders viewed this attempt to codify a professional standard as a proposal that would stifle innovation in health care.

Internal Appeals of Treatment and Coverage Decisions

A second question is whether persons who disagree with the coverage decision of a plan will have the right to an internal review of that decision by the plan. Federal Medicare and Medicaid laws require managed care organizations to provide internal grievance procedures (42 C.F.R. §§422.560–422.590; 42 C.F.R. §434.32). The statutory standards for both programs are relatively minimal, although federal Medicare regulations are more extensive in their requirements for review of treatment decisions (42 C.F.R. §§422.578–422.616). As noted, ERISA (§503; 29 U.S.C. §1133) provides all beneficiaries and participants with full and fair hearing rights before a plan fiduciary (i.e., the entity vested with the authority to make resource allocation decisions regarding the benefits included in an ERISA employee benefit plan). However, as noted, the full and fair hearing process as currently structured in federal regulations is not geared to the consideration of health claims, particularly urgent health claims. Beneficiaries with urgent health care needs can proceed directly to court and request direct judicial review without previously exhausting the appeals procedures, but such direct access is available only in cases of grave medical need (*Adams,* 1991).

The House and Senate legislation pending as of the time of this writing would require plans to develop and make available an internal grievance process that operates rapidly and that includes notice of the adverse decision and the opportunity for review by a plan professional not connected with the original treatment decision. Decisions would have to be rendered in writing and include minimum information requirements regarding the basis for the decision and appeals rights (Borzi & Rosenbaum, 1999).

External Review of Treatment and Coverage Decisions

A far more contentious issue is external appeals, that is, the right to obtain an external review of a plan's decisions. In the case of Medicare and Medicaid, beneficiaries are entitled as a matter of federal law to judicial review of any decision affecting benefits. (In the case of Medicare, judicial review is available only after exhausting all administrative appeals rights [42 U.S.C. §405(g)]. Medicaid beneficiaries who are denied benefits to which they are entitled may proceed directly to court under federal civil rights law [42 U.S.C. §1983], and need not exhaust their fair hearing rights.) Furthermore, both Medicare and Medicaid beneficiaries have the right to external administrative review of health plan decisions. In the case of Medicare, this external review system is federally administered and is subject to minimum federal standards (42 C.F.R. §405.801 et seq.). In the case of Medicaid, the fair hearing requirement discussed above effectively acts as an external review mechanism for all health plan conduct involving benefits, since health plans are considered to be agents of the state (*J.K. v. Dillenberg,* 1993).

In the case of ERISA, current law provides no external review process other than permitting a direct appeal to the court of any claim for benefits. The legislation pending in Congress would address the issue of external review in different ways. The bill passed by the Senate would permit external review only in cases in which the denial by the plan is based on a lack of medical necessity or the proposed treatment's allegedly experimental status. All other cases (i.e., exclusionary and other non-coverage decisions) would have to proceed directly to court.

By contrast, the bill passed by the House would permit external impartial review by an outside expert medical review entity of any treatment decision in which medical evidence is required to resolve the dispute.

Thus, any treatment denials would be appealable if medical facts are involved, regardless of whether treatment is denied on the ground that it is *excluded* because it falls outside the contract (i.e., a macro allocation decision) or is covered but unnecessary. Because so many insurer decisions are couched as exclusions or simple cases of non-coverage, the House bill attempts to extend a simpler medical appeals arrangement to any case in which medical facts are at issue; thus, it provides that health plan decisions that turn to any degree on the assessment of an individual patient's condition should qualify for outside review.

Other issues that arise in debates over the external review process concern the qualifications of, and degree of impartiality to be maintained by, external reviewers; the timelines for review; the types of evidence that reviewers must consider in reaching their decisions; and the right to submit evidence or be present at the external review.

Finally, there is the issue of whether the review is de novo or on the record. In a de novo review, the reviewer can consider the evidence fresh and without regard to the decision reached by the health plan. In a review on the record, the reviewer is limited to a more cursory review of whether in light of the evidence the plan's decision was reasonable (or at least nonarbitrary). In other words, in a de novo review, the reviewer can substitute his or her own medical judgment regarding treatment for that of the plan, even if the plan's judgment was reasonable, or at least not arbitrary and unsupported by the evidence. On the other hand, in a review on the record a reviewer can overturn the judgment of the plan only if the plan's decision was unreasonable and unsupported by the facts. If the issue is simply that the reviewer would have decided the case differently, then the reviewer must in effect let the plan's decision stand. Legislation enacted by the House in 1999 would permit a de novo review; the Senate bill would not (Borzi & Rosenbaum, 1999).

Judicial Review of External Decisions

A basic question of due process is whether the external review by an agency is the final decision or whether individuals who claim the denial or loss of rights under their health plans will have recourse to the courts. As noted, individuals enrolled in Medicare, Medicaid, or ERISA plans all have access to judicial review of claims denials under current law. In the case of Medicare and Medicaid, these rights are grounded in the U.S.

Constitution. With respect to ERISA, the right to judicial review of any claim dispute is part of existing federal law (ERISA §502(a)(1)(B); 29 U.S.C. §1132(a)(1)(B)). As also noted, state courts applying common law principles, as well as many state legislatures as an express statutory matter, permit individuals access to the court to enforce the terms of state-regulated insurance contracts.

Were Congress to create a new external review process for ERISA plan beneficiaries and other privately insured persons, a question would arise as to whether the right to judicial access should remain. Both the House and Senate 1999 legislation would leave judicial access available for ERISA plan beneficiaries, while leaving to state law the question of whether state-regulated insurance decisions are subject to state law. However, the bill passed by the Senate in 1999 would impose new limits on judicial access (Borzi & Rosenbaum, 1999). Similarly, even under a reformed system, existing law, as well as prevailing judicial principles of equity and fairness, would permit claimants who risk death or serious injury as a result of a relatively slow appeals process to seek direct judicial review and bypass the administrative review system.

The Burden of Proof in the Review Process

A fundamental issue in any conduct review proceeding, whether judicial or administrative, is who bears the burden of proof. Under principles of common law, courts typically place the burden of proof on the party who has the easiest access to evidence. At the same time, however, claiming error in a coverage and treatment denial involves the assertion that the plan failed to live up to the coverage agreement and raises questions of both fact and law (e.g., Was the condition serious enough to merit treatment under the terms of the agreement? Does the contract in fact cover the treatment in question?). In such a situation, the burden typically falls to the moving party (i.e., the party alleging the breach of the agreement) to present evidence initially; the opposing party then has the opportunity to rebut the evidence.

Because of constitutional concerns, Medicare beneficiaries receive an external review that effectively shifts the burden of justification to the plan. Information used by the plan is submitted to the external reviewer, which, through a de novo review, places the burden on the plan to submit sufficient evidence to justify its decision. Similarly, in the case of a denial of coverage by the Medicaid agency or its health plan agent, a court or fair hearing officer would effectively be determining whether the agency's decision was justified by the facts it presents.

In the case of ERISA, the burden under current law would fall to claimants to prove coverage at all levels, including during the full and fair hearing and during judicial review. Legislation passed in 1999 in Congress would not shift the burden to the plan to justify its decision before the impartial reviewer, although, as discussed below, the House bill would effectively hold plans to a higher standard of coverage and give reviewers more latitude to reverse their decisions through the use of the de novo process noted above.

Minimum Evidentiary Standards Governing the Review Process

As discussed, the question of evidence can be crucial to the review process. One of the reasons that the professional standard of care has prevailed for more than two centuries is that there is little scientific evidence in the classic sense to govern treatment decision making. Most medical care furnished today is the product of considered professional judgment, because of the costliness and time-consuming nature of clinical trials, as well as their controversy (Borzi & Rosenbaum, 1999). Because treatment decisions turn on medical judgment, the paramount source of evidence is the patient's own record, as evaluated by professional judgment and whatever clinical expertise can be brought to bear on a case. This evidence can be further supplemented with the results of scientific data, where available, if the evidence is relevant and reliable. Relevance is crucial, since a study of effectiveness, no matter how well done, may be irrelevant if the patient's condition places him or her outside the scope of the study. The issue of relevance is particularly crucial in the case of persons with comorbidities, who may not fit a study profile (Borzi & Rosenbaum, 1999). Reliability is critical as well; if the study is poorly designed, the evidence is in effect worthless to the decision-making process. The lack of reliability might work to exclude many industry-developed practice guidelines that rest on actuarial assumptions rather than on scientific rigor (Borzi & Rosenbaum, 1999).

These rules of evidence would apply in judicial proceedings; the further question arises as to whether they should apply in administrative proceedings (i.e., both the internal and external review processes). Federal due process principles would effectively require adherence to rules of good evidence in the case of Medicare and Medicaid appeals. Federal legislation passed by Congress in 1999 also would address this issue, although the House bill would more strictly regulate the evidence that could be considered (Borzi & Rosenbaum, 1999).

The Power To Define the Terms of Treatment and Coverage

Coverage frequently depends on the terms and definitions used in the coverage agreement. In the case of Medicare and Medicaid, federal law typically governs these terms and definitions, thereby binding the federal and state agencies and their health plan contractors. For example, the Medicaid program uses an expansive definition of medical necessity in the case of pediatric care that requires coverage of treatments needed to prevent disabilities, not merely to treat those that already exist (Rosenbaum, Sonosky, Shaw, Zakheim, Shin, & Repasch, 1999). A health plan that contracts to furnish all pediatric care would be governed by these definitions unless the state agency were to exclude certain forms of treatment from the reach of the contract and retain direct coverage liability for the services. This type of exemption is relatively common in the case of children who need extensive mental health services (Rosenbaum, Sonosky, Shaw, Zakheim, Shin, & Repasch, 1999).

As noted, ERISA provides no content standards for health plans. Plan sponsors and the managed care contractors are completely free to negotiate narrow terms and definitions that exclude many forms of care or types of procedures (*Harris,* 1993), limit coverage to specified treatment guidelines, or give the plan administrator nearly unfettered latitude to define medical necessity and apply it.

Pending federal legislation does not step in to define plan terms or provide content to coverage definitions other than the requirement of coverage for emergencies in accordance with a prudent layperson standard. However, the House bill would expressly allow an external reviewer to set aside a plan's definitions of medical necessity in reaching its decision; the Senate bill would not (Borzi & Rosenbaum, 1999).

Penalties for Noncompliance with Treatment Orders

Health plans that fail to comply with treatment orders can be subject to enforcement orders in court under current Medicare, Medicaid, and ERISA law. The House and Senate bills would add penalties for failure to comply (Borzi & Rosenbaum, 1999).

By far the most contentious issue that arises in the managed care debate is whether patients should have the right to sue their plans for injuries suffered as a result of damaging treatment decisions. Both Medicare and Medicaid beneficiaries have such rights if available under state law, as would persons enrolled in non-ERISA private insurance plans. As noted, in the case of ERISA plan participants, the legal right to sue over the quality of care remains untouched by ERISA. However, the right to sue for injuries suffered by substandard coverage decisions is preempted, although the distinction between poor quality and bad coverage decision making is frequently blurred; over the past decade, however, dozens of cases have been dismissed as suits contesting coverage—rather than the quality—of care.

The House legislation passed in 1999 would effectively restore the right to sue for injuries sustained as the right of negligent or bad faith coverage denials; the Senate bill would not. There exists great controversy over the effects of such a provision, with the managed care industry citing the potential for very large premium increases. While existing evidence suggests that the premium effects of such a provision would be very small, extending the right to sue over coverage to ERISA plans could have the effect of unleashing a large investor pullout from the managed care industry, as well as defensive premium increases.

The Regulation of Plan/Professional Relationships

It is arguable that one of the most significant determinants of access to care may be the relationship between a health plan and its network. Federal Medicare and Medicaid laws prohibit physician incentive arrangements that specifically reward health professionals for withholding medically necessary care. However, no such prohibition applies to ERISA plans. Moreover, general incentive arrangements that are not tied to specific patients nonetheless may place physicians at significant financial risk and cause significant reduction in care. Yet, while one federal court held that such incentive schemes by physician-owned health plans violated ERISA because of the conflict of interest it creates between the physicians as owners of their plans and as the individual professionals who treat plan beneficiaries (*Herdrich v. Pegram*, 1998), during its 1999–2000 term the

U.S. Supreme Court reversed the decision (*Pegram v. Herdrich*, 2000), holding instead that treatment decisions made by HMOs through their physician employees are not fiduciary acts within the meaning of ERISA. (For an analysis of this decision, see Rosenbaum, Rosenblatt, Frankford, Teitelbaum, Machiz, Budetti, & Borzi, 2000.)

As insurers increasingly "downstream" financial risk to medical practice groups, and even individual practitioners, an ongoing question arises as to whether protections against health "plans" are sufficient. Of course, in any situation in which a physician is given direct resource allocation decisions and determines to withhold care, the physician would potentially be liable for malpractice. Furthermore, where the physician is specifically retained as a network provider and accorded this type of discretion under a participation contract, the managed care company that retains the physician's services might retain vicarious (i.e., indirect) liability for such decisions. Whether or not corporate vicarious liability exists would be a matter for triers of fact to decide based on the evidence regarding the relationship between the company and its network.

This ultimate issue of the relationship between managed care companies and their physicians has, as noted, begun to receive attention by courts, at least in the ERISA context. It is not an issue, however, in which Congress has chosen to legislate, since the question of what constitutes an acceptable level of financial risk is one that at this point may be unanswerable. Thus it is one that must be left to individual cases as they arise.

THE CONSUMER BILL OF RIGHTS AND RESPONSIBILITIES

On March 26, 1997, President Clinton appointed the Advisory Commission on Consumer Protection and Quality in Health Care Industry to "advise the President on changes occurring in the health care system and recommend measures as may be necessary to promote and assure health care quality and value, and protect consumers and workers in the health care system" (Advisory Commission, 1997). As part of its work, the president asked the commission to draft a consumer bill of rights.

The consumer bill of rights and responsibilities is intended to accomplish the following three major goals:

> First, to strengthen consumer confidence by assuring the health care system is fair and responsive to consumers' needs, provides consumers with credible and effective mechanisms to address

their concerns, and encourages consumers to take an active role in improving and assuring their health. Second, to reaffirm the importance of a strong relationship between patients and their health care professionals. Third, to reaffirm the critical role consumers play in safeguarding their own health by establishing both rights and responsibilities for all participants in improving health status (Advisory Commission, 1997, pp. 10–11).

In furtherance of these goals, the bill of rights speaks to seven areas that are central to providing adequate protections to consumers: information disclosure, choice of providers and plans, access to emergency services, participation in treatment decisions, respect and nondiscrimination, confidentiality of health information, and complaints and appeals. In addition, since "it is reasonable to expect and encourage consumers to assume reasonable responsibilities" in a health care system that protects their rights, the report details several consumer responsibilities (Advisory Commission, 1997, p. 65).

On November 27, 1997, President Clinton accepted the recommendations of the Advisory Commission (a copy of the president's press release accepting the recommendations can be found at www.hcqualitycommission. gov/press/cborimp.html). In so doing, he directed the Departments of Health and Human Services, Labor, Defense, and Veteran Affairs and the Office of Personnel Management to review the programs they administer and the plans they oversee to ensure consistency with the bill of rights. The agencies were instructed to exhaust every administrative action to make the programs they administer and the plans they oversee consistent with the bill of rights and to advise the White House where they needed additional legislative authority to do so. On February 20, 1998, President Clinton released an executive memorandum directing all federal health plans, which serve over 85 million Americans, to come into substantial compliance with the commission's bill of rights (a copy of the executive memorandum can be found at www.hcqualitycommission.gov/press/ pbor.html).

CONCLUSION

This chapter reviewed key patients' rights issues in the context of health care treatment and coverage decision making in managed care. The topic is complex and not amenable to standardized answers to complicated questions. This complexity is due in part to the multipayer nature of the American health care system: each form of coverage—Medicare, Medicaid, employer-sponsored, or private, non-ERISA—operates under its own unique legal framework. (Although beyond the scope of this chapter, still other distinct payment systems and treatment and coverage standards exist for certain populations in this country, including veterans and employees of self-insured state and local governments.) Medicare and Medicaid are constitutionally protected entitlements. Employer coverage is governed by the principles of ERISA, which by the lack of standards, create unique patients' rights issues of their own. Privately purchased non-ERISA coverage is subject to a separate legal framework governed by principles of state statutory law, as well as enduring common law principles.

This complexity also is in good part the result of the sheer complexity of the American legal system, with its constant interplay of federal and state law, each of which comes in three distinct forms: constitutional, legislative/administrative, and judicial. Any single interaction between a managed care company and an individual patient can raise patients' rights issues under all forms of law, and at both levels of government.

There are numerous implications that flow from this maze of laws and programs. First, depending on the source of financing, the rights and protections enjoyed by individuals enrolled in a particular managed care plan offered or administered by a particular health care company may differ significantly, even where individuals are members of exactly the same company in the same locality. The steps that a health care corporation must follow in making coverage determinations in the case of a Medicare beneficiary may be quite distinct from those that it uses in deciding questions of employee health benefits.

Second, this payer-based variation in patients' rights renders debates regarding the development of rights or the establishment of new rights very difficult. Instituting rapid decision-making policies for urgent health problems may be a major advance for persons whose enrollment is sponsored by an ERISA-covered employer. Persons covered by non-ERISA plans, however, may enjoy greater rights and protections under state regulations. Should these rights be preempted in favor of a single standard? Should states be permitted to draw stricter rights for both ERISA and non-ERISA plans? During the 1999 managed care debate in Congress, the question whether Congress would impose a single set of standards and protections at the federal level was fiercely debated. Both the House and Senate bills reflect the intense level of disagreement on this issue. The Senate bill allows states the right to regulate insured products but continues to permit ERISA's special protections for the managed care industry where liability for the consequences of negligent treatment decisions is concerned. The House bill essentially would set minimum patient protection standards for all forms of insurance, while at the same time allowing states to regulate the issue of plan liability.

Underlying both of these issues is perhaps the most fundamental issue of all: the issue of patient protections. It is a debate over whether Americans will have an *enforceable right* to the services and benefits for which they believe they are covered. In a block grant program, for example, individuals may have a general expectation of benefits and services. If the money runs out or the program alters its spending priorities mid-stream, however, persons who use the program simply must accept these realities; there is no legally protected set of expectations about the benefits that they will be able to obtain. Insurance—whether publicly or privately financed—historically has been considered different. Privately insured Americans believe that they have a contractual right to their benefits, having typically forgone significant wages to obtain the benefits on which they and their family members depend. For 35 years the courts have treated publicly insured benefits not as largesse, but as constitutionally protected property that can be denied, reduced, or terminated only in accordance with rigorous due process principles.

The current patients' rights debate, unfolding as it has in an era when many policy makers question Americans' sense of entitlement, is in reality a debate about whether that entitlement is real or merely apparent. To the extent that the law lacks standards that offer meaningful protection of patients against the unfair or arbitrary denial of coverage, the benefits they enjoy are from a legal perspective simply a form of largesse, which can be interrupted at will. The only protections against such interruptions would be social responsibility and the type of "market-induced" protection that could flow from consumer anger over seemingly cavalier treatment at the hands of the health care industry. As coverage has merged with care itself, the issue of whether health benefits are a legal right or a form of a gift in the eyes of the law has taken on a far more urgent quality.

It is perhaps inevitable that unless and until the nation decides to pursue a national health reform policy that insures Americans through a single statutory scheme that governs benefits, rights, and duties within the system, this intense variation in how the nation approaches and resolves this fundamental set of issues will continue.

REFERENCES

Adams v. Blue Cross/Blue Shield of Maryland, Inc., 757 F. Supp. 661 (D. Md. 1991).

Advisory Commission on Consumer Protection and Quality in the Health Care Industry. (1997, November). *Consumer bill of rights and responsibilities.* Washington, DC: Author.

American Medical Security, Inc. v. Bartlett, 111 F.3d 358 (4th Cir. 1997), cert. den., 118 S. Ct. 2340 (1998).

Andrews-Clarke v. Travelers Insurance Company, 984 F. Supp. 49 (D. Mass. 1997).

Arizona v. Maricopa County Medical Society, 457 U.S. 332 (1982).

Bedrick v. Travelers Insurance Co., 93 F.3d 149 (4th Cir. 1996).

Borzi, P., & Rosenbaum, S. (1999, December). *Pending patient protection legislation: A comparative analysis of key provisions of the House and Senate versions of H.R. 2290.* Prepared for the Henry J. Kaiser Family Foundation. Washington, DC: Kaiser Family Foundation.

Bovbjerg, R. (1975). The medical malpractice standard of care: HMOs and customary practice. *Duke Law Journal, 1375.*

Boyd v. Albert Einstein Medical Center, 547 A.2d 1229 (Pa. Super. 1998).

Brook, R. (1989). Practice guidelines and practicing medicine: Are they compatible? *Journal of the American Medical Association, 262,* 3027–3028.

Congressional Research Service. (1993). *Medicaid source book.* Washington, DC: Government Printing Office.

Corcoran v. United Healthcare, Inc., 965 F.2d 1321 (5th Cir. 1992), cert. den., 506 U.S. 1033 (1992).

Corporate Health Insurance, Inc. v. Texas Dept. of Insurance, 12 F. Supp. 2d 597 (S.D. Tex. 1998).

Dukes v. U.S. Healthcare, Inc., 57 F.3d 350 (3d Cir. 1995), cert. den., 116 S. Ct. 564 (1995).

Edelman v. Jordan, 415 U.S. 651 (1974).

Employee Benefit Research Institute. (1999). Managed care confusion. http://www.ebri.org/hcs/1999/fact8-mancareconfus.pdf. Accessed February 2, 2000.

Field, M.J., & Lohr, K.N. (Eds.). (1990). *Clinical practice guidelines: Directions for a new program.* Washington, DC: National Academy Press.

Finkelstein, B.S., Silvers, J.B., Marrero, U., Neuhauser, D., & Cuttler, L. (1998). Insurance coverage, physician recommendations, and access to emerging treatments. *Journal of the American Medical Association, 279*(9), 663–668.

Gabel, J.R. (1999). Job-based health insurance, 1977–1997: The accidental system under scrutiny. *Health Affairs, 18*(6), 62–70.

Gold, M.R., Hurley, R., Lake, T. Ensor, T., & Berenson, R. (1995). A national survey of the arrangements managed care plans make with physicians. *New England Journal of Medicine, 333,* 1678–1681.

Goldberg v. Kelly, 397 U.S. 294 (1970).

Goldfarb v. Virginia State Bar, 421 U.S. 773 (1975).

Goldman, W., McCulloch, J., Cuffel, B., & Kozma, D. (1999). More evidence for the insurability of managed behavioral health care. *Health Affairs, 18*(5), 172–181.

Grijalva v. Shalala, 152 F. 3d 1115 (9th Cir. 1998), vacated and remanded, 199 S. Ct. 1573 (1999).

Gruenberg v. Aetna Insurance Co., 510 P.2d 1032 (Cal. 1973).

Harris v. Mutual of Omaha Co., 992 F.2d 706 (7th Cir. 1993).

Henderson, R.C. (1992). The tort of bad faith in first-party insurance transactions: Refining the standard of culpability and reformulating the remedies by statute. *University of Michigan Journal of Law, 26.*

Herdrich v. Pegram, 154 F.3d 362 (7th Cir. 1998), petition for rehearing en banc denied, 170 F.3d 683 (7th Cir. 1999).

J.K. v. Dillenberg, 836 F. Supp. 694 (D. Ariz. 1993).

Jones v. The Kodak Medical Assistance Plan, 169 F.3d 1287 (10th Cir. 1999) (in which the Tenth Circuit Court of Appeals treated as non-reviewable a company's mental health benefit plan that limited the range of possible treatments available to the plaintiff to interventions that were not appropriate for her condition. The basis for this ruling was that the treatment guidelines themselves were part of the benefit plan design, rather than the result of incompetent treatment decision making by the utilization review company. As a part of the benefit design, the court concluded, the guidelines were effectively non-reviewable by a court.)

Langbein, J., & Wolk, B. (1995). *Pension and employee benefit law* (2nd ed.). Westbury, NY: Foundation Press.

Mathews v. Eldridge, 424 U.S. 319 (1976) (holding that Social Security benefits, while not means-tested and thus not subject to the extraordinary protections available to welfare beneficiaries, nonetheless are constitutionally protected property that cannot be denied, reduced, or terminated without a procedure that meets constitutional requirements). *See Grijalva v. Shalala* (1998).

Metropolitan Life Insurance Co. v. Massachusetts, 471 U.S. 724 (1985).

Moscovitch v. Danbury Hospital, 25 F. Supp. 2d 74 (D. Conn. 1998).

National Conference of State Legislatures. (1999). *State Legislatures Magazine.* www.ncsl.org/programs/pubs/399mancare.htm#standard. Accessed February 2, 2000.

National Guideline Clearinghouse. (2000). *National Guideline Clearinghouse disclaimer.* www.guideline.gov/STATIC/about.disclaimer.asp?view=about.disclaimer. Accessed on February 2, 2000.

Pegram v. Herdrich, 120 S. Ct. 2143 (2000).

Pilot Life Insurance Co. v. Dedeaux, 481 U.S. 41 (1987).

Rosenbaum, S., Frankford, D.M., Moore, B., & Borzi, P.(1999). Who should determine when health care is medically necessary? *New England Journal of Medicine, 340*(3), 229–232.

Rosenbaum, S., Rosenblatt, R., Frankford, D.M., Teitelbaum, J., Machiz, M., Budetti, P., & Borzi, P. (2000). *Pegram v Herdrich:* Implications for managed care law, policy, and practice. Washington, DC: School of Public Health and Health Services, The George Washington University Medical Center.

Rosenbaum, S., Sonosky, C., Shaw, K., Zakheim, M., Shin, P., & Repasch, L. (1999). *Negotiating the new health system: A nationwide study of Medicaid managed care contracts* (3rd ed.). Washington, DC: School of Public Health and Health Services, The George Washington University Medical Center.

Rosenbaum, S., & Teitelbaum, J. (1998, May). *Coverage decision-making in Medicaid managed care: Key issues in developing managed care contracts (issue brief #1).* Managed Behavioral Health Care Issue Brief Series. Washington, DC: School of Public Health and Health Services, The George Washington University Medical Center.

Rosenblatt, R., Law, S., & Rosenbaum, S. (1997). *Law and the American health care system*. Westbury, NY: The Foundation Press.

Rosenblatt, R., Law, S., & Rosenbaum, S. (1999/2000 Supplement). *Law and the American health care system*. Westbury, NY: The Foundation Press.

Sarchett v. Blue Shield of California, 729 P.2d 267 (Cal. 1987).

Schneider, A. (1997, December). Overview of Medicaid managed care provisions in the Balanced Budget Act of 1997. Washington, DC: The Kaiser Commission on the Future of Medicaid.

Shannon v. McNulty, 718 A.2d 828 (Pa. Super. 1998).

Shaw v. Delta Air Lines, Inc., 463 U.S. 85 (1983).

Shea v. Esensten, 107 F.3d 625 (8th Cir. 1997), cert. den., 118 S. Ct. 297 (1997).

Slater v. Baker and Stapleton, 95 Eng. Rep. 860 (King's Bench 1767).

Snoe, J.A. (1998). Under the most popular form of utilization review, the reviewing organization compares the patient-specific diagnosis or treatment request to clinical protocols to ensure the request comports with generally accepted health care practices. *American health care delivery systems*. St. Paul, MN: West Group.

Union Labor Life Ins. Co. v. Pireno, 458 U.S. 119 (1982).

Unum Life Ins. Co. of America v. Ward, 526 U.S. 358 (1999).

U.S. General Accounting Office. (1996, May). *Practice guidelines: Managed care plans customize guidelines to meet local interests.* GAO-HEHS-96-95. Washington, DC: GAO.

Van Vactor v. Blue Cross Association, 365 N.E.2d 638 (Ill. App. Ct. 1977).

Wickline v. State of California, 239 Cal. Rptr. 810 (Cal. App. 1986), petition for review dismissed, 741 P.2d 613 (Cal. 1987).

Wilder v. Virginia Hospital Association, 496 U.S. 498 (1990).

Examples of Medical Necessity Clauses in Employee Health Benefit Contracts

Case Name	*Contractual Definition of Medical Necessity*
Friends Hospital v. MetraHealth Service Corp., 9 F. Supp. 2d 528 (E.D. Penn. 1998)	"A health care facility admission, level of care, procedure, service or supply is medically necessary if it is absolutely essential and indispensable for assuring the health and safety of the patient as determined by the . . . Plan . . . with review and advice of competent medical professionals."
McGraw v. Prudential Ins. Co. of America, 137 F.3d 1253 (10th Cir. 1998)	"To be considered 'needed,' a service or supply must be determined by Prudential to meet all of these tests: a. It is ordered by a Doctor. b. It is recognized throughout the Doctor's profession as safe and effective, is required for the diagnosis or treatment of the particular sickness or Injury, and is employed appropriately in a manner and setting consistent with generally accepted United States medical standards. c. It is neither Educational nor Experimental nor Investigational in nature."
Gates v. King & Blue Cross & Blue Shield of Virginia,	"The Plan defines medically necessary as: Services, drugs, supplies, or equipment

Inc., 129 F.3d 1259
(4th Cir. 1997)

provided by a hospital or covered provider of health care services that the Carrier determines:

a. are appropriate to diagnose or treat the patient's condition, illness or injury;

b. are consistent with standards of good medical practice in the U.S.;

c. are not primarily for the personal comfort or convenience of the patient, the family, or the provider."

Dowden v. Blue Cross & Blue Shield of Texas, Inc., 126 F.3d 641 (5th Cir. 1997)

Services that are "essential to, consistent with and provided for the diagnosis or the direct care and treatment of the condition, sickness, disease, injury, or bodily malfunction," and treatments "consistent with accepted standards of medical practice."

Bedrick v. Travelers Ins. Co., 93 F.3d 149 (4th Cir. 1996)

1. "Services that are appropriate and required for the diagnosis or treatment of the accidental injury or sickness;

2. It is safe and effective according to accepted clinical evidence reported by generally recognized medical professionals and publications;

3. There is not a less intrusive or more appropriate diagnostic or treatment alternative that could have been used in lieu of the service or supply given."

Florence Nightingale Nursing Svc., Inc. v. Blue Cross/Blue Shield of Alabama, 41 F.3d 1476 (11th Cir. 1995)

The services and supplies furnished must "be appropriate and necessary for the symptoms, diagnosis, or treatment of the Member's condition, disease, ailment, or injury; and be provided for the diagnosis or direct care of Member's medical condition; and be in accordance with standards of good medical practice accepted by the organized medical community."

Trustees of the NW Laundry and Dry Cleaners Health & Welfare Trust Fund v.

1. The treatment must be "appropriate and consistent with the diagnosis (in accord with accepted standards of community

Burzynski, 27 F.3d 153 (5th Cir. 1994)	practice)." 2. Treatments "could not be omitted without adversely affecting the covered person's condition or the quality of medical care."
Fuja v. Benefit Trust Life Ins. Co., 18 F.3d 1405 (7th Cir. 1994)	Services that are "required and appropriate for care of the Sickness or the Injury; and that are given in accordance with generally accepted principles of medical practices in the U.S. at the time furnished; and are not deemed to be experimental, educational or investigational."
Lee v. Blue Cross/Blue Shield of Alabama, 10 F.3d 1547 (10th Cir. 1994)	"Appropriate and necessary for treatment of the insured's condition, provided for the diagnosis or care of the insured's condition, in accordance with standards of good medical practice, and not solely for the insured's convenience."
Heil v. Nationwide Life Ins. Co., 9 F.3d 107 (6th Cir. 1993)	Services for which there is "general acceptance by the medical profession as appropriate for a covered condition and [that] are determined safe, effective, and non-investigational by professional standards."
Heasely v. Belden & Blake Corp., 2 F.3d 1249 (3rd Cir. 1993)	Services and procedures "considered necessary to the amelioration of sickness or injury by generally accepted standards of medical practice in the local community."
Dahl-Eimers v. Mutual of Omaha Life Ins. Co., 986 F.2d 1379 (11th Cir. 1993)	a. "Appropriate and consistent with the diagnosis in accord with accepted standards of community practice; b. Not considered experimental; and c. Could not have been omitted without adversely affecting the insured person's condition or the quality of medical care."

Selected Medical Necessity Standards in Medicaid Managed Care Contracts

GENERAL MEDICAL NECESSITY STANDARDS

California

"Medically Necessary means reasonable and necessary services to protect life, to prevent significant illness or significant disability, or to alleviate severe pain through the diagnosis or treatment of disease, illness, or injury." (California Contract, page 8)

Colorado

"TT. 'Medically Necessary' shall mean any health care service required to preserve the Member's health and which, as determined by the Contractor's designated medical representative or medical Director, is:

1. Consistent with accepted standards for the prevention of disease and disability and for treatment of symptoms;
2. Appropriate with regard to standards of good medical practice;
3. Not solely for the convenience of the Member, his or her Physicians(s), Hospital, or other providers; and

Source: Reprinted with permission from S. Rosenbaum, et al., *Negotiating the New Health System: A Nationwide Study of Medicaid Managed Care Contracts, 3rd Edition,* © 1999, School of Public Health and Health Services, The George Washington University Medical Center.

4. The most appropriate supply or level of service which can be safely provided to the Member.

When specifically applied to an inpatient, it further means that the Member's medical symptoms or condition requires that the diagnosis or treatment cannot be safely provided to the Member in any other setting, i.e., home, outpatient, Nursing Facility." (Colorado Contract, page 9)

District of Columbia

"H. Coverage and Benefits
Covered Services.
  b. In making determinations regarding the minimum amount, duration and scope of coverage with respect to any service identified in Attachment I, Provider shall be bound by the same service definitions and coverage requirements which apply to the District Medicaid program under federal and District law, 42 U.S.C. §1396 et seq., 42 C.F.R §431 et seq." (District of Columbia Contract, pages 21, 22)
1. "12. General Rules on Service Coverage
  a. In making coverage determinations under this contract, Provider shall adhere to all applicable federal and District regulations relating to coverage of Medicaid benefits, as well as to specific coverage criteria and procedures set forth in this contract. Decisions must result in a level of coverage that is sufficient to reasonably achieve the purpose, as defined in federal law, of the service or benefit whose necessity is reviewed. Provider may not arbitrarily deny or reduce the amount, duration or scope of a benefit covered under this contract solely because of the diagnosis, type of illness, or condition." (District of Columbia Contract, pages 21, 22, 28)

Florida

"42. Medically Necessary or Medical Necessity—services provided in accordance with 42 CFR section 440.230 and as defined in section

59G-1.010 (167), F.A.C., to include that medical or allied care, goods, or services furnished or ordered must:

(a) Meet the following conditions:

1. Be necessary to protect life, to prevent significant illness or significant disability, or to alleviate severe pain;

2. Be individualized, specific, and consistent with symptoms or confirmed diagnosis of the illness or injury under treatment, and not in excess of the patient's needs;

3. Be consistent with the generally accepted professional medical standards as determined by the Medicaid program, and not experimental or Investigational;

4. Be reflective of the level of service that can be safely furnished, and for which no equally effective and more conservative or less costly treatment is available, statewide; and

5. Be furnished in a manner not primarily intended for the convenience of the recipient, the recipient's caretaker, or the provider.

(b) 'Medically necessary' or 'medical necessity' for inpatient hospital services require that those services furnished in a hospital on an inpatient basis could not, consistent with the provisions of appropriate medical care, be effectively furnished more economically on an outpatient basis or in an inpatient facility of a different type.

(c) The fact that a provider has prescribed, recommended, or approved medical or allied care, goods, or services does not, in itself, make such care, goods or services medically necessary or a medical necessity or a covered service." (Florida Contract, pages 187–188)

1. "27. Medically Necessary—As defined in Rule 10P-1.010, F.A.C., medically necessary is the requirement that the goods and services provided or ordered must be:

a. Calculated to prevent, diagnose, correct, cure, alleviate or preclude deterioration of a condition that threatens life, causes pain or suffering, or results in illness or infirmity;

b. Individualized, specific, and consistent with symptoms or confirmed diagnosis of the illness or injury under treatment, and not in excess of the patient's needs;

c. Necessary and consistent with generally accepted professional medical standards as determined by the Medicaid program, and not experimental or investigational;

    d. Reflective of the level of service that can be safely provided, and for that no equally effective and more conservative or less costly treatment is available; and

    e. Provided in a manner not primarily intended for the convenience of the recipient, the recipient's caretaker, or the provider." (Florida Contract, pages 195–196)

Florida Mental Health

"YY. Medically Necessary—The requirement that the goods and services provided or ordered must be:

1. Calculated to prevent, diagnose, correct, cure, alleviate, or preclude deterioration of a condition that threatens life, causes pain or suffering, or results in illness or infirmity;
2. Individualized, specific, and consistent with symptoms or confirmed diagnosis of the illness or injury under treatment, and not in excess of the patient's needs;
3. Necessary and consistent with generally accepted professional medical standards as determined by the Medicaid program, and not experimental or investigational;
4. Reflective of the level of service that can be safely provided, and for which no equally effective and more conservative or less costly treatment is available; and
5. Provided in a manner not primarily intended for the convenience of the recipient, the recipient's caretaker, or the provider." (Florida Mental Health RFP, pages 16–17)

Georgia

"1.36 Medically Necessary Services—Those services which are reasonable and necessary in establishing a diagnosis and providing palliative, curative or restorative treatment for physical and/or mental health conditions in accordance with the standards of medical practice generally accepted at the time the services are rendered. The services provided, as well as the type of provider and setting, must be appropriate to the specific medical needs of the Member." (Georgia Contract, page 47)

Hawaii

"Health Interventions

1. Health plans are required to cover health interventions within the specified categories that meet the following criteria:
   a. The intervention must be used for a medical condition.
   b. There is sufficient evidence to draw conclusions about the intervention's effects on health outcomes.
   c. The evidence demonstrates that the intervention can be expected to produce its intended effects on health outcomes.
   d. The intervention's beneficial effects on health outcomes outweigh its expected harmful effects.
   e. The health intervention is the most cost-effective method available to address the medical condition." (Hawaii RFP, page B-1)

Iowa

"1.3 Definition
Medical Necessity and Medically Necessary—services covered by the Medicaid program, but not those services which would not be covered by Medicaid pursuant to IAC 441–79.9." (Iowa Contract, page 4)

Iowa Mental Health

"III. Definition of Terms . . .
31. Medically Necessary—The requirement that the goods and services provided or ordered must be:
   a. Calculated to prevent, diagnose, correct, cure, alleviate, or preclude deterioration of a condition that threatens life, causes pain or suffering, or results in illness or infirmity;
   b. Individualized, specific, and consistent with symptoms or confirmed diagnosis of the illness or injury under treatment, and not in excess of the patient's needs;
   c. Necessary and consistent with generally accepted professional medical standards as determined by the Medicaid program, and not experimental or investigational;
   d. Reflective of the level of service that can be safely provided, and for which no equally effective and more conservative or less costly treatment is available; and
   e. Provided in a manner not primarily intended for the convenience of the recipient, the recipient's caretaker, or the provider." (Iowa Mental Health RFP, page 10–5)

Kentucky

"*Medically Necessary Health Services* means age appropriate services reasonable and necessary to diagnose and provide preventive, palliative, curative or restorative treatment for physical or mental conditions in accordance with professionally recognized standards of health care generally accepted at the time services are provided, and in accordance with 42 C.F.R. § 440.230, including services for children authorized under 42 U.S.C. 1396d(r)." (Kentucky Contract, page 14)

"The department shall consider medically necessary health services as those which are reasonable and necessary to diagnose and provide preventive, palliative, curative, or restorative treatment for physical or mental conditions in accordance with professionally recognized standards of health care generally accepted at the time services are provided, in accordance with 42 CFR 440.230 and including services for children authorized under 42 USC 1396d(r)." (Kentucky Contract, Attachment VIII, pages 64–65)

Maine

"II. Definitions . . .

40. Medical Necessity is defined as health care services that are reasonable and necessary to protect life, to prevent significant illness or significant disability, or to alleviate severe pain through the diagnosis or treatment of disease, illness, or injury." (Maine Contract, page 7)

"III. D. . . .

1. Medical Necessity . . .

For purposes of this initiative, medical necessity is defined as health care services which are reasonable and necessary to protect life, to prevent significant illness or significant disability, or to alleviate severe pain through the diagnosis or treatment of disease, illness, or injury." (Maine RFP, page 41)

"Glossary . . .

Medical Necessity—Health care services which are reasonable and necessary to protect life, to prevent significant illness or significant disability, or to alleviate severe pain through the diagnosis or treatment of disease, illness, or injury." (Maine RFP, Glossary)

Maryland

"10.09.67.(94) 'Medically appropriate' means an effective service that can be provided, taking into consideration the particular circumstances of the recipient and the relative cost of any alternative services which could be used for the same purpose.

(95) 'Medically necessary' means directly related to diagnostic, preventive, curative, palliative, or rehabilitative treatment." (Maryland COMAR, page 1736)

Massachusetts

"Medically Necessary Services—those medical services which: (a) are essential to prevent, diagnose, prevent the worsening of, alleviate, correct, or cure Enrollee medical conditions that endanger life, cause suffering or pain, cause physical deformity or malfunction, threaten to cause or aggravate a handicap, or result in illness or infirmity of an enrollee; (b) are provided at an appropriate facility and at the appropriate level of care for the treatment of an Enrollee's medical condition; and (c) are provided in accordance with generally accepted standards of medical practice." (Massachusetts Contract, page 4)

Minnesota

"3.19 Medically Necessary or Medical Necessity. Pursuant to Minnesota Rules, Part 9505.0175, Subpart 25, 'medically necessary' or 'medical necessity' means a health service that is consistent with the enrollee's diagnosis or condition and:
  A. Is recognized as the prevailing standard or current practice by the provider's peer group; and
  B. Is rendered in response to a life threatening condition or pain; or to treat an injury, illness, or infection; or to treat a condition that could result in physical or mental disability; or to care for the mother and child through the maternity period; or to achieve a level of physical or mental function consistent with prevailing community standards for diagnosis or condition; or

C. is a preventive health service defined under Minnesota Rules, Part 9505.0355." (Minnesota Contract, page 3)

Mississippi

"6.17 Medically Necessary Services
Medically necessary services are defined as services, supplies, or equipment provided by a licensed health care professional that:
a. are appropriate and consistent with the diagnosis or treatment of the patient's condition, illness, or injury;
b. are in accordance with the standards of good medical practice consistent with the individual patient's condition(s);
c. are not primarily for the personal comfort or convenience of the Member, family, or provider;
d. are the most appropriate services, supplies, equipment, or levels of care that can be safely and efficiently provided to the Member;
e. are furnished in a setting appropriate to the patient's medical need and condition and when applied to the care of an inpatient, it further means that the Member's medical symptoms or condition require that the services cannot be safely provided to the Member as an outpatient;
f. are not experimental or investigational or for research or education;
g. are provided by an appropriately licensed practitioner; and
h. are documented in the patient's record in a reasonable manner, including the relationship of the diagnosis to the service." (Mississippi Contract, page 22)

Missouri

"Health plans may develop criteria by which the health plan will review future treatment options, set prior authorization criteria, or exercise other administrative options for the plan's administration of medical care benefits. It is the responsibility of the health plan to determine whether or not a service furnished or proposed to be furnished is reasonable and medically necessary for the diagnosis or treatment of illness or injury, to improve the function of a malformed body member, or to minimize the progression of disability, in accordance with accepted standards of practice in the medical community of the area in which the health services are rendered; and the service could not have been omitted without adversely affecting the member's condition or the quality of medical care rendered; and the service is furnished in the most appropriate setting." (Missouri RFP, page 26)

Montana

"Medically Necessary or Medically Necessary Service—a service as defined at ARM 46.12.102(2) which is reasonably calculated to prevent, diagnose, correct, cure, alleviate, or prevent the worsening of conditions in a patient which:
  (a) endanger life;
  (b) cause suffering or pain;
  (c) result in illness or infirmity;
  (d) threaten to cause or aggravate a handicap; or
  (e) cause physical deformity or malfunction.
A service or item is medically necessary only if there is no other equally effective, more conservative, or substantially less costly Course of Treatment medically appropriate for the Recipient requesting the service or, when appropriate, no treatment at all. Experimental services as unacceptable treatment are not medically necessary for purposes of the Medicaid program." (Montana Contract, Attachment 1, unnumbered page)

Nebraska

"1.22: The term 'Medical Necessity' and 'Medically Necessary' with reference to a covered service means health care services and supplies which are medically appropriate and (1) necessary to meet the basic health needs of the Client; (2) rendered in the most cost-effective manner and type of setting appropriate for the delivery of the Covered Services; (3) consistent in type, frequency and duration of treatment with scientifically based guidelines of national medical, research or health coverage organizations or governmental agencies; (4) consistent with the diagnosis of the condition; (5) required for reasons other than the convenience of the Client or his or her Physician; (6) no more intrusive or restrictive than necessary to provide a proper balance of safety, effectiveness, and efficiency; (7) of demonstrated value; and (8) a no more intense level of services than can be safely provided. The fact that the Physician has performed or prescribed a procedure or treatment or the fact that it may be the only treatment for a particular injury, sickness or mental illness does not mean that it is Medically Necessary. Services and supplies which do not meet the definition of medical necessity set out above are not covered." (Nebraska RFP, page 3)

Nebraska Mental Health

"1.19 The term 'Medical Necessity' and 'Medically Necessary' with reference to a covered service means health care services and supplies which are medically appropriate and (1) necessary to meet the basic health needs of the Client; (2) rendered in the most cost-effective manner and type of setting appropriate for the delivery of the Covered Services; (3) consistent in type, frequency and duration of treatment with scientifically based guidelines of national medical, research or health coverage organizations or governmental agencies; (4) consistent with the diagnosis of the condition; (5) required for reasons other than the convenience of the Client or his or her Physician; (6) no more intrusive or restrictive than necessary to provide a proper balance of safety, effectiveness, and efficiency; (7) of demonstrated value; and (8) a no more intense level of services than can be safely provided. The fact that the Physician has performed or prescribed a procedure or treatment or the fact that it may be the only treatment for a particular injury, sickness or mental illness does not mean that it is Medically Necessary. Services and supplies which do not meet the definition of medical necessity set out above are not covered." (Nebraska Mental Health Contract, page 5)

Nevada

"Definitions . . .
Medically Necessary Service: The term 'medically necessary service' is any service performed by, or under the supervision of, a physician, or other provider qualified under Nevada law to furnish medical, dental, or other health services that in his/her professional judgment are necessary to diagnose, treat, or ameliorate a physical defect and/or mental symptom or illness and or other abnormality." (Nevada Contract, pages 15, 18)

New York

"1.19 'Medically Necessary' means health care and services that are necessary to prevent, diagnose, correct or cure conditions in the person that cause acute suffering, endanger life, result in illness or infirmity, interfere with such person's capacity for normal activity, or threaten some significant handicap." (New York Contract, page 8)

North Carolina

"1.41 Medically Necessary Services—Those services which are in the opinion of the treating physician, reasonable and necessary in establishing a diagnosis and providing palliative, curative or restorative treatment for physical and/or mental health conditions in accordance with the standards of medical practice generally accepted at the time the services are rendered. Each service must be sufficient in amount, duration, and scope to reasonably achieve its purpose; and the amount, duration, or scope of coverage, may not arbitrarily be denied or reduced solely because of the diagnosis, type of illness, or condition (42 CFR 440.230). Medicaid EPSDT coverage rules (42 USC *1396 (r) (5) and 42 USC*1396 d(a))." (North Carolina Contract, Appendix I, unnumbered page)

North Dakota

"Medical Necessity—The need for a medically necessary service.
Medically Necessary Service—Medical care and treatment that is:
a. Appropriate for symptoms present and is consistent with the diagnosis, if any;
b. Provided according to generally accepted medical practice and professionally recognized standards;
c. Not generally regarded as experimental or investigational; and
d. Specifically allowed by the licensing laws which apply to the provider of the service." (North Dakota Contract, Attachment C, page C-3)

Oklahoma

"Medically Necessary Service means any service performed by, or under the supervision of, a physician, dentist, or other provider qualified under State law to furnish medical, dental, or other health service that in his/her professional judgment is necessary to diagnose, treat, or ameliorate a physical defect, and/or mental symptom, illness or other abnormality." (Oklahoma Contract, page 6)

Oregon

"(26) Medically Appropriate: Services and medical supplies which are required for prevention, diagnosis or treatment for sickness or injury and which are:
  (a) Consistent with the symptoms of a medical condition or treatment of a medical condition;
  (b) Appropriate with regard to standards of good medical practice and generally recognized by the relevant scientific community and professional standards of care as effective;
  (c) Not solely for the convenience of an OMAP Member or a provider of the service or medical supplies; and
  (d) The most effective of the alternative levels of service or medical supplies that can be safely provided an OMAP Member in Contractor's judgment." (Oregon Contract, page 54)

Pennsylvania

"Medical Necessity—Determinations of medical necessity for covered care and services, whether made on a prior authorization, concurrent, or post-utilization basis, shall be in writing, be compensable under MA, and be based on the following standards. The plan shall base its determination on medical information provided by the individual's family and the primary care practitioner, as well as any other providers, programs, and agencies that have evaluated the individual. Medical necessity determinations must be made by qualified and trained providers. Satisfaction of any one of the following standards will result in authorization of the service:

The service or benefit will, or is reasonably expected to, prevent the onset of an illness, condition, or disability.

The service or benefit will, or is reasonably expected to, reduce or ameliorate the physical, mental, or developmental effects of an illness, condition, injury, or disability.

The service or benefit will assist the individual to achieve or maintain maximum functional capacity in performing daily activities, taking into account both the functional capacity of the individual and those functional capacities that are appropriate for individuals of the same age." (Pennsylvania RFP, pages x–xi)

Rhode Island

"1.14 Medical Necessity or Medically Necessary Service
The term "medical necessity" or "medically necessary service" means medical, surgical, or other services required for the prevention, diagnosis, cure, or treatment of a health related condition including such services necessary to prevent a detrimental change in either medical or mental health status. Medically necessary services must be provided in the most cost effective and appropriate setting and shall not be provided solely for the convenience of the member or service provider." (Rhode Island Contract, page 3)

South Carolina

"'Medically necessary' services include, but are not limited to, services directed toward the maintenance, improvement, or protection of health or lessening of illness, disability, or pain." (South Carolina Contract, page 14)

Tennessee

"Attachment I 'Definitions' shall be revised by replacing and/or incorporating the following definitions into the appropriate alphabetical order in Attachment I of the Agreement and renumbering all definitions accordingly . . .
Medically Necessary—shall mean services or supplies provided by an institution, physician, or other provider that are required to identify or treat a TennCare enrollee's illness, disease, or injury and which are:
   a. Consistent with the symptoms or diagnosis and treatment of the enrollee's illness, disease, or injury; and
   b. Appropriate with regard to standards of good medical practice; and

c. Not solely for the convenience of an enrollee, physician, institution or other provider; and

d. The most appropriate supply or level of services which can safely be provided to the enrollee. When applied to the care of an inpatient, it further means that services for the enrollee's medical symptoms or condition require that the services cannot be safely provided to the enrollee as an outpatient; and

e. When applied to enrollees under 21 years of age, services shall be provided in accordance with EPSDT requirements including federal regulations as described in 42 CFR Part 441, Subpart B, and the Omnibus Budget Reconciliation Act of 1989." (Tennessee Contract, Amendment Number 4, pages 3, 31, 32)

Texas

"II. Definitions . . .

Medically necessary health care services means health care services, other than behavioral health services, which are:

(a) reasonable and necessary to prevent illnesses or medical conditions, or provide early screening, interventions, and/or treatments for conditions that cause suffering or pain, cause physical deformity or limitations in function, threaten to cause or worsen a handicap, cause illness or infirmity of a member, or endanger life;

(b) provided at appropriate facilities and at the appropriate levels of care for the treatment of a member's medical conditions;

(c) consistent with health care practice guidelines and standards that are issued by professionally recognized health care organizations or governmental agencies;

(d) consistent with the diagnoses of the conditions; and

(e) no more intrusive or restrictive than necessary to provide a proper balance of safety, effectiveness, and efficiency." (Texas Contract, pages 6–7)

Utah

"Attachment B
Special Provisions

Article I
Definitions
For the purpose of the Contract: . . .
'Medically Necessary' means any medical service that (a) is reasonably calculated to prevent, diagnose, treat or cure conditions in the Enrollee that endanger life, cause suffering or pain, cause deformity or malfunction, or threaten to cause a handicap, and (b) there is no equally effective course of treatment available or suitable for the Enrollee requesting the service which is more conservative or substantially less costly. Medical services shall be of a quality that meets professionally recognized standards of health care in the community in which services are provided, and shall be substantiated by records including evidence of such medical necessity and quality. Those records shall be made available to the Department upon request." (Utah Contract, Attachment B, pages 1, 2)

Vermont

"Medical/clinical necessity includes a determination that the service(s) is/are medically/clinically appropriate and necessary to meet the medical or clinical needs of the patient; are consistent with the diagnosis or condition; are rendered in a cost-effective manner; and are provided in accordance with accepted professional practice and guidelines regarding type, frequency, duration, amount, and setting of treatment." (Vermont Contract, page 30)

"5.28 Medically/Clinically Necessary (Medical/Clinical Necessity) describes a service or supply that is determined to be:

appropriate for the symptoms, diagnosis or treatment of an enrollee's condition, illness, disease or injury;

provided for the diagnosis or direct care and treatment of an enrollee's condition, illness, disease or injury;

an appropriate, effective clinical preventive health service;

provided in accordance with accepted professional practice guidelines regarding type, frequency, duration, and setting of treatment;

not used primarily for an enrollee's (or their providers) convenience; and

the most appropriate supply or level of service that can safely be provided to the enrollee." (Vermont Contract, pages 60–61)

"Even if a provider prescribes, performs, orders, refers, recommends or approves a service or supply, the Plan may not necessarily consider it medically necessary." (Vermont Contract, page 61)

"Rule 10.000

10.000 Quality Assurance Standards and Consumer Protections for Managed Care Plans

10.100 General Provisions . . .

(BB) 'Medically-necessary care' means health care services including diagnosis testing, preventive services and aftercare appropriate, in terms of type, amount, frequency, level, setting, and duration, to the member's diagnosis or condition. Medically-necessary care must be consistent with generally accepted practice parameters as recognized by health care providers in the same or similar general specialty as typically treat or manage the diagnosis or condition, and

(1) help restore or maintain the member's health; or

(2) prevent deterioration of or palliate the member's condition; or

(3) prevent the reasonably likely onset of a health problem or detect an incipient problem." (Vermont Contract, Attachment H, pages 1, 4)

Washington

Washington State Mental Health

"Medically Necessary/Medical Necessity:

A term for describing a requested service which is reasonably calculated to prevent, diagnose, correct, cure, alleviate or prevent the worsening of conditions in the recipient that endanger life, or cause suffering or pain, or result in illness or infirmity, or threaten to cause or aggravate a handicap, or cause physical deformity or malfunction, and there is no other equally effective, more conservative or substantially less costly course of treatment available or suitable for the person requesting service. For the purpose of this section, 'course of treatment' may include mere observation or, where appropriate, no treatment at all. Mead vs Burdman (3/20/1978)" (Washington State Mental Health Contract, page 10)

Wisconsin

"The term 'medically necessary' means a medical service that meets the definition of HSS 101.03(96m) Wis. Adm. Code." (Wisconsin Contract, page 4)

MENTAL HEALTH– OR SUBSTANCE ABUSE–RELATED MEDICAL NECESSITY STANDARDS

Georgia

"1.36 Medically Necessary Services—Those services which are reasonable and necessary in establishing a diagnosis and providing palliative, curative or restorative treatment for physical and/or mental health conditions in accordance with the standards of medical practice generally accepted at the time the services are rendered. The services provided, as well as the type of provider and setting must be appropriate to the specific medical needs of the Member." (Georgia Contract, page 47)

Hawaii

"The health plan shall make decisions regarding substance abuse client admission, continued stay and discharge criteria based on the most recent edition of the American Society of Addiction Medicine (ASAM) Patient Placement Criteria." (Hawaii RFP Amendment 4.0)

Iowa

Iowa Mental Health

"III. Covered Diagnosis . . .
Coverage is determined by application of the following:
(i) Medical necessity is determined by the Contractor using 'The Medco Behavioral Care Systems Utilization Management Guidelines.'" (Iowa Mental Health Contract, pages 44, 46)
"III. Definition of Terms . . .
32. Medically Necessary or Medical Necessity—The clinical, rehabilitative or supportive mental health services which, as determined by the Contractor, are: 1. Appropriate and necessary to the symptoms, diagnoses or treatment of a mental disorder; 2. Provided for the diagnosis or direct care and treatment of a mental disorder; 3. Within standards of good practice for the service modality; 4. Not primarily for the convenience of the Member or a provider; and, 5. The most

appropriate level of supply of service which can safely be provided."
(Iowa Mental Health Contract, page 4)

Iowa Substance Abuse

"3. Definition of Terms . . .
Service Necessity:
The requirement that the goods and services provided or ordered must
be, pursuant to the criteria of the ICPC:
1. Appropriate and necessary to the symptoms, diagnoses or treatment
   of a substance abuse disorder;
2. Provided for the diagnosis or direct care and treatment of a substance
   abuse disorder;
3. Within standards of good practice within the substance abuse service
   area;
4. Not primarily for the convenience of a plan member or a plan
   provider; and
5. The most appropriate level or supply of service which can safely be
   provided." (Iowa Substance Abuse Contract, page 5)

Kentucky

"*Medically Necessary Health Services* means age appropriate services
reasonable and necessary to diagnose and provide preventive, palliative,
curative or restorative treatment for physical or mental conditions in
accordance with professionally recognized standards of health care generally accepted at the time services are provided, and in accordance with 42
C.F.R. § 440.230, including services for children authorized under 42
U.S.C. 1396d(r)." (Kentucky Contract, page 14)
"The department shall consider medically necessary health services as
those which are reasonable and necessary to diagnose and provide preventive, palliative, curative, or restorative treatment for physical or mental
conditions in accordance with professionally recognized standards of
health care generally accepted at the time services are provided, in accordance with 42 CFR 440.230 and including services for children authorized
under 42 USC 1396d(r)." (Kentucky Contract, Attachment VIII, pages 64–
65)

Massachusetts

Massachusetts Behavioral Health

"Medically Necessary Service—shall mean those mental health and/or substance abuse services which are: 1) reasonably calculated to prevent, diagnose, prevent the worsening of, alleviate, correct, or cure conditions in the Enrollee that endanger life, cause suffering or pain, cause physical deformity or malfunction, threaten to cause or to aggravate a handicap, or result in illness or infirmity, and 2) there is no other equally effective course of treatment available or suitable for the Enrollee requesting the service that is more conservative or substantially less costly. Medical services shall be of a quality that meets professionally recognized standards of health care, and shall be substantiated by records including evidence of such medical necessity and quality. Those records shall be made available to the Division upon request. (*See* 42 U.S.C. 1396a(a)(30), and 42 CFR 440.230 and 440.260.)" (Massachusetts MH/SAP Contract, Appendix A, page 12)

Minnesota

"3.19 Medically Necessary or Medical Necessity. Pursuant to Minnesota Rules, Part 9505.0175, Subpart 25, 'medically necessary' or 'medical necessity' means a health service that is consistent with the enrollee's diagnosis or condition and:
  A. is recognized as the prevailing standard or current practice by the provider's peer group; and
  B. is rendered in response to a life threatening condition or pain; or to treat an injury, illness, or infection; or to treat a condition that could result in physical or mental disability; or to care for the mother and child through the maternity period; or to achieve a level of physical or mental function consistent with prevailing community standards for diagnosis or condition; or
  C. is a preventive health service defined under Minnesota Rules, Part 9505.0355." (Minnesota Contract, page 3)
"3. Mental Health and Chemical Dependency (MH/CD) Services
a. Services

The HEALTH PLAN is responsible for providing MH/CD services as needed by enrollees. Chemical dependency services must be provided in accordance with Minnesota Rules, Parts 9530.6600 to 9530.6660 (CD assessment) and by programs and facilities licensed under Minnesota Rules, Parts 9530.5000 to 9530.6500 (CD licensure). Mental health services must be provided in accordance with Minnesota Rules, Part 9505.0323 (MA payment for outpatient mental health services) and Minnesota Rules, Part 9505.0324 (home-based mental health services). MH/CD services should be directed at rehabilitation of the client in the least restrictive clinically appropriate setting." (Minnesota Contract, Appendix I, page 2)

Missouri

"(n) Behavioral health (mental health and substance abuse) services:
(1) Adults limited to 30 inpatient days and 20 outpatient visits per year for those services listed in Part Two, Section I, Paragraph 5(n)(3). There are no limitations regarding medically necessary services for individuals under age 21.
(2) Services for behavioral health conditions shall be provided based upon medical necessity. This shall be determined by a process of behavioral health assessment that accurately reflects the clinical condition of the patient and the acceptable standards of practice for such clinical conditions." (Missouri RFP, page 8)
"(a) Services for behavioral health conditions shall be provided based upon medical necessity. This shall be determined by a process of behavioral health assessment that accurately reflects the clinical condition of the patient and the acceptable standards of practice for such clinical conditions." (Missouri RFP, page 9A)

Nebraska

"1.22: The term 'Medical Necessity' and 'Medically Necessary' with reference to a covered service means. . . . The fact that the Physician has performed or prescribed a procedure or treatment or the fact that it may be the only treatment for a particular injury, sickness or mental illness does not mean that it is Medically Necessary. Services and supplies which do not meet the definition of medical necessity set out above are not covered." (Nebraska RFP, page 3)

Nebraska Mental Health

"1.19 The term 'Medical Necessity' and 'Medically Necessary' with reference to a covered service means. . . . The fact that the Physician has performed or prescribed a procedure or treatment or the fact that it may be the only treatment for a particular injury, sickness or mental illness does not mean that it is Medically Necessary. Services and supplies which do not meet the definition of medical necessity set out above are not covered." (Nebraska Mental Health Contract, page 5)

Nevada

"Definitions . . .
Medically Necessary Service: The term 'medically necessary service' is any service performed by, or under the supervision of, a physician, or other provider qualified under Nevada law to furnish medical, dental, or other health services that in his/her professional judgment are necessary to diagnose, treat, or ameliorate a physical defect and/or mental symptom or illness and or other abnormality." (Nevada Contract, pages 15, 18)

North Carolina

"1.41 Medically Necessary Services—Those services which are in the opinion of the treating physician, reasonable and necessary in establishing a diagnosis and providing palliative, curative or restorative treatment for physical and/or mental health conditions in accordance with the standards of medical practice generally accepted at the time the services are rendered. Each service must be sufficient in amount, duration, and scope to reasonably achieve its purpose; and the amount, duration, or scope of coverage, may not arbitrarily be denied or reduced solely because of the diagnosis, type of illness, or condition (42 CFR 440.230). Medicaid EPSDT coverage rules (42 USC *1396 (r) (5) and 42 USC*1396 d(a))." (North Carolina Contract, Appendix I, unnumbered page)

Oklahoma

"Medically Necessary Service means any service performed by, or under the supervision of, a physician, dentist, or other provider qualified under State law to furnish medical, dental, or other health service that in his/her professional judgment is necessary to diagnose, treat, or ameliorate a physical defect, and/or mental symptom, illness or other abnormality." (Oklahoma Contract, page 6)

Oregon

"T. Chemical Dependency . . .
(2) Contractor shall make decisions about access to chemical dependency treatment, continued stay, discharges, and referrals based upon Office of Alcohol and Drug Abuse Programs (OADAP) approved criteria, which is deemed to be Medically Appropriate." (Oregon Contract, page 10)

Oregon Mental Health

"Medically Appropriate: Services and supplies which are required for Prevention (including preventing a relapse), Diagnosis or treatment of mental disorders and which are Appropriate and consistent with the Diagnosis; consistent with treating the symptoms of a mental illness or treatment of mental disorders; appropriate with regard to standards of good practice and generally recognized by the relevant scientific community as effective; not solely for the convenience of the OMAP Member or provider of the service or supply; and the most cost effective of the alternative levels of Covered Services or supplies which can be safely and effectively provided to the OMAP Member in the Contractor's judgment." (Oregon Mental Health Contract, page 63)

Pennsylvania

"Medical Necessity—Determinations of medical necessity for covered care and services, whether made on a prior authorization, concurrent, or post-utilization basis, shall be in writing, be compensable under MA, and be based on the following standards. The plan shall base its determination on medical information provided by the individual's family and the primary care practitioner, as well as any other providers, programs, and agencies that have evaluated the individual. Medical necessity determinations must be made by qualified and trained providers. Satisfaction of any one of the following standards will result in authorization of the service:

The service or benefit will, or is reasonably expected to, prevent the onset of an illness, condition, or disability.

The service or benefit will, or is reasonably expected to, reduce or ameliorate the physical, mental, or developmental effects of an illness, condition, injury, or disability.

The service or benefit will assist the individual to achieve or maintain maximum functional capacity in performing daily activities, taking into account both the functional capacity of the individual and those functional capacities that are appropriate for individuals of the same age." (Pennsylvania RFP, pages x–xi)

Pennsylvania Behavioral Health

"Medical Necessity—Clinical determinations to establish a service or benefit which will, or is reasonably expected to:

prevent the onset of an illness, condition, or disability;

reduce or ameliorate the physical, mental, behavioral, or developmental effects of an illness, condition, injury, or disability;

assist the individual to achieve or maintain maximum functional capacity in performing daily activities, taking into account both the functional capacity of the individual and those functional capacities appropriate for individuals of the same age." (Pennsylvania Behavioral Health RFP, page iv)

"4) Provide the criteria to be used to review medical necessity for psychiatric in-patient, residential treatment for children/adolescents, partial hospitalization, outpatient services, and behavioral health rehabilitation services for children and adolescents. Indicate research and/or national models upon which the criteria are based, if other than the Department's guidelines. (N.B.: Department of Health, Office of Drug and Alcohol Services level of care criteria and American Society of Addiction Medicine criteria must be used for drug and alcohol services for adults and adolescents, respectively.)" (Pennsylvania Behavioral Health RFP, page 21)

"Guidelines for Mental Health Medical Necessity Criteria
Adult Psychiatric Inpatient Services . . .
Partial Hospitalization . . .
Psychiatric Outpatient Clinic" (Pennsylvania Behavioral Health RFP,
Appendix T, Part A, unnumbered pages)

"Once the severity of the problem has been determined, the interviewer
must decide the appropriate type and length of care required by the
individual. This decision must be in accordance with the Pennsylvania
Client Placement Guidelines contained in this document addressing each
of the six dimensions or problem areas:

 acute intoxication and/or withdrawal potential
 biomedical condition and/or complications
 emotional/behavioral conditions and/or complications
 treatment acceptance/resistance
 relapse potential
 recovery environment" (Pennsylvania Behavioral Health RFP,
 Appendix T, Part C, page 18)

"Payor organizations that require payor authorization for admission into
treatment must designate facilities/individuals to conduct the intake assessment according to Pennsylvania's guidelines. Placement/continued
stay/authorizations must be made in accordance with criteria contained in
this document. While it is recognized that payors may want to utilize other
nationally recognized criteria, only the Cleveland, ASAM, and the Pennsylvania Client Placement Guidelines for Adults have been approved for
use in Pennsylvania." (Pennsylvania Behavioral Health RFP, Appendix T,
Part C, page 25)

"HealthChoices MCO Readiness Review Program Requirements . . .
Utilization Management . . .
Criteria used for medical necessity are compatible with Appendix T; E,
6, b (p. 71):

 Parts A and B for members receiving mental health services, and
 Part C for members receiving drug and alcohol services." (Pennsylvania Behavioral Health Contract, Exhibit B, pages 8–9)

Rhode Island

"1.14 Medical Necessity or Medically Necessary Service
The term "medical necessity" or "medically necessary service" means
medical, surgical, or other services required for the prevention, diagnosis,

cure, or treatment of a health related condition including such services necessary to prevent a detrimental change in either medical or mental health status. Medically necessary services must be provided in the most cost effective and appropriate setting and shall not be provided solely for the convenience of the member or service provider." (Rhode Island Contract, page 3)

Texas

"II. Definitions . . .

Medically necessary behavioral health services means those behavioral health services which:

(a) are reasonable and necessary for the diagnosis or treatment of a mental health or chemical dependency disorder or to improve or to maintain or to prevent deterioration of functioning resulting from such a disorder;

(b) are in accordance with professionally accepted clinical guidelines and standards of practice in behavioral health care;

(c) are furnished in the most appropriate and least restrictive setting in which services can be safely provided;

(d) are the most appropriate level or supply of service which can safely be provided; and

(e) could not be omitted without adversely affecting the Member's mental and/or physical health or the quality of care rendered." (Texas Contract, page 6)

Utah

Utah Mental Health

"'Medically Necessary' means any mental health service that is necessary to diagnose, correct or ameliorate a mental illness or condition, or prevent deterioration of that condition or development of additional health problems and there is no other equally effective course of treatment available or suitable that is more conservative or substantially less costly." (Utah Mental Health Contract, Attachment B, unnumbered page)

"A. Enrollee's Rights . . .

6. Medical necessity and best practice guidelines—As specifically are developed and accepted by mental health stakeholders to determine medical necessity and best practices, the CONTRACTOR agrees to operate the PMHP program in accordance with these guidelines." (Utah Mental Health Contract, Attachment B, unnumbered page)

Washington

Washington State Mental Health

"State Plan, Title XIX Service Modalities . . .

3. Intake Evaluation:
'Intake Evaluation' means an evaluation initiated prior to the provision of any other services, except crisis services and stabilization services. The intake evaluation must establish the medical necessity for treatment and be completed within thirty days." (Washington State Mental Health Contract, page E–1)

Wisconsin

"In compliance with said provisions, the HMO shall further guarantee all enrolled Medicaid recipients access to all medically necessary outpatient MH/AODA treatment. No limit may be placed on the number of hours of outpatient treatment which the HMO shall provide or reimburse where it has been determined that treatment for mental or nervous disorders or alcohol or drug abuse is medically necessary. The HMO shall not establish any monetary limit or limit on the number of days of inpatient hospital treatment where it has been determined that this treatment is medically necessary." (Wisconsin Contract, page 80)

"2. Mental Health . . . Assessment Requirements—The HMO shall further assure that authorization for MH/AODA treatment to its enrollees shall be governed by the findings of an assessment performed promptly by the HMO upon request of a client or referral from a physician." (Wisconsin Contract, page 80)

DUAL DIAGNOSIS MEDICAL NECESSITY STANDARDS

Iowa

Iowa Mental Health

"B. Medicaid

Determination of coverage under Medicaid funding arrangement is based on logic which examines five (5) variables including the presence of service necessity as determined by the ICPC and for PMIC Substance Abuse Services, the PMIC Admission and Continued Stay Criteria, authorization by the contractor for rendered services at levels IV, V, V–PMIC, VI, and VII as defined by the ICPC and for PMIC Substance Abuse Services, the PMIC Admission and Continued Stay Criteria, by the contractor, the provider of such services, the diagnosis, and the type of services provided. . . .

2. Services are covered at levels IV, V, V–PMIC, VI, and VII when provided by a qualified (participating) provider when services are necessary according to the ICPC and for PMIC Substance Abuse Services, the PMIC Admission and Continued Stay Criteria, and when services are authorized by the contractor. . . .

Exception: PMIC Substance Abuse Services are covered regardless of billing diagnosis when the admission diagnosis is one of the following . . . ." (Iowa Substance Abuse Contract, Attachment 1/1/96, pages 3–4)

Pennsylvania

Pennsylvania Behavioral Health

"Guidelines for Mental Health Medical Necessity Criteria
Adult . . .
A physician has conducted an evaluation that has determined that:

1. The person has a psychiatric diagnosis or provisional psychiatric diagnosis, excluding mental retardation, substance abuse or senility, unless these conditions coexist with another psychiatric diagnosis or provisional psychiatric diagnosis." (Pennsylvania Behavioral Health RFP, Appendix T, unnumbered page)

CHAPTER 6

Private Purchaser Expectations

Veronica V. Goff

Purpose: This chapter provides an overview of what employers desire when they purchase behavioral health care benefits.

Major Topics: This chapter places emphasis on what has "value" to employers in their purchasing decisions. It discusses five elements: Consumer Centered, Health and Optimal Functioning, Evidence-Based Care, Quality and Efficiency, and Accountability for Meeting Population Health Needs in a Cost-Efficient Manner. Depression is used as an example.

INTRODUCTION

Our nation's employers buy health care for 152 million people (Fronstein, 1998). In 1998, large employers spent an average of $4,164 per employee on health care, a 6.1% increase over the previous year's spending and the highest rate of increase since 1993 (William M. Mercer, 1999). Asked what they want for their health care dollars, leading employers, like any smart buyers of a product or service, reply "good value." To many, especially large employers, health care is more than a benefit provided to attract and retain good employees. It is a way to invest in the health, vitality, and productivity of their workforce and the competitiveness of their company. Knowing what they get for their health care dollars is just as important as knowing how much they spend.

The growth of managed behavioral health care is a byproduct of the search for health care value. The first managed behavioral health care

159

initiatives were undertaken to control costs. During the late 1980s, large employers' mental health costs were rising between 40% and 60% annually, with serious care quality concerns (England & Vaccaro, 1991). By the mid-1990s, managed care was taking hold, costs were stabilizing, and employers began to focus on the quality of care provided. In particular, they began looking for evidence of the "value" of their mental health expenditures; that is, what is the outcome of treatment relative to the cost?

Pinpointing value in mental health care is proving to be difficult. Employers are increasingly aware that worker disability, absenteeism, and lost productivity associated with unrecognized and poorly managed mental illness can cost much more than paying for early and appropriate care. In addition, they know that people with untreated mental illness use more general medical care. Several high-visibility efforts have been established to assess and drive quality and value in behavioral health care. Among them are the National Committee for Quality Assurance (NCQA) Health Plan Employer Data and Information Set (HEDIS) measures and behavioral health accreditation standards and the industry-driven Performance-Based Measures for Managed Behavioral Healthcare Programs (PERMS) initiative. Unfortunately, these efforts have fallen short of employers' expectations for health care systems that provide their employees with the right care at the right time, while systematically assessing outcomes such as health status and functioning. While employers are frustrated with health systems' seeming inability to provide meaningful quality information, managed care organizations claim that employers care only about cost, purchasing at the lowest price. They both are right. Most employers cite cost as the most important health care purchasing issue. Until we can systematically demonstrate the value of their investment in health care, the practice is destined to continue.

The purpose of this chapter is to discuss private employer notions about mental health care quality and value, their concerns and expectations for managed behavioral health care, and their role in developing the next generation of managed care. Private employers, as active health care purchasers, have contributed to the rapid growth of managed behavioral health care over the past decade. The core technology of managed care has proved effective at containing costs. But as the 1990s drew to a close, employers were questioning the access, quality, and cost management successes of managed behavioral health care.

There has never been a more promising time in the treatment of mental illness. Improved understanding of brain function and advances in diagnosis and treatment are dramatically improving mental health care outcomes. But problems associated with ensuring appropriate treatments and demonstrating value for consumers and purchasers continue to plague the success of the managed behavioral health care industry and make mental health a public battleground over spending.

PRIVATE PURCHASERS AND THE GROWTH OF MANAGED BEHAVIORAL HEALTH CARE

Managed behavioral health care is a $4.4 billion industry that has seen most of its growth over the last decade. Prior to 1990, most mental health coverage was provided through indemnity insurance. During the late 1980s, a few large private employers signed highly publicized contracts with fledgling managed behavioral health care companies. Over the next five to ten years, many more employers carved mental health and substance abuse care out of their medical plans, changing the way millions of people access services and stimulating a dynamic and highly competitive industry. States began contracting with private managed behavioral health firms during the early to mid-1990s, some in statewide reforms and others for local pilots. By 1998, 177 million people were enrolled in some form of managed behavioral health care (Oss, 1999).

The growth of managed behavioral health care is due largely to its success in controlling costs. A decade ago, behavioral health care was the fastest rising component of employer health care costs. Between 1988 and 1989, costs for large employers rose an average of 47% (Adler, 1990). Employers with the most generous plans saw the largest increases. Managed behavioral health care addressed a number of employers' cost concerns: the cost of behavioral health care, the rate of cost increases, and the predictability of future costs. With managed behavioral health care, employers experienced significant slowing in the rate of increase of mental health costs and in some instances expenditures declined. Future costs became more predictable. Managed care techniques, including utilization review, discounted fee arrangements, and exclusive provider networks, were responsible for the declining costs, with reductions in inappropriate hospitalization the most significant factor. Now, employers do not consider mental health spending the problem that it was a decade ago, and with good reason. A Hay Group (1999) survey found that employers spent an average of $151 per covered life on mental health in 1988. By 1998, spending had dropped to $69 per covered life.

Improvements in care quality associated with managed behavioral health care also contributed to the industry's rapid growth. Compared with traditional indemnity coverage, managed behavioral health care plans enhanced early intervention, offered a broader scope of services, and provided better continuity of care. In case after case of employers shifting to managed behavioral health care, penetration rate (percentage of the population using services) increased due to easy access to outpatient services and the availability of cost-effective alternatives to hospitalization. Employers also began to have access to something missing in traditional indemnity plans—the systematic reporting of data on utilization and cost. Early quality reporting efforts, while not perfect, began to reveal wide variations in treatment practice along with characteristics of good quality care, such as outpatient follow-up after hospitalization and home- and community-based services for adolescents.

TURNING AROUND TRADITIONAL NOTIONS ABOUT MENTAL HEALTH INSURANCE

Prior to the era of managed behavioral health care, employers experienced the conventional problems associated with mental health insurance: moral hazard and adverse selection. Research on insurance practices supported employers' experience that as consumer cost sharing for behavioral health was reduced more services were used. The most generous employer plans saw the largest cost increases. Benefit limits and higher consumer cost sharing were used in an attempt to ensure appropriate service use and control costs. In response to these limits, states enacted mandated mental health benefit laws to constrain the degree to which insurers could limit mental health coverage. As it turned out, state insurance mandates did little to ensure good mental health coverage. Meanwhile, employers wondered about the impact of benefit limits on employees and their families.

Employers began lifting the controversial benefit limits characteristic of traditional mental health and substance abuse coverage due to the success of managed behavioral health care. Administrative, financial, and care management mechanisms used by managed behavioral health care firms held costs down while providing an expanded scope of services compared with unmanaged indemnity plans. Early managed care techniques relied heavily on utilization review, tightly managed provider networks, and discounted fee arrangements. Now, the most innovative programs downplay the use of retrospective reviews in response to concerns about overzealous cost control and third-party decision making. Instead, prospective standards for quality and access are emphasized, as well as individualized treatment planning and case management, albeit with mixed results.

By the time the 104th U.S. Congress passed the Mental Health Parity Act of 1996, the landscape for the provision of behavioral health care had changed dramatically. Managed behavioral health care was helping make clear that good quality behavioral health care was not just a function of benefit design. In fact, in many instances, especially related to hospitalization, benefit design was a problem that helped drive inappropriate care. Many analysts predicted that the impact of the law would be modest because it only addressed annual and lifetime dollar limits. The real impact of the law was unfortunate in that it encouraged the use of day and visit limits, rather than the more global dollar limits. Sturm and McCulloch's 1998 analysis of the Mental Health Parity Act and behavioral health carve-out plans found that many plans are still using deductibles, limits, and other demand-side mechanisms that are potentially not in the best interest of providing quality care.

While there is tacit agreement that benefit design does not drive quality, there is little agreement about how to define quality. Most quality data refer to administrative, customer service, and provider network standards rather than to consumer and purchaser outcomes. A recent survey of employer health plan contracts found that fewer than half contained any performance standards (Deloitte & Touche, 1998). Administrative and customer service standards were most common, while HEDIS measures and provider-related standards were least common. In another study looking at employer purchasing practices, researchers found that many employers are unaware of available clinical quality measures or find the measures irrelevant or difficult to incorporate into their purchasing decisions (Hibbard, Jewett, Legnini, & Tusler, 1997).

EMPLOYERS USE CLINICAL DEPRESSION AS A WINDOW ON QUALITY AND VALUE

Frustrated with the lack of meaningful outcomes-based quality indicators, employers are crafting their own. It is a first good attempt at quantifying health care value from the perspective of employer-purchasers. The indicators are workplace based, relate to health status and functioning, and derive from an understanding about the impact of unrecognized and poorly managed mental illness on workforce absenteeism, disability, and productivity (Frank, McGuire, Normand, & Goldman, 1999; Greenberg, Stiglin, Finkelstein, & Berndt, 1993; Kessler et al., 1999).

Behavioral health disability, and disability due to depression in particular, is a prominent driver of employer indirect costs (those costs associated with lost work time and productivity). Roughly 70% of the more than 17 million adults with depression each year are in the labor force (*Facts about Depression*, 1997). In 1993, a landmark study on the direct and indirect costs of depression was published indicating that annual national spending for depression was $44 billion. Of the total, $12 billion was spent on health care, while more than $24 billion was employer costs associated with absenteeism and lost productivity (Greenberg, Stiglin, Finkelstein, & Berndt, 1993). Employer data, consistent with the study by Greenberg and associates, show that compared with other prevalent conditions such as diabetes, back pain, and heart disease, depression often has the longest average length of disability and the highest probability of a second disability leave within the year (*D/ART National Worksite Program*, 1998).

The devastating impact of depression on productivity is worldwide. A report sponsored by the World Health Organization and the World Bank and produced by researchers at the Harvard School of Public Health projects a steady rise in disability costs due to depression (Murray, 1996). According to the report, depression was the fourth leading cause of disability in the world in 1990. By 2020, it will be the single leading cause (Lopez, 1996). Although most depression can be effectively treated with a combination of medication and psychotherapy, poor recognition and management of depression expose employers to avoidable productivity-related costs.

Over the past several years, many employers have begun to suspect that tightly limited mental health care benefits were contributing to higher psychiatric disability costs and productivity losses. Published studies confirm their suspicions. A 1998 study by the UNUM Life Insurance Company and Johns Hopkins University found that employer plans with good access to outpatient mental health services have lower psychiatric disability claims costs than plans with more restrictive arrangements (Salkever, 1998). In addition, the study found that when front-line supervisors play an active role in disability return-to-work efforts, claims rates were 50% lower than in those companies where supervisors were not actively involved in disability management. As a result, many employers, in partnership with their health plans, are putting less emphasis on managing access to behavioral health care services and more on employee education, early intervention mechanisms, disability prevention and management, and return-to-work programs.

EMPLOYER INNOVATIONS IN MANAGING TOTAL BEHAVIORAL HEALTH COSTS

The recognition of productivity losses associated with unrecognized and poorly managed illness is driving employers to consider total (direct and indirect) costs when designing and administering health care and disability benefits. Two innovative corporate programs are cited below.

First Chicago NBD (FCNBD; now Bank One as a result of a 1998 merger) has used an integrated health data management system, or data warehouse, since 1987 to link direct and indirect costs related to workforce health and disability. A joint effort of the medical, benefits, and information system units, it enables them to track and predict health care and disability costs more accurately and design disease management and other interventions to optimize employee health and establish benchmarks for health care quality improvements (Burton & Conti, 1997).

The employee assistance program (EAP) at FCNBD is part of the medical unit and has managed behavioral health short-term disability (STD) since 1989. The purpose of EAP involvement is to assist employees in receiving appropriate behavioral health care, to manage employees' return to work, and to provide follow-up support after return to work (Conti & Burton, 1999). FCNBD, like other large employers, has experienced an increase in behavioral health disabilities. Between 1989 and 1996, mental illness went from the sixth leading cause of STD to the third leading cause. By 1996, the number of behavioral health STD events per thousand employees rose to 10 from 2.5 in 1985. Between 1985 and 1989, the average duration of the STD increased as well. Since EAP involvement in 1989, the trend has stabilized.

One of the most important aspects of FCNBD's program is that the EAP/medical department works with providers to ensure appropriate treatment. The most frequent concerns discussed with providers about treatment are timely access, inclusion of either medication or psychotherapy, and the step up to a higher level of care (Conti & Burton, 1999). Recommendations for more intense and higher cost treatment are made with knowledge about the interdependence of direct and indirect costs.

At Abbott Laboratories, a task force was formed in 1994 to study opportunities in disability management after several problems were identified. The task force discovered that the firm's approach to managing medical leave was more reactive than proactive. Case management began only after employees entered into extended disability leave or when return-to-work problems arose. Moreover, Abbott was missing opportunities to prevent disabilities. Health care providers were unfamiliar with Abbott Laboratory jobs and the workplace, and therefore were not making appropriate return-to-work recommendations. Finally, employees were becoming psychologically "disemployed" when away from the workplace for an extended period of time. These problems resulted in significant indirect costs. Workers' compensation costs had doubled in the previous five years, extended disability costs were increasing 10% annually, STD costs were higher than average, and there were significant productivity losses associated with delayed return to work (Burgess, Davidoff, & Goff, 1999).

Based on the findings, the task force recommended implementation of a proactive disability management process. The goal of the program is to optimize employee health and performance, not just to return employees to work. Key components of the program include the following:

- Employees on STD leave are identified early.
- Case management is provided during the disability leave. Case managers work directly with employees, their health care providers, and their supervisors. All relevant issues are taken into consideration, and judgment is exercised to balance the needs of all involved.
- Case managers consult with providers regarding the medical leave process and the workplace. This is especially important with providers who need information about the specific requirements of the workplace in order to make recommendations regarding leave, work restriction, and job accommodation.
- Follow-up services continue for the employee after his or her return to work. As needed, case managers maintain contact with the employee to monitor work restrictions as well as to ensure that their medical conditions remain stable. Case managers also educate managers re-

garding return-to-work accommodations and misconceptions regarding illness. For example, a manager may not know how to address job performance problems with an employee who has a psychiatric disability.

- The program is evaluated based on employee satisfaction and lost work time. In addition, quality improvement (QI) monitors are implemented to ensure that the process works as it should. The QI monitors include detailed standards for process and performance. Each quarter, random samples of client files are audited to ensure that standards are met.

The project began with a pilot site. Based on its success, it was fully implemented at three locations by the end of 1998.

These examples of innovative corporate programs provide two lessons for evolving managed behavioral health care practices. First, to show the value of health interventions, the cost paradigm must go beyond direct health care spending to include indirect cost consequences of unrecognized and poorly managed illness. Second, cost control mechanisms commonly used in managed behavioral health care may not enhance service delivery efficiency or patient outcomes.

ONGOING CONCERNS ABOUT MANAGED BEHAVIORAL HEALTH CARE

The growth of managed behavioral health care has dramatically changed the organization and delivery of mental health and substance abuse services. It has prompted large employers to lift the benefit limits typical of traditional coverage, it has changed traditional notions about mental health insurance, and it has opened the way for more relevant research on the impact of mental health parity. Many employers would say that managed behavioral health care has helped them offer generous and protective benefits, reduce cost shifting to individuals, and improve the overall quality of care, all while containing costs.

But as the 1990s drew to a close, the access, quality, and cost successes attributed to managed behavioral health care were being questioned. Advocates for persons with serious mental illness had widespread concerns about managed behavioral health care's effects on access and quality and the relative role of the public mental health system. Medicaid provides health and mental health coverage for approximately 29 million people or 12.5% of all people with health care coverage. People with serious mental illness often must rely on a poorly funded public system of state mental hospitals, community mental health programs, and substance abuse treatment and rehabilitation services that is uncoordinated with other needed services and supports.

In the decade from 1986 to 1996, mental health funding from public sources increased from 49% to 54% of total spending, while funding from the private sector remained relatively flat at 26% (Mark, McKusick, King, Harwood, & Genuardi, 1998). These data cause many mental health advocates to conclude that the responsibility for paying for mental health and substance abuse services is shifting more to the public sector, and the shift is being driven by private sector growth of managed care. Private sector purchasers do not necessarily agree with the conclusion because the data do not account for private sector mental health spending in the general medical sector and for prescription drugs. Roughly 50% of mental health care is provided in primary care, not by the mental health service system. Moreover, managed behavioral health programs typically are not responsible for managing prescription drugs.

A major frustration for employers is lack of information about utilization of general medical care and prescription drugs for behavioral health in relationship to the efforts of managed behavioral health care programs. Pharmaceutical coverage is the fastest rising component of employer health care spending. In 1998, large employers spent an average of 15% more on prescription drugs than the previous year, according to a Washington Business Group on Health (WBGH) survey (1999). Private insurance payments for prescription drugs increased by almost 18% in 1997, after growing 18% in 1996 and 22% in 1995 (Copeland, 1999). The introduction of new antidepressants and antipsychotics in recent years, along with increased awareness of the prevalence of mental illness, has made mental health drugs one of the cost drivers (Browne, 1999).

Rather than resort to conventional component cost controls, employers want to evaluate the growth of prescription drug use in relationship to associated costs (e.g., medical care and disability) and value (e.g., improved workforce health and productivity). Leading employers know it is useless to look at prescription drug expenditures without examining health outcomes and the extent to which drug expenditures impact total costs. A growing number of disease-specific studies demonstrate cost savings due to pharmaceutical use. For example, a recent study of stroke patients found that use of an anti-clotting drug, at a cost of $1.7 million per 1,000 patients saved more than $4 million in rehabilitation and nursing home costs (Fagan, et al., 1998). The impact of prescription drugs on employer costs associated with disability, absenteeism, and lost productivity is a recent area for study. A study on pharmacotherapy and indirect costs for depression by the MEDSTAT Group found a significant increase in absenteeism leading up to depression diagnosis and treatment with antidepressant medication, and a significant decrease in absenteeism after treatment was begun (Claxton, Chawla, & Kennedy, 1999). But evaluations of this kind are rare and are not being done in any systematic way.

The concern noted above is consistent with employer frustrations about health care generally. Other concerns employers have with managed behavioral health care (and health care generally) are lack of provider performance information, wide variations in practice and inadequate use of practice guidelines, poor consumer information, poor coordination of care, and underuse of information technologies.

WHAT DO PRIVATE PURCHASERS WANT?

Employer behavioral health purchasing practices and preferences are subject to much analysis and study. Recent work at the Heller School Institute for Health Policy analyzed behavioral health carve-out practices of Fortune 500 employers against a number of assumptions about health care quality and cost and contract management issues (Hodgkin et al., in press). They concluded that the strongest predictor of an employer's decision to carve out, once other characteristics are controlled for, is size. Employers who value coordination of care are less likely to carve out, while employers who value special expertise are more likely to carve out. Despite the belief that managed behavioral health programs save money, cost savings were more important to employers that did not carve out behavioral health care.

The findings speak to the straightforward manner in which many large employers approach health care purchasing and the uncomplicated nature of their expectations. What do private purchasers want? They want to purchase health care from a consumer-centered, performance-based system, where behavioral health care is fully integrated into the system of care. They also want to be able to quantify the value of their health investments in terms meaningful to their business.

During the early 1990s, members of WBGH, a nonprofit organization of large private and public employers, began thinking about the kind of health care system they wanted. They identified a number of pressing health system problems: fragmented delivery of services, unknowable quality, passive participation by consumers, and little accountability for quality and cost efficiency (Cronin & Milgate, 1993). They began to define characteristics and attributes indicative of the health care system they wanted and to use their purchasing power to influence change. The critical concepts that distinguish such a system are consumer-centered care, integration, accountability, and continuous improvement.

Consumer Centered

Private purchasers want a health care system that is consumer centered in care philosophy and consumer friendly in management approach. The system of care recognizes consumers as partners, educating them about their health and actively involving them in health care decisions. Health care services integrate the physical, mental, and life management needs of consumers and families, and they reflect unique needs of individuals, families, and communities.

Oriented to Health and Optimal Functioning

Private purchasers want a health system, not just an illness system. Optimal health and functioning should be primary goals, with illness prevention and management high priorities. The system recognizes that health is a dynamic state and that all individuals, regardless of age or physical or mental capacity, can improve their health. The system should integrate all the services needed to manage population health and disability and account for the total cost of illness and injury.

Committed to Evidence-Based Care

Private purchasers want a health care system that is committed to evidence-based care and can demonstrate the value of treatments and services. The system uses integrated information systems that enable it to answer, within confidentiality guidelines, key questions about appropriateness, cost, and outcomes of care. Costs are controlled through more effective medical management.

Self-Evaluating for Quality and Efficiency

Private purchasers want a health care system that can adjust its operations and care processes in response to information about performance. It is self-evaluating for quality and efficiency, making utilization review as an oversight mechanism unnecessary. Regular feedback is provided to clinicians, and improvement objectives are developed and implemented.

Accountable for Meeting Population Health Needs in a Cost-Efficient Manner

Private purchasers want a health care system that is accountable to consumers, purchasers, and regulatory organizations and that routinely reports on clinical performance, consumer satisfaction, operations, and year-over-year changes in population health status.

CREATING THE NEXT GENERATION OF MANAGED BEHAVIORAL HEALTH CARE

In 1998, employer health care costs rose in excess of 6%, the largest annual increase since 1993 (William M. Mercer, Inc., 1999). Amid predictions of a return to steep health care inflation, employers are giving unprecedented attention to assessing the value of their investments in workforce health and health care. They are asking not only "How much are we spending?" but also, "What are we getting for those expenditures?" Leading employers are focusing on the second question because they are aware of the impact of health-related absence on workforce productivity and corporate competitiveness. New research and information about the extensive impact of untreated behavioral health problems on the workplace are helping to drive the new focus.

The focus on workforce health as an investment in business success is a new era in corporate health and human resource management. A decade ago, few benefits professionals thought it was possible to demonstrate the value of dollars spent on employee health beyond program cost containment and in terms meaningful to business performance. Health care and disability benefits were seen as costs of doing business and rapidly rising costs at that. Now, advances in disease prevention and management, care management systems, and information technology make it possible for employers to shift from simply managing individual health and disability program costs to more comprehensive strategies focused on optimizing workforce health and performance.

The next generation of managed behavioral health care and the definition of value derived from the health care system will be shaped, in part, by these new, more comprehensive corporate health management strategies. The challenge calls for better coordination of medical and behavioral health care and a new, more integrated way of looking at health care costs and value. First, we must be able to integrate cost and utilization data across medical, behavioral health, and prescription drug services. Then, to show real value, the cost paradigm must go beyond direct health care spending to include indirect costs. Again, pharmaceuticals provide a good example. Purchasers understand the argument that spending more for new pharmaceuticals that enhance treatment compliance can result in better functional outcomes and lower indirect costs. But data from the various "components" of health care must be integrated to make the case. And that is not now being done in any systematic way.

Meeting the challenge also will take a new level of partnership among purchasers, consumers, and the health system and a hard-nosed look at the role of public policy in either facilitating or hampering evaluation of health interventions and system performance. Confidentiality of health information is a hotly debated public policy issue. Yet, the desire for total confidentiality needs to be balanced with good patient care. Successful management of behavioral health conditions requires a multidisciplinary team approach among medical and mental health practitioners. Evaluation of health system performance requires data that often reside with employers. Linking health, disability, workers' compensation, and absence data to better understand the workplace impact of unrecognized and poorly managed health conditions is population based and makes use of aggregated data. Individually identifiable information is used only for functions where it is necessary, such as in the management of disability leave or the processing of workers' compensation claims.

CONCLUSION

Managed behavioral health care is a $4.4 billion industry that has seen most of its growth over the last decade. Private employers, as active health care purchasers, have influenced that growth. The core technology of managed care has proved effective at containing costs. But as the 1990s drew to a close, the access, quality, and cost management successes of managed behavioral health care were being questioned. Employers continue to be frustrated with a lack of provider performance information, variations in practice, inadequate use of practice guidelines, poor consumer information, poor coordination of care, and underuse of information technologies to enhance care delivery and evaluation. A pressing concern is the lack of information about utilization of general medical care and prescription drugs for behavioral health in relationship to the efforts of managed behavioral health care programs.

Employer data show that costs associated with absenteeism and lost productivity when mental health needs are unrecognized or poorly managed far exceed direct spending for mental health care. As a consequence, employers have a strong economic interest in pressing for a health care system that integrates medical and behavioral health care and improves mental health status while reducing inappropriate use of care. Leading employers are beginning to quantify health care value with indicators that are workplace based, relate to health status and functioning, and derive from an understanding about the impact of poorly managed mental illness on the workplace.

A number of changes are needed to better demonstrate the value of behavioral health services. Among them are better integration of cost and utilization data across medical, behavioral health, and prescription drug services and better accounting for the indirect cost consequences of unrecognized and poorly managed illness. New partnerships among health care purchasers, consumers, and the health system will be necessary to make those changes.

REFERENCES

Adler, S. (1990). Psychiatric costs are rising at large firms. *Business Insurance.*

Browne, R.A. (1999). Managing the mental health pharmacy budget: Key messages. *Behavioral Health Management, 19*(3), 18–22.

Burgess, A.G., Davidoff, I., & Goff, V.V. (1999). *Investing in workplace productivity: Innovations in managing indirect mental health costs.* Washington, DC: Washington Business Group on Health.

Burton, W.N., & Conti, D.J. (1997). Use of an integrated health data warehouse to measure the employer costs of five chronic disease states. *Disease Management, 1*(1).

Claxton, A.J., Chawla, A.J., & Kennedy, S.R. (1999). *Absenteeism among employees treated for depression.* Ann Arbor, MI: The MEDSTAT Group.

Conti, D.J., & Burton, W.N. (1999). In J.M. Oher (Ed.), *The employee assistance handbook.* New York: John Wiley & Sons, Inc.

Copeland, C. (1999). *Prescription drugs: Issues of cost, coverage, and quality.* Employee Benefits Research Institute brief no. 208. Washington, DC: Employee Benefits Research Institute.

Cronin, C., & Milgate, K. (1993). *A vision for the future health care delivery system: Organized systems of care.* Washington, DC: Washington Business Group on Health.

D/ART national worksite program. (1998). Washington, DC: Washington Business Group on Health.

Deloitte & Touche LLP. (1998). 1997 employer survey on managed care medical benefits, *15*(10), 1–2.

England, M.J., & Vaccaro, V.A. (1991, Winter). New systems to manage mental health care. *Health Affairs, 10*(4), 129–137.

Facts about depression. (1997). Bethesda, MD: Depression Awareness, Recognition, and Treatment Program, National Institute of Mental Health.

Fagan, S.C., Morgenstern, L.B., Petitta, A., Ward, R.E., Tilley, B.C., Marler, J.R., Levine, S.R., Broderick, J.P., Kwiatkowski, T.G., Frankel, M., Brott T.G., & Walker, M.D. (1998). Cost effectiveness of tissue plasminogen activator for acute ischemic stroke. *Neurology, 50*, 883–889.

Frank, R.G., McGuire, T.G., Normand, S.L., & Goldman, H.H. (1999). The value of mental health care at the system level: The case of treating depression. *Health Affairs, 18*(5), 71–88.

Fronstein, P. (1998, December). *Sources of health insurance and characteristics of the uninsured: Analysis of the March 1998 current population survey.* Employee Benefits Research Institute brief no. 204. Washington, DC: Employee Benefits Research Institute.

Greenberg, P.E., Stiglin, L.E., Finkelstein, S.N., & Berndt, E.R. (1993). The economic burden of depression in 1990. *Journal of Clinical Psychiatry, 54*(11), 1–14.

Hay Group. (1999, April). *Hay Group health care plan design and cost trends 1988–1998.* Washington, DC: Hay Group.

Hibbard, J.H., Jewett, J.J., Legnini, M.W., & Tusler, M. (1997). Choosing a health plan: Do large employers use the data? *Health Affairs, 16*(6), 172–180.

Hodgkin, D., Horgan, C.M., Garnick, D.W., et al. (in press). *Why carve out? Determinants of behavioral health contracting choice among large US employers.* Waltham, MA: Institute for Health Policy, Heller School, Brandeis University.

Kessler, R.C., Barber, C., Birnbaum, H., Frank, R.G., Greenberg, P., Rose, R., Simon, G., & Wang, P. (1999). Depression in the workplace: Effects on short term disability. *Health Affairs, 18*(5), 163–171.

Lopez, A.D. (1996). In C.J.L. Murray (Ed.), *The global burden of disease: A comprehensive assessment of mortality and disability from diseases, injuries and risk factors in 1990 and projected.* Cambridge, MA: Harvard School of Public Health.

Mark, T., McKusick, D., King, E., et al. (1998). *National expenditures for mental health, alcohol, and other drug abuse treatment in 1996.* DHHS publication no. SMA 98-3255. Rockville, MD: Substance Abuse and Mental Health Services Administration.

Murray, C.J.L. (Ed.). (1996). *The global burden of disease: A comprehensive assessment of mortality and disability from diseases, injuries and risk factors in 1990 and projected.* Cambridge, MA: Harvard School of Public Health.

Oss, M. (Ed.) (1999). Over 72 percent of insured Americans are enrolled in MBHO. *Open Minds, 11*(4).

Salkever, D. (1998). *Predictors and descriptors of psychiatric duration, cost, and outcomes study.* Portland, ME: UNUM Life Insurance Company.

Sturm, R.S., & McCulloch, J. (1998). Mental health and substance abuse benefits in carve-out plans and the Mental Health Parity Act of 1996. *Journal of Health Care Finance, 24*(3), 82–92.

Washington Business Group on Health. (1999). *The right prescription for corporate health: Pharmaceutical cost and value.* Washington, DC: WBGH.

William M. Mercer, Inc. (1999). *Mercer/Foster Higgins national survey of employer sponsored health plans 1998.* New York: William M. Mercer.

CHAPTER 7

Public Purchaser Expectations

Martin D. Cohen and Stephen L. Day

Purpose: This chapter provides an overview of what governments—public purchasers—desire when they purchase behavioral health care benefits.

Major Topics: Key variables differentiating between state Medicaid managed behavioral health programs are carve-in or carve-out; statewide, regional, or local; a "make" versus "buy" decision; and who bears how much risk. Major reasons for implementing managed care in the public sector include cost containment, cost savings, improvements in performance and quality, management enhancements, and changes in program-benefit design. Pennsylvania and Washington State are used as examples.

BACKGROUND

In behavioral health care, unlike other segments of health care, government, both state and local, is a major payer *and* provider of care. State and local governments expend $15.9 billion annually in mental health and alcohol and drug abuse treatment services (Frank, McGuire, Regier, Manderscheid, & Woodward, 1994). These services are either provided directly by governments, such as that provided in state-operated psychiatric hospitals and county-run outpatient clinics, or provided by private, often nonprofit, providers through state and local government contracts and grants. This government-supported sector of behavioral health care has come to be known as the "public behavioral health sector."

The public behavioral health care sector is targeted mainly to those who are indigent or lack private insurance to pay for their care. In some jurisdictions services may be further targeted to those who meet strict eligibility requirements such as having a serious and persistent mental illness, or those who may require long-term and continuing care.

Historically, state and local government monies have funded the public sector behavioral health system. These funds were used to care for patients in state hospitals and county homes. There were no financial incentives to operate these institutions efficiently or quality performance measures to ensure that care was appropriate to the patient's individual needs. In the 1960s, the deinstitutionalization movement and the development of community mental health centers changed the locus of care from these largely institutional settings to local communities. Funding for these services continued to come from state and local government and from federal grants provided for the construction and staffing of community mental health centers (CMHCs). Yet, as care moved to these largely nonprofit community settings, there continued to be little financial incentives for productivity or efficiency (Clark, Dowart, & Epstein, 1994). These providers were often the recipients of government grants or contracts that paid for a certain level of capacity, rather than reimbursement for the actual care that was provided. This method of payment began to change in the late 1980s as federal CMHC grants ended, and state and local governments looked for ways to reduce spending. In many cases this resulted in the adoption of fee-for-service contracts where providers were reimbursed on a unit cost basis once the care was delivered (Clark, Dowart, & Epstein, 1994).

In the mid-1980s payments for public sector behavioral health services shifted yet again. Many states sought Medicaid reimbursement for the provision of behavioral services. Since Medicaid is a federal/state program, this allowed states to share the cost (usually between 50% and 75%) of inpatient and outpatient behavioral health services provided to Medicaid recipients with the federal government. As states learned from each other how to maximize federal financial participation (FFP), the amount of Medicaid funding of behavioral health services quickly climbed. The addition of the Medicaid rehabilitation and case management options also expanded the amount of Medicaid reimbursements flowing to states. In addition to these outpatient services, states also sought reimbursement for inpatient care to those under age 22 and over 65, and in some cases for those between 22 and 65 years when this care could be provided in general hospital settings. For example, in 1992, Massachusetts established Department of Mental Health units in several general hospitals to serve as replacement units as it downsized its state hospital system (Commonwealth of Massachusetts, 1995). This allowed these units to seek Medicaid reimbursement for care that could not be reimbursed had it been provided in a state hospital.

As these financing changes were affecting the public sector of behavioral health care, there were formidable changes occurring in the private sector as well. Employers concerned about rising health care costs turned to managed care organizations such as health maintenance organizations (HMOs) to help limit costs and better manage services. Since many of these organizations had no real experience in managing behavioral health care, many sought help from newly formed behavioral health managed care organizations (MCOs). These HMOs and other insurers carved out their behavioral health benefits and contracted with MCOs to manage them sometimes on an at-risk basis. By employing managed care tools such as gatekeeping, utilization management, limited provider networks, and lower rates for volume, these organizations were able to achieve savings that they kept as profit. Since most providers of public sector behavioral health services were largely dependent on government contracts and had limited contracts with these private payers, they did not initially feel the effects of these private sector managed care approaches on their clinical services or finances.

However, in the late 1980s and early 1990s this began to change as states became concerned over rising Medicaid costs. During this time period Medicaid expenditures almost tripled, moving from $52.6 billion in 1988 to $152.4 billion in 1995 (Kaiser Foundation, 1997). Although much of this growth was attributable to changes in enrollment, state use of Medicaid as an alternative to state general fund funding of services contributed to the increase. Since Medicaid is an entitlement, state legislatures or state Medicaid authorities could not arbitrarily limit expenditures. Rather, many state Medicaid agencies were forced to ask for and receive supplemental appropriations from their legislatures to deal with significant Medicaid budget deficiencies. In Massachusetts, the state Medicaid program became known in the legislature as a "budget buster" (Mohl, 1989).

To respond to these increases in costs, states began to explore ways to apply managed care principles and technologies to their Medicaid programs. Although federal regulations made the use of managed care difficult within the Medicaid program, states were able to request waivers from the Health Care Financing Administration (HCFA). There are two types of

Medicaid waivers: Section 1115, which allows for research and demonstration programs where states can test new financing and organization methods, and Section 1915, which allows for the waiver of certain program restrictions, such as a Medicaid beneficiary's freedom to choose his or her care from any Medicaid provider (freedom of choice provision). Although HCFA's waiver authority had been in place since 1981, the use of these waivers was extremely limited. This changed in the 1990s. As an outgrowth of their efforts to pursue health reform, the Clinton administration encouraged states to use waivers to pursue state-level health reform in the Medicaid program.

At first, states applied for waivers to apply managed care principles to physical health care. This led many Medicaid agencies to contract with HMOs for the physical health care of their Medicaid beneficiaries. In these arrangements, behavioral health benefits were mostly carved out of the basic benefit and continued to be paid for on a fee-for-service basis. Gradually, as states realized financial savings and were able to contain the growth of Medicaid spending, these arrangements were expanded to include behavioral health care.

Today, states do not need to apply for waivers to implement managed care plans within their state Medicaid programs. The Federal Balanced Budget Act of 1997 (Balanced Budget Act, 1997) allows state Medicaid authorities to implement such programs by submitting amendments to their existing and approved state Medicaid plans. This change is expected to increase the number of states that will adopt managed care principles for their Medicaid program and expand the number and the array of managed care programs within those states that are already using managed care principles through previously approved waivers.

PUBLIC SECTOR BEHAVIORAL HEALTH MANAGED CARE

The application of managed care strategies to public sector behavioral health care has its earliest roots in four state demonstrations: Arizona, Massachusetts, Iowa, and Utah. These demonstrations, done under HCFA's waiver authority, used rigorous utilization management protocols, the establishment and tracking of outcome and performance measures, the selection and credentialing of provider networks, and the use of risk-based contracts to change utilization patterns and thereby reduce costs. Although these demonstrations have had mixed results, they have been largely viewed as successful in controlling the growth of Medicaid behavioral health expenditures and in creating a certain degree of flexibility and accountability in the use of public funds. As a result, 40 state Medicaid authorities now use managed care to deliver some behavioral health services and 70% of all Medicaid beneficiaries are enrolled in some type of managed care program delivering behavioral health services (SAMHSA, 1999).

Although the application of managed care is fairly consistent across managed care plans, state Medicaid authorities and state and local mental health departments have approached managed care in many different ways. The key variables among most behavioral health managed care plans are: Do they carve in or carve out behavioral health care from physical health care? Are they statewide or is there a regional or local approach to managed care? Do they attempt to "make" or "buy" the provision of managed care? and Do they seek to keep or shift the risk inherent in the provision of care?

Carve In or Carve Out

In a carve-in model of service delivery, behavioral health benefits (mental health and substance abuse services) are included as part of the individual's total health care package. An HMO or other health insuring organization is responsible for all health care, regardless of whether it is behavioral or physical. The HMO also is responsible for ensuring that care is provided and managed appropriately. In a carve-out model of service delivery, behavioral health care is separated or carved out of physical health care, and the responsibility and funds are given to a specialty provider or manager. This provider or manager has the responsibility to ensure that services are provided and care is managed appropriately. The manager could be a behavioral health MCO or could be another government entity such as the state mental health department or a county behavioral health agency. For example, in Pennsylvania's HealthChoices Medicaid managed care program, the state, at the urging of the counties, has elected to carve behavioral health out from physical health, and give the local mental health and substance abuse administrators the opportunity to manage these services, as they do other public mental health and substance abuse funds.

Statewide, Regional, or Local

Some jurisdictions have elected to develop statewide initiatives where a single MCO is responsible for all behavioral health care in the state, while others have elected to develop regional or local approaches to managed care. An example of a statewide program can be found in Iowa, where the state has contracted with a single behavioral MCO to manage care within all 99 counties. At the other end of the spectrum is Arizona, which started its managed care program through the use of regional behavioral health entities. There are currently five such entities in Arizona, each managing care for a defined geographic area of the state.

Make or Buy

Rather than purchase the services of an MCO, some jurisdictions have chosen to "make" their own managed care program. In these cases, the state or county will create its own MCO within its existing state or county mental health and substance abuse agency. This usually involves developing new systems for utilization management and claims processing and hiring new staff who have the expertise to run these systems. An example of a "make" site is Philadelphia, where the city Department of Health created its own behavioral health organization. The organization, Community Behavioral Health (CBH), is a nonprofit corporation formed as a subsidiary of the city's health department. It was capitalized using city funds and operates for the sole purpose of managing the care of Medicaid beneficiaries under the state's HealthChoices program.

Other jurisdictions have chosen to "buy" managed care technology, choosing to procure the services of a specialty MCO to provide the needed technology. There are several national behavioral managed care companies, such as Magellan Health, Inc., ValueOptions, Inc., and United Behavioral Healthcare, that offer these services. Although most of these companies direct their services to the private behavioral health market, each has developed subsidiary groups to provide services to public purchasers. In addition to these national behavioral health MCOs, there are several regional or local organizations that also offer such services. These include some that are subsidiaries of hospitals or providers of behavioral health care within local communities.

Retention, Sharing, or Shifting of Risk

A key aspect of managed care is the assumption of clinical and financial risk. A principle in many managed care plans is to cap the amount of money that is available to provide care. In these types of "capitation" contracts, the program, usually a unit of government such as the state or county mental health agency or MCO, receives a set amount of funds to cover the cost of care for those eligible to receive care. The amount is usually based on historical expenditures and adjusted to account for how much "management" of care is expected. This becomes the capitation rate, and the program must live within the capitation rate for the total number of beneficiaries for whom it must provide. If the amount of care provided exceeds the total cap rate for all beneficiaries, then the program is responsible for making up the difference. If the program is able to spend less than the total cap rate through good management, then the MCO is allowed to keep some, if not all, of the savings. As with any type of insurance risk, there will always be those who will use more care than expected, the cost of which is made up for by those who use little or no services. This is the risk inherent in managed care.

One way programs protect themselves in a managed care environment is to shift or share the risk with others, such as to an HMO or MCO or to providers. Risk can be shifted entirely, whereby any loss or any gain stays with the managed care entity, or it can be shared, whereby any savings or loss can be shared on a percentage basis between the program and the MCO. Another way a program can minimize its risk is through the purchase of reinsurance, whereby the program buys an insurance policy protecting it from losses that exceed its capitation rate. The Commonwealth of Pennsylvania has shifted all the financial and clinical risks for care to county governments. Some counties, such as Philadelphia, have decided to keep the risk within the county but have purchased reinsurance to protect itself from catastrophic losses. Other counties, such as Chester and Montgomery, have opted to shift risk to a private MCO. Some jurisdictions, such as Massachusetts, have decided to share the financial risk with an MCO. Under this arrangement, the state limits the upside and downside financial exposure of the MCO. Savings are shared between the two, as are losses up to the agreed upon profit/loss cap.

WHAT PUBLIC PURCHASERS WANT TO PURCHASE

The advent of managed care in the public sector has meant considerable change in how government, in particular public behavioral health agencies, views its role in a managed system of care. The most fundamental change is the distinction of moving from being a payer—an organization that provide funds or reimburses providers for care—to that of being a purchaser of care—an organization that provides funds to another party to manage or provide the care to a designated set of beneficiaries. This is a subtle but important distinction as it changes how government views its role in the provision of public sector behavioral health services.

Public purchasers, be they state mental health, Medicaid, or substance abuse agencies or local (county) mental health and substance abuse authorities, have generally looked at managed behavioral health to meet specific needs within their Medicaid, mental health, or substance abuse programs. While these needs vary and each program's managed care request for proposals is unique, these needs have generally included the establishment of cost controls, the achievement of cost savings, improvements in performance and quality, management enhancements, changes in programming, and a reduction in the level of administrative and political burden.

Cost Containment

Most state and local behavioral health authorities have looked to managed care to help control escalating costs in the provision of behavioral health services, particularly in their state Medicaid programs. While behavioral health care expenses are generally a small percentage of all state Medicaid expenditures, nationally, behavioral health expenditures were 15% of all Medicaid expenditures (Congressional Research Service, 1988). These expenditures have risen at a higher rate in recent years due to the increased use of the Medicaid rehabilitation and case management options, as well as increased public awareness of the benefits of seeking care for mental health and substance abuse problems. Although the rise in these expenditures was in some part the result of explicit state policies to maximize federal Medicaid reimbursements for behavioral health expenditures, the impact on state funds caused many state Medicaid directors to look at how these costs could be controlled through the use of managed care.

Building on the success that MCOs had had in the private sector, several state Medicaid programs (Tennessee, Iowa, and Massachusetts) decided to contract with these organizations for the management of their Medicaid behavioral health programs. In the bidding process leading up to these contracts, MCOs were given historical cost and utilization information in the form of a data book, which allowed these firms to make actuarially sound estimates of projected expenses and how these expenses might be altered through the use of managed care principles. The resulting contracts with these organizations were structured so as to shift responsibility for expenditure growth from the state to the MCO. Essentially, these contracts put the MCO at risk for expenditures that exceeded current or agreed-upon funding levels. In some cases this was at full risk or shared risk with the state. MCOs were not at risk for expenditure increases that were attributable to increases in enrollment.

By employing basic managed care techniques such as prior authorization for expensive procedures, discounted rates, and the creation of limited provider networks, it was possible for these MCOs to bring the behavioral health expenditures in these states within budget. The behavioral health budget will now include the MCO's own expenses and profit margin.

For the state agency, controlling expenditures through the use of managed care gave it distinct advantages that it did not have otherwise. First, since its costs were now controlled, the agency could accurately project its budget needs, which was difficult to do when costs were open ended. Second, since the risk for overexpenditure now rested with the MCO, the state agency would not be in a position of having to seek a deficiency budget from the state legislature if expenses exceeded what was in the state budget. Finally, by controlling costs in the behavioral health area, the state agency could put its time and energy into controlling costs in areas that had a greater impact on state costs, namely acute care and long-term care.

Cost Savings

For many states, controlling expenditures through the use of managed care was not good enough. These states looked to managed care as a way to reduce their behavioral health expenditures and enable them to use the resulting savings to expand their Medicaid program in other directions, meet deficits in other care areas, or redirect savings within their behavioral health budgets. Several states (Massachusetts, Pennsylvania, Iowa, and Michigan), either in their first or second procurement for managed behavioral health care services, took savings off the top of their behavioral health budget before putting the program out for bid, or created significant incentives within their program to achieve savings.

Many behavioral health requests for proposals for managed care firms create risk corridors. Within these corridors, managed care firms can accumulate savings that they are entitled to keep, share with the purchaser (state or county), or reinvest in the behavioral health program. In some instances (King County, Washington), all three objectives can be found in the purchaser's request for proposals.

Iowa's first mental health managed care contract called for the MCO to use savings to increase rehabilitation services within the state. Other jurisdictions have targeted their savings for improvements in services to people with a dual diagnosis of mental health and substance abuse, or to create new community services, such as non-hospital-based detoxification services. Some states also have targeted savings as a way to increase Medicaid eligibility, raise the minimum income thresholds, or add new beneficiary groups.

Purchasers must be careful as to how they structure programs designed to achieve savings. The temptation to generate savings must not become an incentive for the MCO to act irresponsibly and limit or deny care to needed beneficiaries. Conversely, purchasers do not want there to be too little incentive, which would have the potential of not using the tools of managed care to their optimal advantage. Ohio chose to create a very limited risk/savings corridor of only ±4% in its managed care design so as to ensure that expenditures and utilization remained close to their historical levels while creating some, albeit limited, potential for the MCO to achieve some savings (State of Ohio, 1996).

A major complaint by advocates is that savings achieved from the use of managed care in behavioral health ought to remain within the behavioral health budget. While some states, like Iowa, have done this, other states, like Tennessee, have used these savings to support deficiencies in other program areas. Very often the complex financing of Medicaid and other public behavioral health care makes tracking savings and the reallocation of funds difficult.

Improvement in Performance and Quality

Public purchasers also have looked to managed care as a way to improve the overall performance of their behavioral health care program and the quality of services provided in their behavioral health programs. Many public sector managed care procurements and contracts detail specific performance objectives from prospective bidders and contractors. These range from such items as increasing the number of beneficiaries served by the program (penetration rate measure) and decreasing the time a patient must wait to be seen by a qualified clinician (access measure) to how quickly claims must be adjudicated and paid.

Although every managed care procurement and contract is unique, improvements in performance usually fall into three classes: (1) system performance—those areas that relate to how well the public behavioral health care system is working; (2) clinical performance—how well the program is improving clinical outcomes for participants; and (3) administrative performance—how well the MCO is meeting its performance expectations. Public purchasers have included many performance and outcome measures within their managed care contracts. For example, Tennessee established 192 performance indicators in its first managed care contract (The TennCare Partner Program Vendor Contract). These indicators ranged from such things as how fast the telephone was answered to improvements in the level of functioning for patients. Table 7–1 shows some of the domains typically used by public purchasers in their managed care contracts to improve performance within their behavioral health programs. Very often there are incentive bonuses or financial penalties associated with each of these performance measures. In some instances, the MCO's profit level is tied to its ability to achieve certain defined performance objectives.

While performance contracting in behavioral health care is not new, many of the domains and measures found in state and county managed care contracts are new to the field, or they are at a level of detail and measurement that is new to most publicly funded mental health and substance abuse providers. They also require changes in data management systems so that this level of data can be regularly collected and analyzed. Ohio scrapped the data systems used by the state and county mental health and substance abuse authorities in favor of a managed care information system so it could better track expenditure, utilization, and performance data.

Table 7–1 Domains Used To Improve Performance

System Performance	Clinical Performance	Administrative Performance
• Penetration levels	• Functioning levels	• Call pickup
• Expenditure levels	• Admission rates	• Call abandonment
• Utilization levels	• Hospital diversion rates	• Hold times
• Service admittance rates	• He-hospitalization level	• Wait for appointments
• Unavailability of service	• Sobriety	• Claims payment rate
• Time between inpatient discharge and first outpatient appointment	• Involvement with criminal justice system	• Service appeals
• Consumer participation in treatment	• Participation in school (children)	• Service denials
• Consumer involvement in program planning	• Employment/income levels	• Complaints
• Consumer-run services	• Stable housing	• Network turnover
• Use of best practices	• Level of safety	• Transaction times
• Cultural competency	• Change in health status	• Consumer satisfaction
• Level of unusual incidents	• Placements outside the home (children)	• Delinquency in data reporting

In addition to improvements in performance, public purchasers also are looking to MCOs to improve the quality of care. This is done largely by requiring MCOs to institute clinical protocols and guidelines that recognize industry best practices, such as the use of newer atypical antipsychotic medications, and programs, such as assertive community treatment. In addition, public purchasers also have insisted on accreditation for the MCO by the National Committee for Quality Assurance (NCQA) and requirements that the MCO contract only with accredited providers. Other quality enhancements required by purchasers have included rigorous readiness reviews, clinical qualifications for utilization managers and care coordinators, and periodic evaluations of the program by an independent body.

One common complaint about the expectations of public purchasers in the area of performance and quality is that the desired level of performance is often pegged higher for MCOs than for the public purchaser's own provider systems. Since the MCO must contract with these same provider systems, there are often unreasonable expectations that performance will dramatically change under a managed system of care. Another complaint is that certain performance measures may be very desirable, but outside the direct control of the MCO or its behavioral health providers. For example, the ability of consumers to have meaningful employment may be dependent not only on their level of functioning, but also on the nature of the local economy where they live. Although gaining employment and an income for beneficiaries is an important objective, the ability of the MCO to impact this objective may be slight.

Management Enhancements

A significant expectation of purchasers is that the move to managed care will bring new technology to their mental health and substance abuse services that will enhance their management and delivery. These enhancements and improvements can include changes in clinical decision making, service utilization management, data and information management, financial management and accounting, provider network development and contracting, and quality management.

Many public purchasers are looking for the technology and principles of managed care to "modernize" their mental health and substance abuse systems. Typically, this involves the use of standardized clinical guidelines in determining who is in need of service and the use of sophisticated utilization management criteria and processes to determine the amount, duration, and scope of treatment that should be authorized on behalf of the client. While many public mental health and substance abuse systems use clinical criteria to determine eligibility and screen for the need for certain services, they typically do not engage in this type of rigorous utilization management. These types of procedures have proved beneficial in directing those in need of service to the most appropriate level of care, thereby reducing costs. Purchasers also have looked at these methods as ways to reduce waiting lists or long wait times for services.

In addition to management enhancements in clinical decision making, public purchasers often look to purchase enhanced management information capacity. Most public mental health and substance abuse systems have limited data processing capacity. By using a managed care vendor, these purchasers often hope to capture higher levels of utilization, expenditure, and performance data that they can use for their own management and planning purposes. In some cases, purchasers (e.g., San Diego County, California, and King County) have gone to managed care to replace their own or contracted claims payment systems that were limited in scope. Paying claims in a timely manner has become one of the single most important expectations of public purchasers.

Purchasers also have looked to MCOs to help them refine their provider networks. MCOs have developed provider credentialing and provider contracting systems that are designed to shape the provider network around the needs of beneficiaries. This typically means that substandard providers are removed from these systems and new and different types of providers are brought in depending on local circumstances. In the public behavioral world, making these types of decisions is often difficult, but can be made more difficult when there are insufficient data on either client needs or provider performance from which to base such decisions. This is one reason why public purchasers use MCOs to shape their provider networks.

Some purchasers also are looking for their managed care vendor to bring to their systems new ideas about how to finance care. This includes the use of capitated payments to providers, new rate-setting methodologies, and contracting methods that provide incentive bonuses and financial penalties for providers based on performance.

Public purchasers often are limited in how they contract with providers and for how long. By moving to an MCO, the purchaser can make use of more market-driven payment methodologies found in other health insurance sectors. These include techniques such as capitation payments, case rates, risk-adjusted rates, disease state management programs, and volume discounts.

Enhancements in management technology also extend to the people MCOs can attract to run their systems. Low public pay scales make it difficult for public purchasers to recruit people with the expertise needed to carry out many of the functions listed here. By using an MCO that is outside the constraints of government, it is assumed that these organizations can pay more to recruit people with the expertise and experience needed to manage these programs. As so many MCOs have recruited managers away from state and local governments to run their public sector behavioral managed care programs, one may not be sure that this is indeed the case.

Changes in Programming

Public purchasers also have looked to MCOs to change or modify the nature and types of services being provided to those in need of mental health and substance abuse services. Procurements for managed care services also have included requirements that MCOs add new services, such as in Tennessee where new case management and housing coordination services were requested. Another example is Iowa, where the procurement required the vendor to use savings to develop new psychosocial rehabilitation services. Nine new rehabilitation services were added after the first year of operation in Iowa (U.S. General Accounting Office, 1999).

Other programmatic enhancements requested by public purchasers have included the development of social drop-in centers and clubhouses (Colorado), a focus on recovery and rehabilitation services (Ohio, King County), consumer-run services (Ohio, King County, New York), and better integration and coordination of mental health services with substance abuse services (Pennsylvania, Ohio). Many public purchasers also have set expectations of managed care plans for the coordination of physical health benefits for their behavioral health beneficiaries, especially in those communities where a carve-out model of managed care was chosen.

Some purchasers have used the move to managed care as a way to manage other elements of their behavioral health care system. Massachusetts shifted responsibility for all acute care mental health services, including those not under the state's Medicaid program, into its managed care plan. This included responsibility for outpatient, emergency, and inpatient care to people with serious mental illness, which had been under the jurisdiction of the state's mental health agency. Montana and Tennessee also included payment for and management of state hospital utilization within their managed care procurements.

Public purchasers have used their managed care procurements to increase eligibility for services. Under San Diego County's managed care plan, the county increased by approximately 10,000 the number of beneficiaries eligible to receive limited outpatient mental health services (Croze & Coakley, 1999). King County used its mental health managed care procurement to enable a limited number of non-Medicaid-eligible mental health consumers to receive benefits under their prepaid mental health (Medicaid) plan. Other jurisdictions have used their managed care plans to target special populations within the behavioral health population. These could include heavy users of care (New York), or the general assistance/ indigent population (Connecticut).

Easing the Burden

Perhaps the most important, although not explicit, expectation of public purchasers who contract for managed behavioral health care is that in doing so they will ease the administrative and political burden they have in trying to manage publicly financed behavioral health systems. Since many of these systems are creatures of 40-plus years of public policy, they have become enmeshed in Byzantine systems of public finance, contracting, and civil service, coupled with multiple layers of legislative scrutiny and oversight. Contracting with an MCO gives these public purchasers some freedom from these systems by stepping down day-to-day responsibility for management, while exacting a high degree of reporting and internal control. In some instances, this allows the public purchaser to free up staff or management for other assignments or cease certain operations such as the payment of claims. In some cases, contracting with an MCO also may save the state/local agency the expense of having to upgrade or replace aging computer systems used to support the purchasing of public behavioral health care services.

More important than the management and administrative relief achieved through the use of managed care is the political relief that these public purchasers gain. As public systems, state and local mental health and substance abuse agencies often have to make difficult decisions regarding contracts and funding of community treatment organizations, including decisions to no longer contract with certain providers. By using a third-party intermediary, in this case a managed care firm, the public administrator may be relieved from having to deal with angry legislators who may want to know why a particular program in their district is not being funded. The onus of responsibility for these decisions now conveniently moves from the state agency administrator to the MCO. This is not to say that the state agency is not ultimately responsible for public funds given to a managed care firm to manage, but as the level of day-to-day management responsibility that the state agency has begins to lessen, so does the political burden.

Limitations

Public purchasers also have placed significant limitations on what managed care contractors may do within the scope of their public sector programs. In the public sector it is common for contracts to have limitations on administrative costs and profits. For example, Pennsylvania limits all administrative costs and profits within its managed care contracts to approximately 11%. Ohio established a ceiling of 15% in its managed care design. This is done to prevent organizations from taking too much of the available health resource out of the service delivery system. It also is a way for public purchasers to display due diligence in protecting the public interest from those organizations that may be interested in profit at the expense of the behavioral health program.

Public purchasers also may place restrictions on the provider network. In King County, all existing providers must be part of the new MCO's network for at least the first year. This provides a degree of continuity of care for patients, while also ensuring that the network providers are given a chance to compete. Other limitations that states and counties have placed on their managed care programs include such things as sign-off on the hiring of key staff positions, approval of office locations, or the types of corporate entities that are eligible to bid (profit versus not-for-profit) on the contract. Some contracts have even stipulated prior approval of press releases and other public pronouncements about the program.

While these types of limitations are designed to exercise various levels of control over the MCO by the public sector, public purchasers need to be careful that these and other types of limitations on the MCO do not adversely affect the ability of these organizations to do their work. Limitations on how the program is implemented may have consequences on the price that these MCOs bid to perform the work, or on how aggressively they are able to meet the other expectations of purchasers.

CASE STUDIES

The following case studies provide examples of the expectations of public purchasers who have used managed care in their public behavioral health care programs.

Case Study 1: Pennsylvania's HealthChoices Program

Building on its success with a physical health managed care demonstration in the west Philadelphia area, the Commonwealth of Pennsylvania Department of Public Welfare (DPW) made a decision in the early 1990s to seek the mandatory enrollment of Medicaid beneficiaries into managed care plans, mainly HMOs. These plans would have control over both behavioral and physical health care. County officials responded to this decision with disdain because they felt the management of public mental health funds was a county responsibility as outlined in Pennsylvania State Code. Pursuant to the Commonwealth's 1966 Mental Health/Mental Retardation (MH/MR) Act, 1976 Mental Health Procedures Act, and 1972 Drug and Alcohol Services Act, counties administer or provide for the delivery of a broad array of publicly funded drug and alcohol and mental health services for both medical assistance (MA) or non-MA populations. After considerable debate and legal challenge, DPW elected to carve behavioral health out of the HMO benefit and give counties the "right of first opportunity" to serve as the manager of care for behavioral health services under the Medicaid program.

DPW opted to implement the program on a staggered basis, starting first in the large population areas of the southeast, and slowly moving to the southwest, central, Lehigh, and remaining areas of the state on a yearly basis. This managed care program is referred to as the HealthChoices Behavioral Health Program (HealthChoices).

On May 24, 1996; DPW issued its first request for proposals (RFP) for a mandatory medical assistance behavioral health managed care program for Bucks, Chester, Delaware, Montgomery, and Philadelphia counties. On October 22, 1997, a subsequent request was issued for the southwest region of the state. Roll out of HealthChoices for the rest of the state is expected to occur over the next three years.

The goal of HealthChoices is to improve accessibility, continuity, and quality of services for Pennsylvania's MA populations, while also controlling the program's rate of cost increases (Commonwealth of Pennsylvania). The behavioral health managed care program is being implemented consistent with a vision of service systems of the future and a set of expectations about what managed behavioral health will accomplish. This includes the following: (1) to facilitate the efficient coordination and continuity in the provision of behavioral health services, (2) to coordinate the provision of behavioral health services with the physical health services component of the HealthChoices Program, and (3) to coordinate behavioral health services with the broader array of publicly funded human service programs (Commonwealth of Pennsylvania). Such broad-based coordination is essential to assuring appropriate access, services utilization, and continuity of care for persons with serious mental illness, children with serious emotional disturbances, substance-abusing adolescents, and persons with addictive diseases.

A county's acceptance of the Commonwealth's right of first opportunity for contracting is contingent on the county's agreement to enter into a full-risk capitation contract at an actuarially sound rate, as determined by the DPW, and demonstrated capacity to meet the program and fiscal requirements detailed in the Commonwealth's RFP. Under the first opportunity provision, counties, either individually or in groupings, are afforded the option to manage the behavioral health program directly or to subcontract with a private sector MCO. Such subcontracts do not relieve counties of ultimate responsibility for compliance with the RFP's program and fiscal requirements. Counties may, however, impose additional requirements and incentives on subcontractors as may be needed to effect appropriate management oversight and flexibility in addressing local needs.

Although counties are required to account for service utilization and all expenditures specific to the managed care program separately, the Commonwealth is encouraging counties to use this opportunity to effect integrated program and fiscal management of the managed care program and the other county-administered mental health and drug and alcohol services programs. However, counties or other contractors will be required to ensure that Medicaid funds are spent only for Medicaid-eligible recipients. Savings achieved from HealthChoices can be used to support mental health and drug and alcohol service enhancements and expansions for both Medicaid and non-Medicaid beneficiaries.

Case Study 2: King County's (Washington) Mental Health Program

Since 1995, King County has operated a prepaid health program for outpatient mental health services provided under the state's Medicaid program. The program, operated by United Behavioral Health (UBH) on a non-risk basis, provides a tier rate to providers based on the level of clinical acuity of patients seeking outpatient care. UBH's work involves the creation of the provider network, retrospective review of tier rate authorizations, and utilization management. Claims also are paid by UBH using King County's data system. Inpatient care is not under the county's managed care system, but utilization of inpatient care is monitored by UBH on behalf of the state.

In 1999, the King County Mental Health Division (KCMHD) set out to re-procure its managed health care system from a new MCO. This re-procurement was necessitated by the state's desire to move risk for inpatient care from the state to the county and integrate its management with outpatient care. The goals of this new integrated system are:

- To assume both the financial risk and management of inpatient services with enough administrative control so that transition will be clinically and financially successful
- To continue to improve the quality of care for populations served by KCMHD
- To assure culturally appropriate services
- To move to a performance-based system rather than a service-monitoring system
- To continue the process of system and policy simplification in order to achieve greater administrative efficiencies
- To coordinate and integrate mental health and chemical dependency services for those with dual treatment needs (King County, 1999)

To accomplish these goals, KCMHD issued an RFP in January 2000 for the purchase of managed care services on a shared-risk basis with a behavioral health organization. The RFP called for a "single contractor to manage an integrated system of inpatient, outpatient, crisis and residential services for children and adults who have emotional disturbances/mental illnesses and are dependent on the publicly funded mental health system for services" (King County, 2000).

The RFP presented both a detailed description of the types of services desired from the managed care vendor, as well as a conceptual model for clinical services hoped to be developed as a result of the procurement. The RFP calls for the vendor to be responsible for the provision (through contracts with providers) of crisis, inpatient, outpatient, and residential services. In addition to these services, the MCO will manage client grievances and complaints; establish a provider network; educate consumers, families, and providers; provide billing and reimbursement; and maintain a management information system to standards set by the county. The county's responsibilities are to maintain oversight of the system and to monitor the performance of the managed care vendor.

In its RFP, the county also established a series of desired system changes expected from the implementation of the managed care program. These changes include the movement toward a rehabilitation and recovery orientation for its mental health service delivery system and the eventual integration of mental health and substance abuse service. While the specifics on how these will occur are not necessarily spelled out in the RFP, the RFP does ask prospective bidders to describe how they would see these occurring should they be the successful bidder.

Another unique feature of the King County RFP is that the county is looking for the vendor to assume contractual and management responsibility for some of the services that are typically not found in managed care contracts. The RFP asks bidders to assume contractual authority on behalf of the county for a series of programs and special initiatives such as grants to advocacy groups, special demonstration programs, and residential contracts. The county previously contracted for these services directly. By moving them under the auspice of the managed care vendor, it hopes to reduce its administrative burden while also ensuring that these initiatives are well integrated into the rest of the mental health care system.

The King County managed care design includes a shared financial risk with the managed care vendor. The design calls for the establishment of a risk corridor in which the managed care vendor will be totally at risk for all service and administrative expenditures. Beyond this threshold, the managed care vendor and the county will share the risk or gain derived from the managed care program. The proposed model also includes a series of performance objectives that are established for the vendor. Incentive payments are tied to these objectives, allowing the vendor to reap additional remuneration should it achieve appropriate performance levels.

CONCLUSION

What are the expectations of public purchasers as they develop their managed care procurements and contracts? There is no standard answer. Each jurisdiction has shaped its managed care program differently to meet a broad array of needs and local circumstances. The common thread in all these managed care plans is the potential to use new technologies and principles that have been developed in the private managed behavioral health care sector and apply them to their public sector purchase of behavioral health care systems.

However, the public sector is different from the private health care sector. Because the purchase of services is being done with public funds, and because the beneficiaries of care are largely indigent or have a serious and persistent illness and must rely solely on the government for their care, the use of managed care principles and technologies may have to be tempered in the public sector. Recent fervor over managed care in general shows little public tolerance for dramatic changes in how health care is provided or at what rate and how providers are paid.

In the public sector, there is heightened concern that dramatic change in these areas could threaten an already overburdened and underfunded system of care. It is therefore incumbent on public managers in the behavioral health care field to be very realistic about their expectations for the use of managed care. They also must educate the public, especially consumers, families, and providers, as to what these expectations are and how they might change this already delicate system of public behavioral health care.

REFERENCES

Balanced Budget Act of 1997. (1997). Public Law 105–33.

Clark, R.E., Dowart, R.A., & Epstein, S.S. (1994). Managing competition in public and private mental health agencies: Implications for services and policy. *Milbank Quarterly, 72,* 653–678.

Commonwealth of Massachusetts, Executive Office of Human Services. (1995, September 22). *Request for proposals for mental health/substance abuse program.* Boston, MA: Author.

Commonwealth of Pennsylvania, Department of Public Welfare, Office of Mental Health and Substance Abuse Services. Behavioral HealthChoices Program. (www.dpw.state.pa.us/omhsas/omhchoices.asp)

Congressional Research Service. (1988). *1984 Medicaid expenditures.* Washington, DC: Library of Congress.

Croze, C., & Coakley, T. (1999, November). Case study: The County of San Diego's mental health services ASO contract administered by United Behavioral Health. *Behavioral Health Tomorrow.*

Frank, R.G., McGuire, T.G., Regier, D.A., Manderscheid, R., & Woodward, A. (1994). Paying for mental health and substance abuse care. *Health Affairs, 13,* 337–342.

Kaiser Foundation Commission on the Future of Medicaid. (1997, November). *Medicaid facts.* Washington, DC.

King County, Department of Community and Human Services, Mental Health Division Integrated System Management. (1999, May). *The proposed model for inpatient and outpatient mental health service integration in King County.* Seattle, WA: Author.

King County, Mental Health, Chemical Dependency Services Division. (2000, January). *Inpatient and outpatient mental health services integration request for proposals.* Seattle, WA: Author

Mohl, B. (1989, November 8). Five accounts threaten to swamp state budget. *Boston Globe.*

State of Ohio, Department of Mental Health. (1996, September). *Request for proposals for behavioral health care services to Medicaid recipients.* Columbus, OH: Author.

Substance Abuse and Mental Health Services Administration. (1999, August). *SAMHSA managed care tracking report.* Vol. II, No. 2. Rockville, MD: Author.

U.S. General Accounting Office. (1999, September). *Medicaid managed care: Four states' experiences with mental health carveout programs.* Washington, DC.

CHAPTER 8

Persons with Serious Mental Illness, The Public Sector, and Managed Care

E. Clarke Ross

Purpose: This chapter discusses four areas in which public-sector managed care has performed poorly and consequently failed to provide appropriate care for persons with serious mental illness.

Major Topics: This chapter discusses Seamless Systems of Care, Adequacy of Services, Public Accountability, and Consumer-Family-Enrollee Participation in the context of behavioral health care services for the severely mentally disabled.

INTRODUCTION

Advocates of managed care have promised to improve delivery of services to persons with serious mental illness by focusing on effectiveness and accountability. With the exception of a few beacons of success, experience shows that managed care has not delivered on its promises. Many of the flaws hindering adequate provision of services are not the cause of managed care organizations (MCOs) but are associated with historic problems in the nation's public mental health system. This chapter also focuses on the adequacy and methodology of establishing capitation rates within the public sector.

Source: Adapted with permission from E.C. Ross, Will Managed Care Ever Deliver its Promises? Managed Care, Public Policy, and Consumers of Mental Health Services, *Administrative Policy in Public Health*, September 2000, pp. 7–21, © 2000, Kluwer Academic/Plenum Publishers.

THE PUBLIC INTEREST

In the light (or shadow) of President Clinton's first-term health care reform initiative, the leading companies in managed behavioral health care formed an association called the American Managed Behavioral Healthcare Association (AMBHA). One objective of AMBHA at that time was to initiate a dialogue with many of the long-standing interest groups associated with mental health care in order to better define the public interest in an era where more than one half of the American population was covered for mental health care by privately owned or publicly traded managed behavioral health care firms.

In 1997, AMBHA representatives and public mental health officials (National Association of State Mental Health Program Directors, National Association of County Behavioral Health Directors, and National Council for Community Behavioral Health) formally articulated five components of the public interest in managed behavioral health care in the public sector that arose out of these dialogue meetings (Dixon & Croze, 1997). These five components were citizen participation, public accountability, equity, efficiency, and results. This document was produced during a time when state- and county-managed care initiatives involving contracts with private managed care companies were a highly controversial enterprise, fraught with litigation and grass-roots agitation from consumer advocates and others suspicious of the "profit motive" in public programs designed to serve those in poverty with chronic and persistent mental illness.

This 1997 publication built on an earlier work (Harbin, Hogan, Mayberg, Shusterman, & Croze, 1995) by the leading managed behavioral health care organizations and the state mental health directors (American Managed Behavioral Healthcare Association and the National Association of State Mental Health Program Directors). The 1995 publication identified four issues of particular concern to public system advocates: services to adults with serious mental illness and children with serious emotional disturbance, state and local government responsibility for indigent care, the critical interrelationship of public funding streams in their support of a seamless system of care, and development and application of appropriate performance standards for managed behavioral health care. In short, significant open discussion, argument, and attempts at policy formulation have taken place over the past several years with respect to managed behavioral health care in the public-sector delivery system.

Attempts to define managed care have been an important part of this process. AMBHA established five "core" attributes of managed behavioral health care: (1) services are provided through integrated and coordinated delivery systems; (2) health plans, their management agents, and their contracted or employed providers document their accountability for positive clinical outcomes and consumer satisfaction; (3) managed behavioral health care should produce an expansion of services and also a substitution of services (e.g., outpatient for inpatient care); (4) managed care plans are obligated by payers to constrain costs; and (5) decisions on the appropriateness, setting, and medical necessity of services are driven by explicit and well-defined standards (AMBHA, 1997; Ross, 1997; Ross, 1998–1999).

This chapter focuses on the application of managed behavioral health care to public sector mental health programs. In this regard, the attributes and statements of public interest by both managed behavioral health care firms and public mental health officials are consolidated; evidence that suggests that, other than constraining costs, most managed behavioral health care programs have not lived up to their promises is cited. While there are beacons of success that offer hope for the future, even within these beacons of success major flaws in the public mental health system continue.

In poorly performing public managed care systems, often the managed care vendor lacks a social commitment because of primary obligations to private shareholders or the bottom line. The absence of a fundamental social commitment contributes to the flaws and problems faced by consumers, families, and enrollees. In beacons of success, it is often not the managed care vendor that limits the full potential to serve consumers adequately, but the underlying system itself that is flawed and limiting in its effect on what the managed care company can do. This, hopefully, will become clearer, when the evidence is cited. Lessons learned from both the disasters and beacons of success provide clues for realizing hope in the future.

So, in consolidating these previously announced principles, this chapter analyzes and comments on the following four elements of the public interest:

1. Seamless systems of care that include integrated and coordinated delivery

2. Adequate services to persons with severe mental illnesses
3. Public accountability, which includes publicly documented performance measurement, positive clinical outcomes, and publicly documented consumer satisfaction
4. Meaningful and authentic consumer, family, and enrollee participation in all aspects of services planning, implementation, and evaluation

SEAMLESS SYSTEMS OF CARE THAT INCLUDE INTEGRATED AND COORDINATED DELIVERY: LINKAGE BETWEEN MEDICAID AND PUBLIC MENTAL HEALTH HAS FAILED

Managed care for persons with mental illness in the governmental sector has been initiated through the Medicaid program. Medicaid is the single most significant payer of public mental health services. And yet, there has been little linkage between the state Medicaid and state mental health agencies. Absent such linkage, failure in providing appropriate treatment and support services will and does occur. This is a fundamental systemic and structural flaw that is pervasive throughout the United States.

This is true in the state-managed mental health programs considered by the national experts to be the most positive. Some experts (Sturm, 1999) consider Massachusetts one of the more positive experiences, but here linkage fails. The Medicaid managed mental health program is responsible for "acute" care while the Department of Mental Health is responsible for "continuing" care. But where is the linkage between the two? There are no clear linkages. For example, consumers and families wait for services and providers refuse to serve until complex billing procedures between the two agencies are clear. Colorado Health Networks is considered by some observers (Sturm, 1999) to be a positive program. But the Medicaid managed mental health program is not responsible for persons requiring state psychiatric hospital care. As a consequence, numerous Medicaid-enrolled persons are transported to state hospitals (suggesting that financial incentives are, perhaps, as alive and well in the public sector as they are in the private). Because Fort Logan, near Denver, is a smaller hospital with typically 100% occupancy, many persons in north and central Colorado are transported, at a cost of $450 a ride in an ambulance or in shackles by police, to the southern hospital in Pueblo. Even when state hospitals are included in the managed care program, such as in Tennessee, other linkage problems continue.

Any public managed care program for persons with severe mental illness must have precise boundaries established between the Medicaid managed care entity and the state mental health agency—or no boundaries at all (i.e., consolidation). Minimally, all consumers, families, and providers must know which agency is responsible for which services under which conditions. If boundaries and responsibilities are not clear, or agencies remain fragmented structurally or functionally, persons will wait for treatment, and this could be extremely dangerous. Those waiting are, by definition, the more severely ill population.

Frank and Morlock (1997) observed, "When multiple parties exert partial authority, act according to different rules, and respond to incentives from a variety of financing sources, the result is unlikely to be coordination among complementary community institutions" (p. 3). They conclude that "simple strategies that just manipulate either the organizational or the financial arrangements do not enhance systemic coordination" (p. 29). Frank and Morlock propose "mixed strategies" of "blending centralized organizational structure" and "aggressive management in the form of monitoring, feedback, and education at the provider agency level" (p. 29). Irrespective of the particular expertise of a managed care vendor, and even in the face of an overwhelming social commitment from these private organizations, service will continue to be abysmal if public fiscal and administrative agencies are unable to collaborate on a plan of action.

The U.S. Department of Health and Human Services Office of Inspector General (DHHS OIG, 2000b) observed that in seven Medicaid managed mental health programs "responsibility for care is fragmented with possible cost shifting" (p. 2). The DHHS OIG recommended the development of interagency agreements to promote coordination.

ADEQUATE SERVICES TO PERSONS WITH SEVERE MENTAL ILLNESSES: "APPROPRIATE PAYMENT IS A CRITICAL SAFEGUARD"

"Appropriate payment is a critical safeguard" is a recommendation and conclusion from the July 1999 draft Health Care Financing Administration (HCFA)–National Academy of State Health Policy (NASHP) report on special needs populations enrolled in Medicaid managed care. Managed care capitation payment rates are often arbitrary and are set in such a way that total funding is lower than previous private insurance or Medicaid fee-for-service base. Managed care uses capitation to pay health plans. According to Dubin (1995), capitation is: "The paid assumption of risk by a provider for delivery of a defined set of services to a designated population over a specified time period, with the payment calculated on a per-person basis" (p. 29). The typical purchaser request for proposal (RFP) specifies three items: global budget range, defined population and benefit, and list of performance expectations.

During the 1990s behavioral health costs in a "typical" private insurance "indemnity plan" were reduced from 12% to 25% of total medical costs to 4% to 7% in a "highly managed PPO [preferred provider organization] plan" (Mercer, 1997). During the 1990s, fee-for-service private rates, when translated into per member per month (PMPM) units of $16.00, were reduced to a range of $1.00 to $10.00 PMPM health plan payment rate (American Psychiatric Association, 1997).

Melek (1998) provides an example of payments and costs in an integrated managed behavioral health organization (MBHO) benefits management and employee assistance program (EAP) private employer program. EAP was capitated at $2.25 PMPM, while actual costs were $2.34, and MBHO benefits were capitated at $4.00 PMPM, while actual costs were $3.60 PMPM. Word of mouth is that these private employee capitation rates are much lower in 2000 than these 1998 published rates.

Most public mental health systems in the nation have historically been underfunded. So cap rates determined on discounts from past funding are usually inadequate to fund quality care. National Institute of Mental Health (NIMH) researcher Dr. Roland Sturm (1999) recently observed: "Financial viability of managed behavioral health ventures in the public system has been difficult to achieve" (p. 18).

Montana, perhaps the worst public managed mental health program in the nation (subsequently terminated by the state legislature following 23 months of implementation), is an example. The five-year managed care contract of $380 million was $6 million less in the first year than the previous year fee-for-service (FFS) spending. In addition, Montana added a pharmacy benefit for non-Medicaid uninsured persons to the capitation contract, and the MCO then absorbed $4 million in outlays, $2.8 million over the previous year's FFS pharmacy outlays. The MCO, by contract, was obligated to continue current funding to the state hospital in Warm

Springs thereby limiting community-based services (Faulkner & Gray, 1999; Kanapaux, 1998a, 1998b, 1999a–f; Rudd, 1998).

Montana added uninsured persons to the Medicaid managed care program. This group had never been served before, so another $11 million in expenditures were incurred by the MCO. So, the MCO received $6 million less than the previous year's spending and incurred $13.8 million in extra and unbudgeted (and thus deficit) expenses in 23 months. Provider payments were substantially squeezed and consumers were denied services. The MCO was not entirely blameless. From the outset, the original vendor (subsequently sold to another company) had difficulties paying claims in the first place, a capability the state inadequately evaluated during the bidding and a problem that alienated providers and fostered hostility to the program. In one instance, the claims payment issue bankrupted a community mental health center highly regarded by local consumers and their families.

Kapur and associates (1999) concluded, "Previous research has not yielded a fail-safe formula for implementing a publicly funded capitation program" (p. 1). Inadequate resources will lead to program failures. They describe the 1993 Los Angeles County Department of Mental Health capitated care program for persons with the most serious mental illness. Six not-for-profit community providers were given between $14,000 and $21,000 per client per year to serve persons whose previous year expenditures averaged $30,000 and were in the top 15% of mental health services expenditure utilizers. Providers could disenroll clients and return them to the FFS system. The result was that 1,188 of 1,563 assigned clients were disenrolled. Those disenrolled had average previous year expenditures of $24,500 while those retained in capitation had previous year average expenditures of $17,510.

Kapur, Young, and Murata (2000) concluded that for persons with severe mental illness, "risk adjustment methods, as developed to date, do not have the requisite predictive power to be used as the sole measure in setting capitation rates" (p. ii). They further concluded that payments to providers for persons with severe mental illness should not be fully capitated but rather involve risk sharing between payers and providers. They also found that risk adjustment models that contain good historic data on rehospitalization rates have a "higher predictive power." They went on to explain that "a consistent finding in the research so far is that past diagnostic information has little predictive power" (p. 3).

Kapur, Young, and Murata's (2000) conclusion about prior rehospitalization experience supplements research by Sullivan and associates (1995, 1997) that a large share of the treatment costs of persons with severe mental illness frequently rehospitalized is associated with comorbid alcohol abuse, medication noncompliance, and dangerous or aberrant behaviors.

For purposes of estimating capitation rates, Kapur and colleagues (2000) found that 83% of 1,956 high-cost, severely mentally ill persons served in Los Angeles County between 1991 and 1994 averaged $25,294 in treatment costs. Of these persons, 78% had a diagnosis of schizophrenia, implying that at least this diagnosis may have higher predictive ability. Basic demographics—sex, age, race/ethnic, marital status, and primary language—had no predictive power.

Proper targeting—matching targeted clients and targeted services—can be effective. Magellan's Iowa managed mental health care program targeted an extra and special payment of $900 PMPM for programs of assertive community treatment (PACT) for the most severely ill population. This targeting has resulted in marked improvement in consumer functioning and average annual treatment costs dropping from $18,000 to $11,000 (Zwillich, 1999).

Determining adequate payment levels for public mental health services is difficult, particularly when comparing state to state (Table 8–1). But some state-specific information has to be used to make an initial judgment of adequacy. Massachusetts capitation rates are $100 PMPM for persons with mental illness on Supplemental Security Income (SSI) and $70 PMPM for non-SSI-eligible persons with mental illness enrolled in Medicaid and also served by the state mental health department. Compare this with Arizona's Maricopa County rate of $44.49 PMPM for persons with serious mental illness. Are the costs of living between Arizona and Massachusetts really that much different? What accounts for these dramatic differences? In a federal class action lawsuit against Arizona, the parties, including the state, agreed that at least $316 million was required by Maricopa County to finance its public mental health system adequately (Snyder, 1999). Currently, $112 million is spent.

In Massachusetts, 100% of the capitation goes to direct clinical care. Pharmacy is not part of the capitation. A separately funded administration budget is independently negotiated. Massachusetts uses for-profit vendors. So, where is the profit? Profit is exclusively tied to the achievement of performance goals. In year 1, the vendor receives a bonus for achieving performance targets. In year 2, the previous bonus target becomes a

Table 8–1 Examples of State Medicaid Mental Health Capitation Rates for Non-Elderly Adults with Mental Illness Receiving Supplemental Security Income

State	Rate (PMPM)	Reference Year
Arizona–Maricopa County (Davis, 2000; Open Minds, June 1999; Rudd, 2000c)	$44.49*†‡§	2000
Iowa (Faulkner & Gray, 1999; Open Minds, June 1999; GAO, 1999)	$70.85–$103.98*†‡	1999
Massachusetts (GAO, 1999; Open Minds, June 1999; Sheola & Lane, 1999)	$100.00‡	1999
Tennessee	$22.93*†‡ (blended for all mental health)	1996–1997
Tennessee (Kanapaux, 1999g, 1999i; Open Minds, June 1999; Wooldridge & Mitchell, 2000; Yennie, 1998; Yennie & Birch, 1999)	$319.41*†‡	1997–1998
Texas–Dallas North Star (Bagwell, 2000; Kanapaux, 2000; Rudd, 2000a, 2000b, 2000c)	$45.61*†‡§	1999

PMPM, per member per month.
*Includes administrative costs.
†Includes profit.
‡Includes direct clinical treatment costs.
§Includes pharmacy.

contractual obligation with financial penalties. New performance targets are introduced each year, so the program continuously improves. Massachusetts also uses risk corridors to limit profit and loss. Massachusetts' capitation financing is unique in the nation.

Capitation rates can be designed as incentives or disincentives in serving the most disabled of the population with mental illness. Tennessee is an example. In 1996 and 1997 the state used a blended behavioral capitation rate of $22.93 PMPM. The result was that persons with serious mental illness were largely unserved. In 1997 the capitation rate was adjusted. Persons served with serious mental illness received a PMPM rate of $319.41. By the end of 1999, the proportion of the population with severe and persistent mental illness and serious mental illness actually served was identical to Center for Mental Health Services (CMHS) estimated prevalence (2.6% and 5.4% of the enrolled population). But in an inadequately financed system operating under a global budget, the amount left over for persons without serious mental illness was $8.83 to $10.35 PMPM. Community mental health providers entered the year 2000 demanding an end to the "two-tiered" capitation system so that they could serve more persons with less serious mental illness. The problem is that if the desired change is enacted, then persons with serious illness would again be underserved.

The Dallas, Texas "North Star" managed behavioral health care program has come under recent criticisms for underserving the population. The capitation rates used in North Star are $3.06 PMPM for SSI aged recipient, $10.24 PMPM for SSI child, $45.61 PMPM for SSI adult, $23.99 PMPM for Temporary Assistance to Needy Family (TANF) adult, and $9.25 PMPM for a TANF child.

After a bumpy first two years, national experts generally view the Iowa managed behavioral health care program as a positive one. The SSI child PMPM cap rate varies geographically from $78.84 to $117.72, while the SSI adult PMPM cap rate varies geographically from $70.85 to $103.98.

A study of expenditures in three states (Larson et al., 1998) demonstrates that serving persons with mental illness is more expensive than serving the rest of the Medicaid population. In Michigan, the average Medicaid expenditure was $1,726 for persons with mental illness and $583 for other Medicaid persons. In New Jersey, the differential was $3,143 for Medicaid-eligible persons with mental illness compared with $1,301 for others. In Washington, the differential was $1,119 and $570, respectively. Are the capitation rates paid to serve persons with mental illness reflective of such differential expenditure histories? The 1997 managed care report of the National Alliance for the Mentally Ill (NAMI) found that managed care programs failed to provide persons with serious mental illness with adequate hospital length of stay, programs of assertive community treatment, access to the newest classifications of medications, psychiatric rehabilitation, and supported housing (Hall, Edgar, & Flynn, 1997). To what degree is funding a root cause of this failure?

Adequate payment is a complex and difficult subject. There are at least eight strategies that can be advanced to address this issue:

1. Develop a clear definition of eligible member, an idea of what constitutes a sufficient volume of covered members, an understanding whether the amount of services promised are manageable, a definable scope of services, a view of potential cost shifting across provider groups, a plan to control consumption, a commitment to fair negotiations, a system of reasonable links between capitated population and providers, and an actuarially sound basis for adjusting capitation rates (American Psychiatric Association, 1997).

2. Do not add a pharmacy benefit to the basic capitation rate. Where this has been tried (e.g., Montana and initially Tennessee), this has been a financial nightmare. Pharmacy is the fastest-growing health care component expense, yet often proper medication can offset more expensive hospitalization. Keep it out of the cap rate since the principles of underwriting the financial risk of psycho-pharmaceuticals is so poorly understood. The DHHS OIG (2000a) studied seven Medicaid managed mental health programs. None included pharmacy "primarily because states were unsure of how to accurately determine the cost for this benefit. . . . States believed that if they did not set the capitation rate for prescription drugs at a correct level, managed care organizations would have an incentive to restrict access" (p. 8). This led the DHHS OIG to recommend that drug formularies be excluded from managed care.

3. Make sure that there is an unduplicated count of persons served by the public mental health system, so that actual per person utilization can be documented. Unfortunately, only 27 state mental health systems in the nation can currently do this (SAMHSA, 2000). Without a real utilization history base, cap rates will be gambles. In such gambles, persons with severe illnesses often lose.

4. Do not add the uninsured into capitated managed care until a historic utilization pattern is known, as tempting as the goal of universal coverage is. That means financing the uninsured through FFS or special risk arrangements until actual experiences are known. Where this has been tried (e.g., Montana and Tennessee), financial nightmares have occurred.

5. Do not cut the budget at the beginning if anticipating savings, such as Montana did. Implement managed care; if there are savings, make a judgment after the savings have accrued about whether to invest in additional services or return the savings to the state treasury. Reinvestment is always a possibility, such as what Colorado and Iowa

require. Iowa required, for three consecutive years, profits of $1 million each year be invested in mobile counseling and therapeutic socialization programs. Colorado required that $1.3 million in year 1 profits and $1.9 million in year 2 profits be invested in telemedicine, 24-hour intensive care, and respite care (U.S. General Accounting Office, 1999).

6. Compare your state's capitation rate with those of other states. Yes, local costs and composition of professional services differ, but not to the degree reflected in current state capitation funding levels for these types of programs. As a state official, you need comparisons.

7. Do not gamble and guess capitation rates as Montana and many other states did when historic utilization was not known. Use a risk corridor. Risk corridors set limits on the amount of profits and losses that are realized by MCOs. Risk corridors apply whether or not the MCO is a for-profit or a nonprofit. Eight states (California, Hawaii, Massachusetts, Nevada, Ohio, Oklahoma, Utah, and Wisconsin) currently use risk corridors (HCFA-NASHP, 1999); one (Massachusetts) uses risk corridors in its mental health program.

8. Do not be inflexible. The results of a federally funded study of managed mental health care in Tennessee (Hoag, Wooldridge, & Thornton, 2000) concluded that states avoid overestimating cost savings and underestimating the difficulty of setting capitation rates when implementing managed care. The authors argued that capitation rates cannot be inflexibly set for a fixed contract period but must be updated periodically: "The true test of rate setting comes only after programs have been implemented and after plans provide program benefits for the specified capitation rates. . . . Thus, the initial rate setting must be followed by an active process of monitoring and adjustment that relies on the delicate process of judgment calls, based on available information and indices such as care quality, service availability and MCO profits" (p. 131).

When Tennessee's original use of an average aggregate cost approach (dividing estimated total costs by estimated annual enrollment) to determine PMPM capitation failed in serving persons with serious mental illness, the state did adjust its rate setting. However, rather than adjust rates based on precise actuarial analyses, the state responded to political, media, provider, and MBHO complaints within a fixed or global budget. Tennessee encountered a variety of problems including difficulty in estimating medical costs because of an overreliance on FFS Medicaid claims data rather than total public mental health system experience, failure to attend to the cost impact of additional services mandated under the managed care contract, and a failure to anticipate the need to reassess the capitation rate.

Even following these strategies, capitation rates remain problematic. Studies by the New York and Ohio Departments of Mental Health (National Association, 1993, 1994, 2000; Roth, Snapp, Lauber, & Clark, 1998) documented significant client movement in and out of Medicaid and out of community mental health programs. This movement makes use of risk-adjusted capitation plans based primarily on past service utilization questionable. On the other hand, the New York data showed that even though a third of the 212,000 Medicaid-eligible persons with severe mental illness annually leave the program rolls, both the aggregate number of eligible persons and utilization of similar patterns of care remained generally constant, affirming capitation rates based on prior utilization. As Roth and associates (1998) concluded, "clearly there is a critical need for more systematic, longitudinal information about people with severe mental disabilities and their service utilization" (p. 243).

Inflexible reliance on prior utilization also brings problems. As New York unveils its special needs plans (SNPs) for adults with serious mental illness, counties with better reform track records are being financially penalized. New York City, which has a recent history of moving persons out of hospitals and into community treatment, will receive a per member per year capitation of $8,479. But Westchester County, which has historically relied much more on inpatient care, will receive a per member per year capitation of $12,087 (Kanapaux, 1999h).

Many families and consumers are concerned that profit motive undermines the delivery of adequate services. One response has been ideological—ban all profit in human service delivery. A more realistic and workable strategy is to replicate the Massachusetts Medicaid managed behavioral health care experience. In Massachusetts, 100% of the capitation goes to direct clinical care. Pharmacy is not part of the capitation. A separately funded administration budget is separately negotiated. Massachusetts uses for-profit vendors. So, where is the profit? Profit is exclusively tied to the achievement of performance goals. In year 1, the vendor receives a bonus for achieving performance targets. In year 2, the previous bonus target becomes a contractual obligation with financial penalties. New performance targets are introduced each year, so the program continuously improves. Because Massachusetts uses risk corridors, profit and loss are limited.

Most managed care contracts—public and profit—hide both the administrative and profit amounts. MCOs claim just a little, and a reasonable amount goes to administration and profit. Critics claim most dollars go to administration and profit. The public does not know. With MCOs reluctant to reveal these data publicly—and even more reluctant to be independently audited within the context of a public forum—the Massachusetts contract offers a model. At least in Massachusetts everyone knows how much precisely goes to clinical care, administration, and profit. In fiscal year 1998, the managed care vendor—Massachusetts Behavioral Health Partnership—was awarded $4.819 million in performance bonuses, out of a possible $6.7 million in budgeted allowable bonuses (Robinson, 1999).

John Ruskin, a 19th century businessman, observed: "It is unwise to pay too much, but it is worse to pay too little. When you pay too much, you lose money. That is all. But when you pay too little, you sometimes lose everything because the thing you bought was incapable of doing the thing it was bought to do" (Dewan, Daniels, & Greenberg, 1999, p. 112).

ACCOUNTABILITY IS RARELY PUBLIC

Managed care advocates claim that their approach is an improvement over the previous FFS system because they make judgments based on positive clinical outcomes, documented performance measurement, and documented consumer satisfaction. Some MCOs do, but rarely are these publicly available.

A handful of states and their MCO vendors develop, use, and make publicly available documented performance measurement. Colorado Health Networks has done an outstanding job at documenting its performance in developing self-help groups, in developing drop-in centers, and in publicly documenting average time for first appointments, penetration rates, hospital readmission rates, average hospital length of stay, waiting list elimination, mental health and physical health follow-up services within 30 days from inpatient discharge for both adults and children (note that the National Committee for Quality Assurance [NCQA] Health Plan Employer Data and Information Set [HEDIS] standards now use seven days), and involvement of family and guardians in discharge planning. Iowa state officials have published in numerous journals and newsletters about all the performance data they require of their MCO vendor; yet the public's access to actual data has been difficult. Massachusetts has structured its entire profit scheme to the attainment of performance data. Michigan has said that it will be collecting a wide array of data but no data are currently available to the public. These are the more positive states, the "beacons of success."

While 36 states can track clients between state psychiatric hospitals and community services using client identifiers (National Association, 2000), only 27 state mental health agencies in the nation are able to provide an unduplicated count of persons served and the services that they utilize (SAMSHA, 2000). How can meaningful performance information be collected if a state cannot even provide an unduplicated count of persons served?

Consumers want plan-by-plan comparisons using performance data. But where does this exist in the nation? The NCQA developed HEDIS, but the data set is grossly inadequate in terms of meaningful measures for serving the most seriously mentally ill population. It derives, as its name suggests, from the needs of employers and employed persons—not the indigent or those whose disabilities preclude employment. Yet, HEDIS has value to consumers because it is a nationwide standard performance system, data are posted on the NCQA Web site (www.ncqa.org), and the data contain two measures of importance—antidepressant medication management experiences and follow-up of care after hospitalization within seven days. But HEDIS is a voluntary process, and few MCOs and MBHOs in the nation make public their HEDIS reporting. Maryland, New Jersey, and Utah publish consumer guides using plan-by-plan comparisons that rely on HEDIS data. Several states, such as New York, require MCOs to provide the state with HEDIS data but then refuse to release such data to the public.

To date, it largely requires special finance and long-term analysis to document cross health plan comparisons. The U.S. General Accounting Office (GAO, 1999) recently documented the range of penetration rates (the proportion of an enrolled population actually receiving mental health services) between four state-managed mental health programs: Massachusetts, 25.1%; Iowa, 12.8%; Colorado, 11.9%; and Washington, 7.0%.

Four states (Colorado, Iowa, Massachusetts, and Washington) studied by GAO required their managed care vendors to collect encounter data but none of the four systematically used the data. GAO (1999) concluded that data from MBHOs "were untimely, incomplete, or inaccurate" (p. 26). Sturm (1999) concluded: "While all companies claim to measure outcome, none are systematically examining key outcomes for people with serious mental health problems" (p. 17).

NAMI's managed care report card for 1997 failed the leading MBHOs for not maintaining scientifically up-to-date and comprehensive treatment guidelines and for failing to use measurable patient outcomes used to determine coverage policy (Hall, Edgar, & Flynn, 1997). Most MCOs publish consumer satisfaction surveys that consistently show that roughly 80+% of enrollees are satisfied. The surveys are usually done by internal MCO marketing departments and occasionally by contracted public opinion firms or universities. These studies often do not reveal levels and areas of dissatisfaction. Even this generalized satisfaction is changing. In a June 1999 survey by Hewitt Associates (Bureau of National Affairs, 1999), 22% of consumers in managed care plans reported they were dissatisfied, an increase from 17% in 1997.

The use of independent, third-party consumer- and family-staffed organizations is basic to NAMI's evolving agenda to ensure accountability by all participants in the health care arena—payers, purchasers, health plans, management agents, delivery systems, and providers. Several public mental health systems have launched and are using consumer- and family-staffed independent consumer interview teams that focus on consumer dissatisfaction and mechanisms for resolving such dissatisfaction. Alabama, Georgia, Massachusetts, Ohio, and Pennsylvania operate such consumer satisfaction teams (CSTs). None are ideal in their independence. All have had to accommodate themselves to purchaser and political realities. Some involve providers. One uses focus groups rather than actual individual consumer interviews. One is financed by the MCO, calling into question its true independence. Yet all offer more independence and a greater consumer/family focus than normal MCO operations.

Few public purchasers have contracted with external evaluators at the beginning of a managed care contract and retained a commitment to continually using such external evaluators to assist them in judging vendor performance. Massachusetts (Beinecke & Lockhart, 1998) started such an external evaluation but did not maintain it. Florida (Shern & Robinson, 1999) has such an evaluation agreement in its Tampa Bay and Jacksonville demonstration projects.

The Florida evaluation (Shern & Robinson, 1999) has been a very public process and has provided much useful information. In comparing HMOs that either contracted with MBHOs or internally managed benefits with MBHOs, the University of South Florida documented that MBHOs far outperformed HMOs in the performance areas of penetration rates, proportion of adults with serious mental illness who reported receiving mental health services, persons with schizophrenia who received atypical antipsychotic medications, and individuals who were discharged from inpatient settings and seen within 30 days. HMOs and MBHOs performed about equally in terms of persons with major depression who received selective serotonin reuptake inhibitors (SSRIs). MBHOs performed somewhat better than HMOs in providing day treatment and targeted case management.

The use of independent, third-party entities to promote accountability continues to grow. In 2000, NCQA began to require independent validation of all HEDIS data provided by health plans. Twenty-nine states now mandate independent external clinical appeals (National Conference of State Legislatures, 1999). A centerpiece of all major legislative proposals before the U.S. Congress is mandatory, independent, third-party clinical review. Four states—Delaware, New Hampshire, Oklahoma, and Pennsylvania—currently use independent, third-party consumer and family monitoring teams in their state psychiatric hospitals. Two state Medicaid managed mental health care programs—Colorado and Washington—use independent ombudsman programs (GAO, 1999).

Clearly, much more needs to be done in the area of public accountability, but the trend is toward more accountability. Johnston and Romzek (1999) concluded: "There is a tendency in privatization efforts, and especially in contracting relationships, to assume that contract management and accountability will take care of themselves or that they can be relatively easily achieved through contract monitoring. The reality is that contract management and accountability do not take care of themselves" (p. 394).

MEANINGFUL AND AUTHENTIC CONSUMER, FAMILY, AND ENROLLEE PARTICIPATION IS RARE

Many public purchasers and their management agents fail to meaningfully involve consumers, families, and enrollees in their operations. Consumers lack necessary information. In an October 1998 NAMI survey of its members' experiences with managed care, 55% of respondents did not know how to file an appeal with their MCO. Respondents to the survey were those members who took the initiative to send in a survey response, so one would think they are the more involved and knowledgeable of citizens (Hall, 1998). This demonstrates that all parties involved in health care must make a greater effort to educate citizens about their rights as health plan enrollees. CSTs, as previously discussed, are vehicles for education as are consumer and family organizations, such as NAMI, and ombudsman programs.

NAMI's 1997 managed care report card (Hall, Edgar, & Flynn, 1997) failed the leading MBHOs regarding consumers and their family members being effectively engaged in their care. Not only can consumer and family organizations, ombudsmen, and purchasers help, but also health plans themselves can actively involve consumers and families. In a representative democracy, citizens expect representation, which includes the important principle of meaningful and substantial involvement in the design, delivery, and monitoring of the system. Authentic public participation includes not only this representation, but also the citizens' confidence that their input has an impact. Impact determines whether the involvement was authentic. Sitting through quarterly advisory meetings and listening to whatever the health plan wants to say is not authentic involvement. Health plans are at a disadvantage because they have not experienced what authentic involvement really is. Since 1986 and the Public Law 99-660 federal Mental Health Block Grant requirement, every state has had to operate a citizens' mental health planning and advisory council. Some of these have been shams, but many have been forums for meaningful and authentic involvement. Health plans will have to learn from their state council counterparts.

Pires, Armstrong, and Stroul (1999) studied how MCOs and MBHOs involve families in their operations. By and large, MBHOs significantly involve families more than MCOs. Regarding initial planning and implementation activities, families were significantly involved in 36% of MBHOs compared with 13% of MCOs; 14% of MBHOs and 47% of MCOs did not involve families at all. Involvement in current refinements were even more striking: 47% of MBHOs significantly involved families while only the same 13% of MCOs involved families. Regarding organizations that had no family involvement, MBHOs were 0% while MCOs were 7%. While 77% of MBHOs provided a training and orientation program to families, only 23% of MCOs provided such training.

Some states have attempted more meaningful family and consumer participation. Some examples follow:

- Oregon's Medicaid staff held weekly meetings with health plan representatives, beneficiary representatives, and state social services agencies for more than a year before bringing beneficiaries with disabilities into managed care. These meetings covered topics such as building a common understanding of case management and case workers. Following implementation, Medicaid staff met regularly with MCO management, medical directors, and advocacy and social service agency representatives to discuss payment rates, data reporting, and other matters relating to health care (HCFA-NASHP, 1999).

- In Colorado, the Medicaid Managed Care Contracting Disability Working Group, composed of individuals who are disabled and their family members, MCO administrators, and state personnel, formulated recommendations to assess risk-adjusted rates and choice of home health agency (HCFA-NASHP, 1999).
- In Vermont, a Quality Improvement Advisory Committee, composed of consumers, advocates, MCO representatives, providers, and state staff, was established to assist the state with ongoing and comprehensive improvements of its managed care program (HCFA-NASHP, 1999).
- In California, a 13-member committee is composed of community advocates (one seat is reserved for a representative of persons with disabilities), MediCal beneficiaries, and representatives of the county social services agency and health care agency (HCFA-NASHP, 1999).
- The Massachusetts Medicaid managed mental health program has both a consumer advisory council and family advisory council that meet monthly with both state officials and the managed care vendor (Sabin & Daniels, 1999): "When asked about the councils' most important accomplishment, council members cited their work to influence the annual performance standards for the carve-out company" (p. 884).

Sabin and Daniels (1999), advocates of meaningful and important consumer and family involvement, conclude: "Consumers, families, and the public cannot be expected to trust health care systems that do not hold themselves accountable for demonstrating that their limit-setting policies are reasonable and fair" (p. 883). The DHHS OIG (2000a) recommended that Medicaid-managed mental health programs involve beneficiaries and families in both the conversion process from fee-for-service plans and in treatment planning.

CONCLUSION

Before the advent of managed care, the public mental health system was beset with fundamental problems, including inadequate resources, lack of accountability, and limited documentation of the health outcomes achieved. Managed care promised greater effectiveness and accountability. Some managed care organizations were able to deliver, others could not overcome fundamental flaws in the organization and financing of public mental health services, especially in the case of persons with serious mental illness.

This chapter looks at four areas of managed care to determine how well it has performed in providing adequate services for the severely mentally disabled. First, whereas managed care supposedly is integrated care, the linkage between state Medicaid and state mental health agencies has been tenuous. As a result, appropriate treatment and support services for the severely mentally disabled sometimes fail to be provided.

Second, appropriate payment for services provided to special needs populations is a critical safeguard to ensure that the services are indeed adequate. However, public mental health systems have traditionally been underfunded, so capitation rates based on past funding levels are often too low to support the provision of high-quality care. Some researchers have concluded that coverage payments for persons with severe mental illness should not be fully capitated and that the payers and providers should share the risk of underpricing. In any case, some methods of setting capitation rates are more accurate than others, and proper targeting (matching clients and services) can help reduce the gap between payment levels and service needs.

Making managed care organizations and providers publicly accountable for the services they deliver is thought to be a good way of getting them to improve their services, and in fact consumers want performance data to use in their decision making. Nonetheless, only a few states make performance data publicly available, and in addition few managed care organizations are measuring outcomes or using the outcomes data to help determine the coverage they offer or improve the services they provide to the severely mentally disabled.

Finally, managed care organizations are failing to involve enrollees and their families in their operations and in decisions regarding treatment options. However, it is true that managed behavioral health care organizations do a better job of involving families than other types of managed care organizations. In addition, some states have set up special committees or councils to increase the amount of enrollee and family participation that does occur. It is a fact that the more enrollees and families are able to participate in the operations of a managed care organization, the more likely they are to trust the organization to provide high-quality care.

REFERENCES

American Managed Behavioral Healthcare Association. (1997, July 7). *Managed behavioral healthcare: Five core approaches*. Washington, DC: AMBHA.

American Psychiatric Association. (1997). *The psychiatrist's guide to capitation and risk-based contracting*. Washington, DC: American Psychiatric Association.

Bagwell, J. (NAMI Regional Director). Internal NAMI communication, March 2000.

Beinecke, R.H., & Lockhart, A. (1998, March). Provider assessment of the Massachusetts Medicaid managed behavioral health program: Year four. *Administration and Policy in Mental Health, 25*(4), 411–426.

Bureau of National Affairs. (1999, June 2). Customer service problems lead to rise in dissatisfaction with managed care plans. *Managed Care Reporter*, 528.

Davis, S. (NAMI Arizona Executive Director). Personal communication with E. Clarke Ross, January 2000.

Dewan, N., Daniels, A.S., & Greenberg, P. (1999, September 23–25). Quality, outcomes, and benchmark measures for behavioral healthcare. In *Behavioral Healthcare Tomorrow conference syllabus* (pp. 111–146). Tiburon, CA: Institute for Behavioral Healthcare.

Dixon, K., & Croze, C. (1997, February). Improving public/private partnerships in managed behavioral healthcare. *Behavioral Healthcare Tomorrow, 6*(1), 67–75.

Dubin, M.D. (1995). Grasping capitation. In G. Zieman (Ed.), *The complete capitation handbook* (pp. 29–36). Tiburon, CA: CentraLink Publications.

Faulkner & Gray. (1999). Appendix B: Capitation rates of selected state/county contracts. In *Medicaid managed behavioral care sourcebook, 1999* (pp. 489–493). New York: Faulkner & Gray.

Frank, R., & Morlock, L. (1997). *Managing fragmented public mental health services*. New York, NY: Milbank Memorial Fund.

Hall, L.L. (1998). Managed care—Survey of the NAMI members. Arlington, VA: National Alliance for the Mentally Ill, October 1998 internal staff summary. Never published.

Hall, L.L., Edgar, E., & Flynn, L. (1997, September). *Stand and deliver: Action call to a failing industry—The NAMI managed care report card*. Arlington, VA: National Alliance for the Mentally Ill.

Harbin, H., Hogan, M., Mayberg, S., Shusterman, A., & Croze, C. (1995, September/October). Public mental health systems, Medicaid restructuring, and managed behavioral healthcare. *Behavioral Healthcare Tomorrow, 4*(5), 63–69.

Health Care Financing Administration–National Academy of State Health Policy. (1999, July 2). *Report to Congress: Safeguards for individuals with special health care needs enrolled in Medicaid managed care* [Draft]. Portland, ME: NASHP.

Hoag, S., Wooldridge, J., & Thornton, C. (2000, July–August). Setting rates for Medicaid managed behavioral health care: Lessons learned. *Health Affairs*, 121–133.

Johnston, J., & Romzek, B. (1999, September/October). Contracting and accountability in state Medicaid reform: Rhetoric, theories, and reality. *Public Administration Review*, pp. 383–399.

Kanapaux, W. (Ed.). (1998a, September 28). Magellan gives Montana carve-out program 30 days to improve. *Mental Health Weekly*, 1–2.

Kanapaux, W. (Ed.). (1998b, November 2). Montana, Magellan officials reach agreement on carve-out. *Mental Health Weekly*, 1, 3–4.

Kanapaux, W. (Ed.). (1999a, February 8). Montana lawmakers consider options for ailing carve-out. *Mental Health Weekly*, 1–2.

Kanapaux, W. (Ed.). (1999b, February 15). Montana lawmakers move toward canceling carve-out contract. *Mental Health Weekly*, 1, 4–5.

Kanapaux, W. (Ed.). (1999c, February 22). Montana lawmakers vote to end carve-out. *Mental Health Weekly*, 1–3.

Kanapaux, W. (Ed.). (1999d, March 1). Montana lawmakers pull reins on Magellan carve-out contract. *Mental Health Weekly*, 1, 4–5.

Kanapaux, W. (Ed.). (1999e, March 8). Magellan wants out of Montana carve-out contract by April 1. *Mental Health Weekly*, 3–5.

Kanapaux, W. (Ed.). (1999f, March 15). Magellan, Montana agree company will pull stakes on June 30. *Mental Health Weekly*, 1.

Kanapaux, W. (Ed.). (1999g, May 17). Budget crunch could force changes in Tennessee MH system. *Mental Health Weekly*, 1–3.

Kanapaux, W. (Ed.). (1999h, September 20). NYC providers say carve-out offers too much for too little. *Mental Health Weekly*, 1, 4.

Kanapaux, W. (Ed.). (1999i, December 13). Governor prepares major changes for Tennessee carve-out program. *Mental Health Weekly*, 1–2.

Kanapaux, W. (Ed.). (2000, March 6). Dallas-area centers feel carve-out's financial squeeze. *Mental Health Weekly*, 1–3.

Kapur, K., Young, A., & Murata, D. (2000, July). *Risk adjustment for high utilizers of public mental health care*. Working paper no. 195. Los Angeles, CA: UCLA and RAND Research Center on Managed Care for Psychiatric Disorders.

Kapur, K., Young, A.S., Murata, D., Sullivan G., & Koegel, P. (1999, March). *The economic impact of capitated care for high utilizers of public mental health services: The Los Angeles partners program experience*. Working paper no. 150. Los Angeles, CA: UCLA and RAND Research Center on Managed Care for Psychiatric Disorders.

Larson, M.J., Farrelly, M., Hodgkin, D., Miller, K., Lubolin, J.S., Witt, E., McQuay, L. Simpson, J., Pepitone, A., Kama, A., & Manderscheid, R. (1998). Payments and use of services for mental health, alcohol, and other drug abuse disorders: Estimates from Medicare, Medicaid, and private health plans. In *Mental health, United States, 1998* (pp. 124–142). Washington, DC: U.S. Department of Health and Human Services, Center for Mental Health Services.

Melek, S. (1998). Behavioral health care risk sharing and medical cost offsets. In *Guide to managed care strategies*. New York: Faulkner & Gray.

Mercer, W.M. (1997). *Case studies: A guide to implementing parity for mental illness*. New York: Marsh and McLennon Companies.

National Association of State Mental Health Program Directors, President's Steering Committee on Health Care Reform. (1993, December 6). Medicaid data analysis [Internal analysis]. Alexandria, VA: NASMHPD.

National Association of State Mental Health Program Directors, President's Steering Committee on Health Care Reform. (1994, June 13). Medicaid data analysis [Memo to Clinton Administration Officials]. Alexandria, VA: NASMHPD.

National Association of State Mental Health Program Directors. (2000, August). Clients served and the use of unique client identifiers by state mental health agencies. In *State profile highlight* [Draft]. Alexandria, VA: NASMHPD.

National Conference of State Legislatures. (1999, July 26). New report shows states making strides to protect consumers in managed care plans [Press Release]. Denver, CO: NCSL.

Open Minds. (1999, June). *Examples of capitation or case rate approaches by state*. Gettysburg, PA: Author, 10.

Pires, S., Armstrong, M., & Stroul, B. (1999, January). *Health care reform tracking project: Tracking state managed care reforms as they affect children and adolescents with behavioral health disorders and their families*. Tampa, FL: University of South Florida (in collaboration with Human Service Collaborative and Georgetown University Child Development Center).

Robinson, G. (1999, September 23–25). Characteristics of public behavioral managed care. In *Behavioral Healthcare Tomorrow conference syllabus* (pp. 63–72). Tiberon, CA: Institute for Behavioral Healthcare.

Ross, E.C. (1997, June). Managed behavioral healthcare premises, accountable systems of care, and AMBHA's PERMS. *Evaluation Review, 21*(3), 318–321.

Ross, E.C. (1998–1999, Winter). Psychosocial rehabilitation in a managed care world. *International Journal of Mental Health*, pp. 73–87.

Roth, D., Snapp, M.B., Lauber, B.G., & Clark, J.A. (1998, January). Consumer turnover in service utilization patterns: Implications for capitated payment. *Administration and Policy in Mental Health, 25*(3), 241–255.

Rudd, T. (Ed.). (1998, September 17). Magellan threatens early exit; state prepares fee-for-service backup. *Managed Behavioral Health News*, 1.

Rudd, T. (Ed.). (2000a, January 27). Dallas center's money troubles prompt closer look at North Star. *Managed Behavioral Health News*, 5.

Rudd, T. (Ed.). (2000b, April 10). North Star money troubles could make vendors ready to leave. *Managed Behavioral Health News*, 4–5.

Rudd, T. (Ed.). (2000c, April 27). State Medicaid capitation rates. *Managed Behavioral Health News*, 6–7.

Sabin, J.E., & Daniels, N. (1999, July). Public-sector managed behavioral health care III: Meaningful consumer and family participation. *Psychiatric Services*, 883–885.

Sheola, R., & Lane, N. (1999, January 22). Massachusetts Behavioral Health Partnerships. Meeting with staff of the National Alliance for the Mentally Ill, Arlington, VA.

Shern, D.L., & Robinson, P. (1999, April). *Evaluation of Florida's prepaid mental health plan: Year 2 report*. Tampa, FL: University of South Florida, Louis de la Parte Florida Mental Health Institute.

Snyder, J. (1999, August 17). Judge agrees $316 million needed to improve care. *The Arizona Republic*.

Sturm, R. (1999, July). *Tracking changes in behavioral health care: How have carve-outs changed care?* Working paper no. 162. Santa Monica, CA: RAND and UCLA.

Substance Abuse and Mental Health Services Administration. (2000, February). *Fiscal year 2001: Justification of estimates for appropriations committees*. Rockville, MD: SAMHSA.

Sullivan, G., Wells, K.B., Morgenstein, H., & Leake, B. (1995). Identifying modifiable risk factors for rehospitalization: A case-control study of seriously mentally ill persons in Mississippi. *American Journal of Psychiatry, 152*, 1749–1756.

Sullivan, G., Young, A.S., & Morgenstein, H. (1997). Behaviors as risk factors for rehospitalization: Implications for predicting and preventing admissions among the seriously mentally ill. *Social Psychiatry and Psychiatric Epidemiology, 32*, 185–190.

U.S. Department of Health and Human Services Office of Inspector General. (2000a). *Mandatory managed care: Early lessons learned by Medicaid mental health programs*. OEI-04-97-00343. Washington, DC: DHHS.

U.S. Department of Health and Human Services Office of Inspector General. (2000b). *Mandatory managed care: Children's access to Medicaid mental health services*. OEI-04-97-00344. Washington, DC: DHHS.

U.S. General Accounting Office. (1999, September). *Medicaid managed care: Four states' experiences with mental health carveout programs*. HEHS-99-119. Washington, DC: GAO.

Wooldridge, J., & Mitchell, J. (2000, May 8). Mental Health Services under Managed Care: What Have We Learned So Far? Evaluations of Section 1115 Medicaid managed care demonstrations. Presentation to the Center for Mental Health Services, SAMHSA. Baltimore, MD.

Yennie, H. (1998, February). A look at the new TennCare partners financing model. *Open Minds*, 4–5.

Yennie, H., & Birch, S. (1999). Medication costs significant share of TennCare partners. In *Managed behavioral care sourcebook, 1999*. (pp. 225–226). New York: Faulkner and Gray.

Zwillich, T. (1999, September). PACTs poised to spread nationally. *Clinical Psychiatry News*, 1, 5.

CHAPTER 9

Persons with Addictive Disorders, System Failures, and Managed Care

David Mee-Lee

Purpose: This chapter discusses the status and barriers confronting persons with addictive disorders in managed care programs. The text describes the coexistence of both "primitive" and "advanced" generations of care and care management.

Major Topics: Managed care has a bias focused on the primary addictive disorder diagnosis rather than dealing with associated complications, aftercare, and continuing care. A framework for the successful treatment of addiction is offered in an attempt to overcome program-driven treatment models, bias in favor of self-/mutual-help recovery groups, relapse, and discriminatory private insurance benefit design. Managed care has the potential to promote outcomes-driven protocols and evidence-based care and utilization management.

INTRODUCTION

When it comes to providing and managing care for persons with addictive disorders, the evolution of care and the systems designed to manage addiction treatment represent a curious mix of Neanderthal man and Homo sapiens. Primitive ideologies of care and care management coexist with more advanced generations of treatment and managed care apparently oblivious to new knowledge and refinements. Many health care systems still assess and treat only the secondary medical and mental health complications of addictive disorders isolated from knowledge about the

225

advantages of early diagnosis and intervention. Many managed care systems still manage cost through first-generation utilization review methodologies, avoiding more sophisticated strategies that are both more effective and more efficient (Institute of Medicine, 1997).

This coexistence of primitive and advanced generations of care and care management provides the framework and context for a discussion about the systems failures in addiction treatment and managed care. It also provides the opportunity for suggesting hopeful strategies and systems for realizing the true potential of managed care to transform how care is delivered, funded, evaluated, and improved. Instead of managed care being viewed and experienced as a barrier to access and utilization of resources, advanced generations of care skillfully managed can, on the contrary, increase access to care and improve efficiency of care and effectiveness of outcomes (Institute of Medicine, 1997). What then are these generations of care for addictive disorders, and what might be the vision of new generations of managed care?

GENERATIONS OF CARE FOR ADDICTIVE DISORDERS

While the following generations of care are outlined, as if chronologically discrete, the unfortunate reality is that all of these "generations" still operate concurrently. That fact represents an ongoing failure of the health care system to provide appropriate addiction treatment. Not only is this costly in human terms, but also it represents misguided public, private, and fiscal policy. Inadequate addiction treatment ultimately "shoots us all in the foot" when it comes to public safety, health care costs, criminal justice and public welfare impacts, and the bottom line in business and industry. Yet despite clear data on the economic, health, and societal advantages of early detection of and intervention in addictive disorders as a primary disorder, the nature of stigma and the lack of training perpetuate a focus on complications—not primary disorder treatment.

In 1994, the Department of Alcohol and Drug Programs in California reported on a statewide evaluation of treatment outcomes and cost-effectiveness (*Evaluating Recovery*, 1994). The California Drug and Alcohol Treatment Assessment found that $1 invested in alcohol and other drug treatment saved taxpayers $7 in future spending associated mainly with criminal justice and health care costs. In 1996, an Ohio statewide study of the costs and benefits associated with treatment found a $4 return for every

$1 spent, even when treatment achieved only a 50% abstinence rate (*Initial Cost-Offset*, 1996).

The first generation of complications-driven treatment persists even in this day of accountability and performance expectations.

COMPLICATIONS-DRIVEN TREATMENT

Recognition of alcohol and substance dependence as primary disorders predates the development of managed care as we currently understand it (Keller, 1976). Good medical and health care focuses on the treatment of primary disorders rather than on the repeated treatment of the secondary complications. Good fiscal policy and utilization of health care resources do no less than this. Indeed, secondary complications require care and attention, but to focus only on the secondary complications and needs wastes both human and health care resources.

The complications-driven generation of care gives cursory attention to the diagnosis of the primary addictive disorder even in cases when it is included in the list of disorders coded in the medical record. Instead of vigorous pursuit of the real cause for the gastrointestinal, psychiatric, orthopedic, trauma, or emergency-related presentation, only the patient's bleeding or gastritis is addressed, depression is medicated, or fractures are splinted or pinned while the continuing care for the addictive disorder is superficial or nonexistent. When the patient returns for detoxification, recurring gastrointestinal bleeding, suicidality, or repeated trauma, the complications are again faithfully treated. This time, however, there is perhaps greater disdain and judgment for the patient's weak will than was first harbored or expressed.

Besides the wastefulness of using health care resources on the repeated care of complications instead of a proactive plan for the treatment of the primary addictive disorder, the sense of futility and hopelessness that accompanies complications-driven care has its own clinical and fiscal implications. Instead of conveying a sense of hope and vigorous treatment, a focus on complications breeds a passive preparation for referral for primary addiction treatment. When the addictive disorder diagnosis is poorly screened for and no diagnosis is made, complications are treated and continuing care fleetingly suggested, if at all. Relapse is poorly addressed and the cycle of complications-driven care starts again (Figure 9–1).

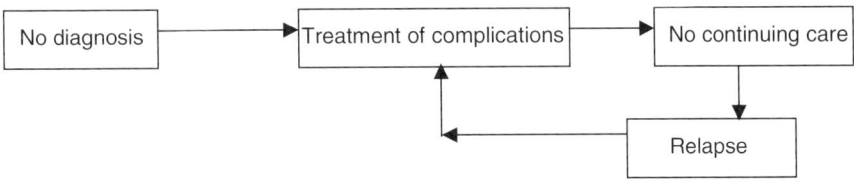

Figure 9–1 Complications-Driven Treatment

Health maintenance organizations and mature managed care organizations that are at risk for all health care costs, not just the carved-out behavioral health benefit, have recognized the implications of a complications-driven system of care management. The early detection and diagnosis and primary care of the addictive disorder meant that the savings on the medical, orthopedic, and trauma side made such outreach efforts worthwhile. The "opportunity" for managed behavioral health care organizations is no less worthwhile. Intensive case management for the high utilizer of detoxification, mental health, or crisis services can have a positive impact and begin to break the cycle of the complications-driven generation of care. Mental health and general health care professionals may continue to miss the diagnosis of addiction and focus on the care of complications. Managed care has the opportunity to track, highlight, and intervene on a system that has failed before to detect or impact inefficient and ineffective preoccupation with secondary complications.

The failure to see substance use disorders as primary disorders deserving of parity not only with other mental health problems but also with other medical disorders negatively compromises benefit plan design, flexible managed care strategies, access to care, and sufficient health care coverage to ensure effective outcomes. Benefit plans explicitly exclude addictive disorders or severely limit numbers of sessions, episodes of care, or lifetime caps. For example, the Mental Health Parity Act of 1996, which became effective on January 1, 1998, requires health insurance issuers (including self-insured plans with more than 50 employees) to adopt the same annual and lifetime dollar limits for mental health that apply to medical benefits. However, substance abuse is not covered under the law, and it does not apply to Medicare and Medicaid programs, both of which serve a large number of people with addictive disorders. While over 30 states have enacted parity laws with varying approaches to prohibit discrimination in insurance and managed care coverage of mental illness, only a handful of states have extended parity to the treatment of addictive disorders (American Psychiatric Association, 2000).

Managed care organizations and those with addictive disorders have to contend with a benefit that barely covers acute care needs. A more adequate benefit would allow flexible care and disease management that could minimize relapses and actualize the cost offsets so well and repeatedly documented. Besides the problem of a limited benefit for addiction treatment, individuals also face access problems with care managers who refuse authorization for those they perceive are so well motivated that all they need is attendance at self-/mutual-help recovery groups. Or, they refuse authorization for those coerced or mandated for treatment on the grounds that they are too unmotivated to justify care. Having now provided training to care managers and other staff in all of the major managed behavioral health care organizations who manage a total of over 120 million lives, the author has encountered these attitudes and policies frequently. Personal experience in private practice and repeated anecdotes from providers bemoaning these access problems reinforce the fact that what is reflected in the attitudes and questions of care managers during training events is often acted on in day-to-day utilization review and care management decisions.

Between 1988 and 1998, the total value of employer-provided health benefits decreased, in constant dollars, by 11.5%. During the same period, however, substance abuse benefits declined by 74.5%. Substance abuse accounted for 0.7% of a health care plan's value in 1988, but the percentage dropped to 0.2% in 1998 (The Hay Group, 1998). Data like these highlight how systems of care and managers of care have repeatedly failed persons with addictive disorders.

DIAGNOSIS, PROGRAM-DRIVEN TREATMENT

In the 1970s, a variety of factors led to a significant increase in the establishment of programs for alcoholism, the most prevalent addictive disorder then and now. The public began to accept alcoholism as a "disease" through public education even though it had been declared such by the American Medical Association a couple of decades earlier (Keller, 1976). Celebrities and other public figures began to disclose their own alcoholism, which served to reduce some of the stigma associated with addictive disorders. In business and industry, employee assistance programs (EAPs) began to identify employees with alcohol problems, and companies were convinced or "coerced" by unions to invest in treatment for their most valuable resource, their employees. Finally, mandated benefits in a number of states and changes in health care benefit plans made third-party reimbursement more available.

All these factors increased demand for services, which was met in certain areas of the country with the creation of additional inpatient beds and freestanding residential treatment centers. This was especially true in states that mandated hospital level of care, for example, for 30 days of inpatient care annually. The expansion of outpatient services was limited because of the disincentive created by the reimbursement mechanisms and mandates. Thus began the generation of diagnosis, program-driven treatment. Now, at least, persons with addictive disorders could be diagnosed as knowledge and training improved and as the financial incentives facilitated primary addiction treatment.

Curiously, however, just as society began to accept alcoholism and addiction as treatable disorders, it revealed its ambivalent attitudes and double standards about drinking, drugging, and addiction as a disease. This society repeatedly calls for a war on drugs and supports an emphasis on supply reduction. Broader strategies of harm reduction, public health initiatives, and increased access to treatment are underfunded comparatively, despite a growing awareness, at least in the scientific literature, of the relative ineffectiveness of supply reduction (Wodak, 1998). There are general attitudes that contribute to such policy directions and emphases. Despite the fact that most Americans drink, and do so without problem, many use alcohol with a mixture of ambivalence, guilt, and anxiety. There is still fiery debate between those advocating teaching children and young people about responsible drinking and those who are just as sure about teaching abstinence, banning underage drinking, and raising the drinking age.

All of this is to say that how persons with addictive disorders are viewed and treated is significantly influenced by the cultural ambivalence and attitudes about use, abuse, and dependence, not just research data. Despite favorable health care utilization and cost offset data and impressive returns on investment in treatment versus data on the relative ineffectiveness of supply reduction, society dictates opposite policies. Limited benefits, expanded resources for drug interdiction over treatment, and loss of disability benefits for primary diagnosis of substance dependence all move in the opposite direction to the research data. Even in the treatment field in the United States versus Europe, Canada, and Australia, the debate still rages hot between advocates of harm reduction and abstinence-based treatment despite the effectiveness of needle-exchange programs and methadone treatment in a range of important outcomes (Wodak, 1998).

Ideology about fixed length of stay, intensive primary treatment, and rehabilitation for alcoholism and other addictive disorders followed by aftercare and self-/mutual-help groups was incentivized by reimbursement mechanisms that were and still are program driven. In a diagnosis-driven system of care, it is the diagnosis that determines the level and length of care (e.g., the diagnosis of alcoholism required 28 days of residential rehabilitation followed by two years of aftercare). People were fit into programs designed more around program specifications, often influenced by the prevailing reimbursement, than based on the specific assessed needs of the client. Should a client relapse after the primary care and aftercare program, the client was readmitted to another 28 days or whatever the program's ideology prescribed (Figure 9–2). Some clients became so familiar with the program philosophy and schedule that they could function almost as a junior counselor espousing platitudes, slogans, and therapeutic admonitions in a manner that "talked the talk" much better than they "walked the walk."

The diagnosis, program-driven treatment generation advanced the cause for persons with addictive disorders by heightening awareness of the importance of diagnosis and early intervention. The proliferation of programs for addictive disorders, especially in hospitals and freestanding residential centers, broadened access to care for individuals with addictive disorders. But what this generation of care also did was to set the framework and fertilize the groundwork for the introduction and expansion of managed behavioral health care organizations: "Between 1984 and 1990, the number of freestanding psychiatric and substance abuse hospitals increased 84 percent. The beds were filled through sophisticated market-

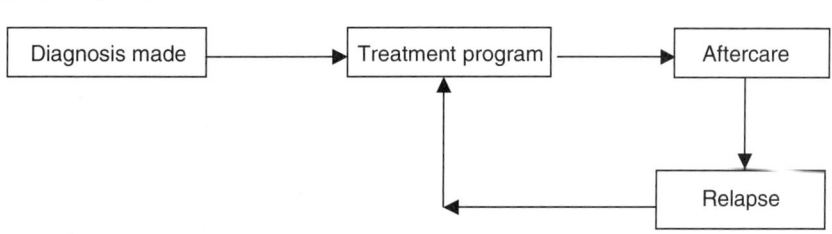

Figure 9–2 Diagnosis, Program-Driven Treatment

ing campaigns targeting adolescents and substance abusers, resulting in many unjustified and even harmful hospitalizations as well as sharply increased costs" (England & Goff, 1993, p. 7). A National Center for Health Services Research study found that 45% of all substance abuse hospitalizations between 1980 and 1985 could have been managed in outpatient settings (Hewitt Associates, 1989).

Alarmed by spiraling health care inflation and the overcapacity of inpatient beds, at least in the private sector, payers and funders sought mechanisms and methods to ratchet down health care costs and reduce inpatient utilization (Iglehart, 1992). The very generation of care that legitimized and advanced direct care of addictive disorders also precipitated managed care's closer scrutiny and demands for accountability. Some excesses such as long lengths of fixed stay in hospitals or residential treatment centers that focused on filling beds added fuel to the managed care fire. Demands by payers for more flexible care in the 1980s and 1990s advanced the generation of individualized, clinically driven treatment.

INDIVIDUALIZED, CLINICALLY DRIVEN TREATMENT

As the health care inflation rate began to escalate, the increased access to inpatient and residential treatment came under increasing scrutiny. This was true not only in the addiction treatment field, but also in health care in general. In the 1980s, there was more scientific research on the effectiveness of treatment, especially comparisons of inpatient versus outpatient care. The findings of controlled studies that randomly assigned patients to more or less intensive settings consistently found "no differences in outcome based on the duration or intensity of treatment or setting (e.g., inpatient versus outpatient)" (Institute of Medicine, 1990, p. 529). Such findings raised considerable doubt about the widespread use of inpatient and residential care for long, fixed lengths of stay—the nation's predominant model of addiction treatment (Miller & Hester, 1986). The diagnosis, program-driven generation of care was now under attack, and appeals to well-meaning tradition, experience, personal recovery, and good intentions could no longer justify decisions about appropriate treatment type and level of care.

Throughout the 1980s, payers thrust on practitioners and programs utilization review and placement criteria that clinicians found increasingly objectionable. Inpatient care was becoming restricted to those with only the most severe of signs and symptoms. Lengths of stay were expected to be flexible, not fixed according to program model or philosophy, and "failed first" criteria began to push for a trial of outpatient care before inpatient care could be authorized. Payers were armed with research findings that supported the demand for more use of outpatient services in place of, or at least before use of, inpatient care. They also were under increasing pressure from benefit design managers and business and industry that wanted lower or less sharp increases in health care benefit premiums. Payers sought new ways to slow the growth in the cost of health care, and managed care as we know it now began impacting providers increasingly throughout the 1990s.

The addiction treatment field was both reactively and proactively coming to grips with the shift to an individualized, clinically driven model of care. Most providers extolled the virtues of individualized treatment, but unfortunately this often appeared to be individualized, financially driven treatment. The treatment level and length of stay are driven more by what can be authorized and approved than by an assessment of what the client needs. Thus this generation of care gained momentum from both practitioners and payers and managed care organizations. Programs sought to survive by becoming more flexible, guided by research that placed more focus on treatment matching than just on the differences between inpatient versus outpatient care (Mee-Lee, 1995). Also, the field began to develop placement criteria for multiple levels of care.

The Northern Ohio Chemical Dependency Treatment Directors Association sponsored the development of the *Cleveland Admission, Discharge, and Transfer Criteria: Model for Chemical Dependency Treatment Programs* (Hoffmann, Halikas, & Mee-Lee, 1987). Also in 1987, the National Association of Addiction Treatment Providers published *Admission, Continued Stay and Discharge Criteria for Adult Alcoholism and Drug Dependence Treatment Services* (Weedman, 1987). The joint efforts of these organizations with the American Society of Addiction Medicine (ASAM) eventually led to the first set of consensus national criteria, *Patient Placement Criteria for the Treatment of Psychoactive Substance Use Disorders* (Hoffmann, Halikas, Mee-Lee, & Weedman, 1991). These criteria played a significant role in moving the treatment field toward more individualized, clinically driven care that recognizes the importance of careful assessment and diagnosis of addictive disorders, but sees diagnosis as a necessary but not sufficient determinant of treatment plan and placement.

Unlike diagnosis-driven care, this generation of care emphasizes multi-dimensional assessment; problem and priority identification within the context of severity of illness and the client's level of function; treatment matching of needs to services and an intensity of service within a broad continuum of care; and ongoing assessment of progress and treatment response. This continuous quality improvement cycle of assessment, treatment matching, level of care placement, and progress evaluation (Figure 9–3) represents a generation of care that the addiction treatment field still struggles to implement.

Besides the ideological difficulty of moving away from a program-driven model of care, payers, funders, and managed care organizations also often disincentivize practitioners from providing more flexible care. Benefit packages are frequently still program driven. They set out benefits in rigid levels of care for fixed numbers of days or sessions and are unsupportive of a variety of levels of service. A broad continuum of covered services would be ultimately less expensive than acute care–oriented plans. For example, there is little funding for supportive living environments that allow detoxification to be done on an ambulatory basis. Instead, detoxification in an acute inpatient setting is covered at a daily rate much higher than the cost of "unbundled" living and detoxification services. Add to this

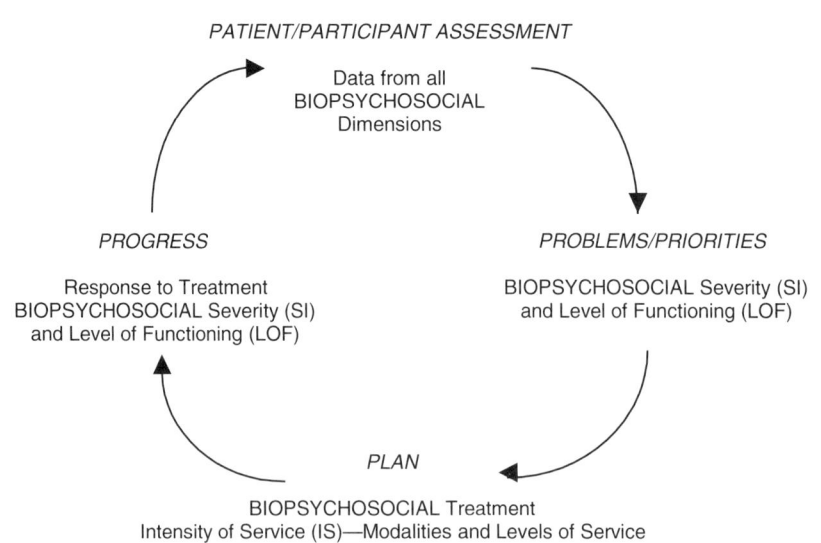

Figure 9–3 Individualized, Clinically Driven Treatment

the fact that more flexible levels of care are not available. The implementation of broad placement criteria and flexible, individualized treatment becomes a struggle in a policy and funding world that seems still caught in a diagnosis, program-driven generation of care.

Managed care committed to truly managing care and not just cost could be a significant catalyst to facilitating the transition to this generation of care. When managed care organizations are restricted to managing a rigidly predefined benefit structure, the potential for a working alliance for individualized, clinically driven care is greatly diminished. Programs are understandably frustrated with their inability to provide time-tested services because of denial of entry to that level of care or because of authorizations for care with limited lengths of stay. Yet, even if they are willing to be more flexible, they are faced with a managed care company that will not or cannot flex the benefit so they can provide a supportive living bed in conjunction with a partial hospital service. Or authorization for further residential care may be denied, yet there is no easy outpatient level available to the client or the sudden discontinuity jeopardizes the therapeutic gains so far achieved. Instead of authorizing a flexible compromise to continue outpatient care at the facility, the program is forced to refer a barely stabilized client to a distant clinic that is both unfamiliar with the client and unfamiliar to the client.

If managed care is to get providers to be more flexible and to deliver individualized treatment plans over placement into fixed programs and levels of care, attention must go to examine and change funding and benefit plans. When funders and care managers automatically restrict authorizations to a fixed number of days or sessions for any one particular level of care, this can be as formulaic as care providers who place a client in a fixed, 28-day inpatient program or in a 24-session intensive outpatient program.

CLINICAL, OUTCOMES-DRIVEN TREATMENT

The previously described generations of care still coexist to varying degrees depending on the regional differences. These may encompass differences in managed care penetration, in historical insurance mandates, and in the prevailing addiction treatment ideologies (e.g., social model versus medical model); they also may involve rural and frontier issues among other policy, licensure, cultural, and ethnic variations. This next generation of care is only just beginning to be articulated and actualized despite a broad clamor for outcomes, performance measures, and accountable and data-driven services.

The 1990 Institute of Medicine (IOM) report, *Broadening the Base of Treatment for Alcohol Problems*, posed a comprehensive and complex question that remains too inadequately answered a decade later: "Which kinds of individuals, with what kinds of alcohol *(or other drug)* problems, are likely to respond to what kinds of treatments by achieving what kinds of goals when delivered by which kinds of practitioners?" (IOM, 1990, p. 143, italics added). If definitive answers at this level of specificity could ever be achieved, care providers and care managers would have the kind of outcomes data to drive decisions about the type, level, and "dose" of care needed to achieve particular outcomes. Even without definitive, specific data at this point, the question highlights the elements that serve to guide the treatment field and managed care in the transition to clinical, outcomes-driven treatment. There is a lack of a common approach and classification system meaningful to a diverse set of clinicians and client populations, as regard to the kinds of (a) individuals treated; (b) alcohol or other drug problems identified for treatment; (c) treatment modalities and models utilized; (d) goals targeted in treatment plans; (e) practitioners trained in which disciplines and methodologies, with what therapist characteristics; and (f) outcomes sought.

Current conflicts between practitioners and managed behavioral health care organizations over client placement are a direct result of the fact that criteria, placement decision making, benefit plan design, and measures of service reimbursement and funding are not data driven. More extensive and specific treatment outcomes data and a body of literature that clarify which kinds of individuals do well in which treatments provided by which clinicians providing which services for which expected outcomes are needed. Managed care organizations have been under increasing pressure by accreditation bodies such as the National Committee for Quality Assurance (NCQA) to measure the effectiveness of their care management. Managed behavioral health care organizations, at least those in the American Managed Behavioral Healthcare Association (AMBHA), realized in the mid-1990s their growing responsibility for accountability and meaningful, measurable, and manageable performance measures. This began the development, in a self-regulatory manner, of their own outcomes and performance measures.

Performance Measures for Managed Behavioral Healthcare Programs (PERMS) arose out of recognition that NCQA's performance measures,

HEDIS (Health Plan Employer Data and Information Set), did not adequately address the area of behavioral health. With the development of PERMS 2.0 (AMBHA, 1998) and HEDIS 3.0 (NCQA, 1998), both NCQA and AMBHA have improved performance measures for behavioral health and merged many of the measures. While performance measures do not necessarily translate into effective outcome measures, it remains a significant step in advancing the generation of clinical, outcomes-driven treatment. The next step for outcomes-driven addiction treatment is to improve measures that provide some indication of access to care and quality of care, but yet do not capture effectiveness of addiction treatment.

For example, one measure for chemical dependency utilization—the percentage of members receiving inpatient, day/night, and ambulatory services (AMBHA, 1998)—provides utilization data. However, it is difficult to assess the appropriateness of those percentages without some correlation with the range of severities of the target member population. If the membership whose care is being managed consists of predominantly healthy, young adults and adolescents, a low inpatient utilization rate for detoxification may be appropriate. However, if the member population is a Medicare population of older adults and those on permanent disability, then the same data may be most inappropriate. Other measures come closer to the kind of outcomes data that go beyond utilization and tap into quality of care that can influence outcome effectiveness. For example, the measure of engagement rates for substance abuse treatment seeks the percentage of ambulatory patients who have at least three total substance abuse ambulatory visits within four weeks of the initial diagnosis (AMBHA, 1998). If it is assumed, as this PERMS measure does, that the assessment process in which the diagnosis is made should take no longer than two visits, the subsequent third visit would constitute the initiation of therapy. This operational definition of engagement identifies a performance measure that can speak to how well a clinician or program establishes sufficient engagement with the patient that he or she returns. However, it does not distinguish between those who come voluntarily versus those mandated for care through referral of an employer, probation officer, or judge. For a measure of engagement to provide a better indication of likely outcome, it would need to measure, for example, the level of empathetic contact established and the degree of patient satisfaction and confidence in the therapist. Such ratings as the Session Rating Scale (Johnson & Miller, 2000) provide a model for performance measures that can assist providers and managers of care with data that promote outcomes-driven treatment.

In both the addiction treatment field and within managed care organizations, the tilt to outcomes- and data-driven systems of care and care management has more to do with future intentions than with using any existing factual information to drive decisions about care. It may be that only if and when payment is based on outcomes achieved will the move toward outcomes-driven treatment gather the kind of momentum needed to realize its full potential (Bickel & McLellan, 1996). The conceptual principles that can guide this generation of care begin with data gathering on the kinds of individuals receiving care (Figure 9–4). These data would describe individuals based on profiles arising from multidimensional assessment information from all biopsychosocial dimensions. Following that data is an inventory of the kinds of problems and priorities that represent the range of needs in the target population served. This inventory includes psychosocial and societal factors such as child care needs, transportation, or specific ethnicity concerns. Next is the range of modalities ("The specific activities that are used to relieve symptoms or to induce behavior change . . . advice, psychotherapy, self-help groups, aversive counter-conditioning, anti-anxiety medication, self-control training, stress management" [IOM, 1990, p. 73]) and levels of service that meet the

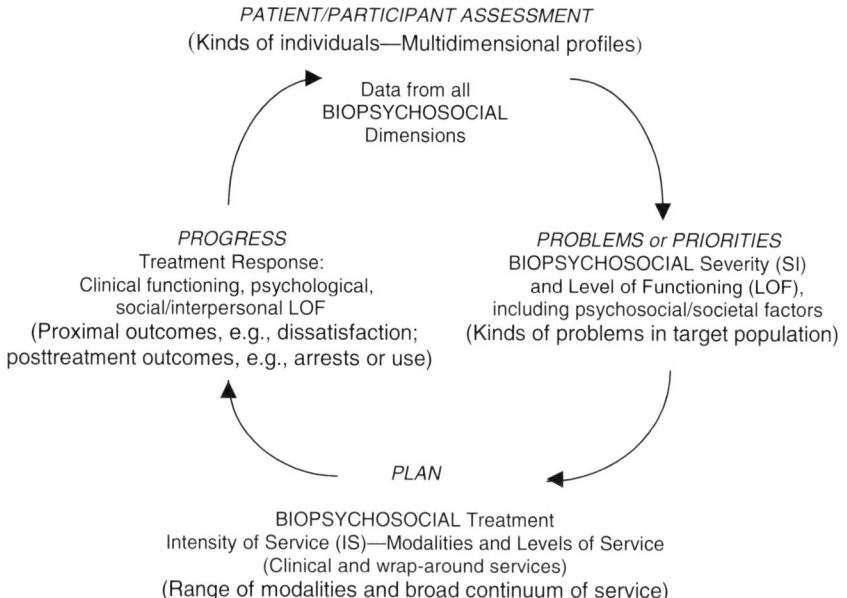

PATIENT/PARTICIPANT ASSESSMENT
(Kinds of individuals—Multidimensional profiles)

Data from all
BIOPSYCHOSOCIAL
Dimensions

PROGRESS
Treatment Response:
Clinical functioning, psychological,
social/interpersonal LOF
(Proximal outcomes, e.g., dissatisfaction;
posttreatment outcomes, e.g., arrests or use)

PROBLEMS or PRIORITIES
BIOPSYCHOSOCIAL Severity (SI)
and Level of Functioning (LOF),
including psychosocial/societal factors
(Kinds of problems in target population)

PLAN

BIOPSYCHOSOCIAL Treatment
Intensity of Service (IS)—Modalities and Levels of Service
(Clinical and wrap-around services)
(Range of modalities and broad continuum of service)

Figure 9–4 Clinical, Outcomes-Driven Treatment

specific needs of the inventory of problems in the target population. The research literature, as well as local outcomes data, would assist in the scope, comprehensiveness, and content of the modalities and levels of service chosen. Finally, data on the client's response to treatment would involve both "proximal" (outcomes measured close to actual treatment [e.g., attendance at all treatment sessions, level of satisfaction or trust in the counselor, follow through on treatment plan strategies and assignments]) and posttreatment or recovery outcomes (outcomes measured after the initial treatment episode [e.g., health care utilization at one year sobriety, alcohol or other drug use six months after detoxification]).

All of the generations of care have served their purpose in their own time and place in the care of persons with addictive disorders. Treatment of the complications of addiction was better than no treatment at all for a stigmatized population of alcoholics and addicts. The proliferation of residential programs opened access, hand in hand with mandated insurance benefits, to primary addiction treatment. Previously, persons with addictive disorders were caught in the revolving door through medical and surgical units in the generation of complications-driven care. Individualized, clinically driven treatment has begun to inspire practitioners and programs to design services around clients' needs rather than to plug them in predesigned programs for fixed lengths of stay regardless of their specific, assessed needs. Last, the hope for outcomes-driven treatment is that decisions about care will be less arbitrary and capricious and that data-driven care will improve the recovery of persons in cost-effective, client-centered, continua of care. If managed care and practitioners could form an alliance with that vision in mind, the adversarial atmosphere that sadly pervades current care providers and care managers could gradually dissipate. With a focus on the specific clinical and social support needs of persons with addictive disorders there can begin a reversal of systems failures of the past and continual improvement in the generations of care. Managed care has an important role to play in that evolution.

WHAT DO PERSONS WITH ADDICTIVE DISORDERS NEED?

As the generations of care in the addiction treatment field have progressed, there has been a shift from reactive care of complications toward proactive management of diseases. Over recent years "disease management" has become a buzzword that represents a combination of a list of other buzzwords that were not heard much during the era of traditional fee-for-service health care—cost-effective, continuous quality improvement, outcomes, practice guidelines, best practices, and patient satisfaction to name a few. Clinicians feel they have been managing diseases for years and in large numbers resent a third party insinuating themselves into the confidential and previously sacred and untouchable patient-doctor or client-clinician relationship. However, as the generation of outcomes-driven, evidence-based care expands, there is an urgent need for consensus between care provider and care manager about what persons with addictive disorders need and how such disorders should be managed. One such effort has been the development of joint statements on treatment, parity, practice guidelines, credentialing, and privileging of professionals and outcomes evaluation (AMBHA & ASAM, 1997a, 1997b, 1999, 2000, in press).

Disease management seeks to bring together the best knowledge concerning diagnosis, treatment, and control of a specific illness or disease through an information-based process. The goal is to achieve the best clinical results with optimal patient satisfaction in the shortest time at the most reasonable price (Baum, 1996). Managed care, whether in the form of a health maintenance organization (HMO), preferred provider organization (PPO), point-of-service plan, or managed behavioral health care organization (MBHO), has similar goals. These goals are "to control costs through improved efficiency and coordination, to reduce unnecessary or inappropriate utilization, to increase access to preventive care, and to maintain or improve the quality of care" (IOM, 1997, p. 15).

When the goals of disease management and managed care are seen together, there is the potential for a productive alliance (Table 9–1). The data needed and collected by care providers and care managers are either identical or at least complementary (e.g., readmission rates and circumstances are data that measure outcome; they help evaluate the validity and effectiveness of a practice guideline). But data are equally important in coordinating care and tracking utilization of services and in performing cost-effectiveness and cost-efficiency studies to manage costs.

Thus, there are more commonalities than conflicts between care providers and care managers committed to evidence-based, outcomes-driven systems of care. This reframes the focus on the needs of persons with addictive disorders from an adversarial struggle between practitioner and care manager fighting over more hospital days to a collaborative discussion about care, resources, community alternatives, and research data.

Table 9–1 Comparison of Goals of Disease Management and Managed Care

Aspect of the Goal	Disease Management	Managed Care
1. Quality of care	Best knowledge concerning diagnosis, treatment, and control of a specific illness or disease	Maintain or improve the quality of care through outcomes monitoring
2. Processes to achieve goals	Information-based: Collection and analysis of data on the clinical and financial results of managing disorder across the continuum of care	Coordination of care; reduce unnecessary or inappropriate utilization; increase access to preventive care
3. Efficiency of care	Achieve best clinical result in shortest time at the most reasonable price	Control costs through improved efficiency and control of access to care
4. Patient satisfaction	Optimal satisfaction using guidelines or protocols for certain patients	Optimal satisfaction using levels of clinical review and appeal to challenge nonauthorizations

Source: Data from N. Baum, How to Better Manage Care By Managing Disease, *American Medical News*, September 9, 1996, p. 21, © 1996.

There can be a common goal for effective care delivered in the most efficient but safe and satisfying manner to the patient, provider, and payer. However, even if there could be a joining of purpose and vision between providers and managed care, the question of what those with addictive disorders need remains complex and fraught with conflicting opinions; philosophies and models of care; prejudices; and varying attitudes about use, abuse, and dependence. Among both practitioners and programs and within the managed care field there are often opposite views about what clients need. For example, for a client resistant to an abstinence-based recovery program, opinion in the provider community runs the gamut. One approach may be to turn the client away until he or she is ready to accept the unmanageability of his or her life and commit to trying abstinence, if only for the duration of the program. Another approach may be to admit the client to an intensive level of care for education, peer support, and confrontation to break through denial over a four-week stay in a structured, residential chemical dependency treatment program.

Still other providers may see the problem as clear demonstration that the client is at an early stage of readiness to change, which warrants motivational enhancement therapy. This would take place at a low-intensity outpatient service designed to meet clients where they are in their readiness to change and to engage them in treatment. Such outpatient interventions may be "discovery" services only to explore their substance use and first "discover" if they have a substance problem. They are not yet ready to commit to abstinence and an abstinence-oriented recovery plan. When such "real-world" situations arise, not only are practitioners divided on the best clinical management strategies, but also managed care comes to the process with its own set of models and biases. For example, one company may consider any treatment plan that does not include active attendance at Alcoholics Anonymous (AA) meetings with the selection of a sponsor less than adequate and refuse authorization of care.

Another managed care organization may be supportive of motivational interviewing and enhancement strategies and stand ready to authorize services that utilize stages of change work; at this point in care it may not even require AA attendance, let alone choosing a sponsor. As a foundation for developing more consensus on treatment needs and eventually more effectiveness and outcomes data that could guide decisions based on evidence not ideology, it is useful to discuss assessment of needs for persons with addictive disorders. How assessment occurs and what is assessed are colored by theoretical models of addictive disorders, perspective as a provider of care or manager of care, personal life experience with recovery, traditional insurance models within a private insurance system versus funding and grants experience within the public sector, and real-world availability of and access to services.

Many providers were raised in the diagnosis-, program-driven generation of care where the principal concern was the identification of an addiction disorder that would qualify the client for a funded slot or an empty residential bed. They view assessment more as documentation of comprehensive substance use history and psychosocial data for licensure, accreditation, and insurance or funding expectations rather than driving the treatment plan and service intensity. Managed care has its views of medical necessity based on traditional insurance concepts of assessment dimensions within an acute care model of services. Even just these two perspectives indicate why and how consensus is difficult to achieve and why the adversarial environment between practitioners and managed care will likely persist until evidence-based decision making diminishes the gap.

With that day still far off, a beginning point is the examination of some instruments and approaches that have already provided a basis for consensus on assessment dimensions that can define more specifically and comprehensively the range of needs of persons with addictive disorders. Because substance use disorders are biopsychosocial disorders in etiology, expression, and treatment, assessment must be comprehensive and multidimensional to plan effective care. The common language of the six assessment dimensions of the *Patient Placement Criteria for the Treatment of Substance-Related Disorders* (ASAM, in press) can be used to target priorities and define the variety of needs of both individuals and population groups. These six dimensions are:

1. Acute intoxication and/or withdrawal potential
2. Biomedical conditions and complications
3. Emotional/behavioral/cognitive conditions and complications
4. Readiness to change
5. Relapse/continued use/continued problem potential
6. Recovery environment

Since the publication of the first edition of the ASAM criteria in 1991, there has been almost a decade of experience with these criteria (ASAM, 1991). The second edition of the criteria is mandated to be used with publicly funded populations in 20 states, within the Department of Defense worldwide, by a national MBHO that manages over 20 million lives, and by a national HMO. While universal acceptance of these criteria does not exist, they have provided a common language for both care providers and care managers to communicate about the multidimensional assessment of those with alcohol and other drug dependence (Gregoire, 1998). This has enabled a more focused discussion about the biopsychosocial needs of clients that has yielded greater efficiency in the care management process. It also has moved discussion of cases away from a recitation of historical information to a succinct, organized, focused, targeted identification of priorities and problems to be addressed at this point in time within the particular level of service of a broad continuum. At least three MBHOs have found this effective in improving communication and collaboration with providers.

IMPROVING SERVICES BY LEARNING FROM PAST SYSTEMS FAILURES

Whether a provider or care manager uses the common language of the ASAM criteria assessment dimensions or not, these six aspects do provide a useful structure for examining where and how systems of care and care management have failed persons with addictive disorders in the past. These failures provide direction on opportunities for improving how care provider and care management systems might form alliances that serve the goals of both disease management and managed care.

It is difficult, if only for a moment, to put aside the real world of benefit design constrictions; limited levels of care in a continuum of services; competing funding streams and bureaucracies; ideological and training obstacles within the addiction treatment field and between managed care and practitioners; and lack of parity of coverage for substance use disorders. Consider the possibilities for a shared vision of what holistic care that advances cost-conscious, effective care might encompass in future generations of care provision and care management (Table 9–2).

Comparing the early generations of care and managed care with the potential of advanced generations and coordinated systems, the principal difference lies in the fragmented way old systems treated and managed persons with addictive disorders. This was disruptive for clients who were often bounced between different agencies, funding sources, and treatment philosophies. It also was an inefficient and wasteful use of resources as repeated use of acute care services depleted limited annual or lifetime benefit limits without the desired kinds of return on investment of the health care dollar. Outcomes regarding abstinence or fewer using days, improved vocational or social functioning, or decreased legal recidivism or health care utilization cannot be impressive when clients drop out of treatment or have their biomedical problems addressed but live in a drug-infested, urban ghetto with few psychosocial, vocational, and significant other supports.

Even if many real-world obstacles to holistic, person-centered care that values outcomes data and cost-effective results remain, the opportunity exists, even today, for managed care to collaborate with practitioners and programs to realize as much of the advanced generations of care as possible. For example, a managed care reviewer should have a better overall perspective on what supportive living environments are available in the network (dimension 6: recovery environment resources) than a

Table 9–2 Comparison of Generations of Care Provision and Care Management

Assessment Dimensions	Early Generations of Care and Managed Care	Advanced Generations of Care and Managed Care
1. Acute intoxication/ withdrawal potential	Detoxification and discharge; authorization for brief hospital detoxification	Link detoxification to addiction and biopsychosocial services; coordination of care beyond just withdrawal management to ensure continuity of care and engagement into recovery
2. Biomedical conditions and complications	Treat complications of addiction only; view the stay as a medical benefit isolated and unrelated to concerns about the behavioral health benefit	Biomedical care integrated into the treatment plan; increase primary care knowledge and interventions; consider carve-in strategies to promote early identification and intervention
3. Emotional/behavioral and cognitive conditions and complications	Treat complications only and/or "underlying psychological conflict"; poor collaboration between mental health and addiction treatment professionals; care managers frequently from the mental health tradition and training— less knowledgeable about addiction	Treat any co-occurring problems and integrate with mental health needs; care management truly becomes "behavioral health" and manages coordination and collaboration of mental health and addiction services to diminish fragmented care and bouncing between systems
4. Readiness to change	If not ready for recovery, send away, ignore, or nag patient; little understanding or use of stages of change or motivational strategies; no	Motivational strategies and engagement; stages of change understood and utilized; managed care authorizes such motivational therapy

continues

Table 9–2 continued

Assessment Dimensions	Early Generations of Care and Managed Care	Advanced Generations of Care and Managed Care
	authorization of "discovery" services; patient seen as "unmotivated" or mandated to care and therefore unworthy of treatment resources or authorization of care	as treatment that is low intensity; effective in preventing intensive, restrictive, expensive services for a person not yet ready to embrace abstinence and recovery
5. Relapse/continued use/continued problem potential	Ignore or reject from treatment; treat and fund repeated treatment of complications with no accountability for failure to address the primary diagnosis	Relapse is a learning opportunity in a chronic, relapsing illness; prevent dropout and retain client in care to minimize repeated readmission to acute services; intensive case management
6. Recovery environment	No or little individualized family or significant other care; fixed programmatic family week (family meets with treatment team at least once a week for multiple weeks) and aftercare; poor discharge planning; no funding for recovery environment services	Careful assessment of this dimension; "wrap-around" services; individualized family work; collaborative coordination of systems work; proactive care and case management

Source: Data from M. Edmunds, et al., eds., *Managing Managed Care—Quality Improvement in Behavioral Health*, Committee on Quality Assurance and Accreditation Guidelines for Managed Behavioral Health Care, Division of Health Care Services, © 1997, National Academy Press.

single practitioner. The care manager could work with the practitioner and be as focused on coordinating transfer to a safe postdetoxification environment as on how many more days are medically necessary in the hospital detoxification unit (dimension 1: acute intoxication or withdrawal potential detoxification needs).

Or, a therapist with a court-mandated client (dimension 6: recovery environment component; i.e., the court judge) may be well aware that the client is at a very early stage of readiness to embrace abstinence and recovery, arguing that he or she does not have a problem and can stop anytime he or she wants (dimension 4: readiness to change problem). In addition, the client feels certain that he or she could stop without groups and self-/mutual-help meeting attendance as he or she has strong will-power (dimension 5: relapse/continued use/continued problem potential). In advanced generations of care, the managed care reviewer's concurrent review calls are focused on the practitioner's assessment of what leverage exists in the client's family, work, living, and legal situations. The collaboration is then about how this leverage can be used to incentivize the client's movement through stages of change (dimension 4: readiness to change; dimension 6: recovery environment strategies).

The care management process in this advanced generation of care revolves now around how many and what kinds of outpatient sessions are needed. The focus is on motivational enhancement sessions and legal and significant other interventions to sharpen the incentives for change. Rather than a managed care reviewer's insistence on the client's attendance at a Narcotics Anonymous meeting before further authorization of service, or denial of care unless the client complies with a structured abstinence-oriented, recovery program, practitioner and care manager work together on an accountable "discovery" treatment plan. This motivational enhancement approach matches the assessed client's stage of change, uses only the resources most likely to be assimilated by the client, and strives to prevent the client dropout that only costs more in human and financial terms.

If a client should have co-occurring mental and substance-related disorders, managed care can be more aware of what "dual diagnosis" programs would accept the client and help coordinate admission to a service more skilled in addressing the emotional, behavioral, or cognitive problems (dimension 3: emotional/behavioral/cognitive conditions and complications). Should a provider be preoccupied with more acute issues, the managed care reviewer can expect and also assist in facilitating appropriate discharge or transfer planning so that a client does not face discharge from an inpatient or residential setting with no outpatient session scheduled. Such coordination of care can provide the support those with addictive disorders need to minimize relapse, especially when moving from structured settings to face the pressures of peer drug use, readily available substances, poor job possibilities, and financial pressures.

When practitioners and programs acted as isolated parts of a fragmented continuum of care, the continuity needed for improved outcomes was severely compromised. Managed care has realized the initial relatively easy goals of controlling inpatient utilization costs and reducing unnecessary or inappropriate utilization in a fee-for-service system that had incentivized inpatient utilization. The jury is still out on improved efficiency, increased access to preventive care, and improvement in the quality of care. The easy reductions in costs and utilization are reaching their limit as more and more markets are becoming managed care mature. The recent increases in health benefit premiums underscores this more difficult phase in the evolution of managed care (*Tracking Health Care*, 2000).

Providers, too, have made some progress in achieving the goals of disease management. Through an increase in knowledge from treatment services research over the previous predominance of "laboratory rat" basic science research, more programs now incorporate more models of care and diversity of approaches. The focus on best practices, practice guidelines, clinical pathways, and standardized diagnostic and placement criteria continues to build consensus on the best knowledge concerning diagnosis and treatment. Publicly funded programs are increasingly required to do common assessments such as the addiction severity index (McLellan, Luborsky, Woody, & O'Brien, 1980) and collect client and management information data. As states seek to quantify more precisely what it actually costs to provide care and how to justify the value of funds appropriated to legislatures demanding of accountability and outcomes, collection and analysis of data will be the rule, not the exception ("Developing State," 1995). Partly in response to managed care, but also in response to the use of placement criteria such as the ASAM criteria, providers have developed and are utilizing a broader continuum of care with more flexibility in lengths of stay. Some providers are even taking on at-risk contracts that propel them even more decidedly toward finding how to achieve the best clinical results in the shortest time at the most reasonable price.

Finally, programs have long had clients fill out quality assurance satisfaction surveys. However, the influence of customer-focused care and consumer satisfaction in the business, free-market environment is beginning to influence behavioral health providers and managed care organizations in ways that are perhaps long overdue. The opportunities to adjust and make mid-course corrections in the evolution to outcomes-driven information and evidence-based systems of care are ripe. However, both practitioners and managed care, upon some self-reflection and self-evaluation, may well find areas and issues to be improved. There are no simple solutions, but highlighting major areas for attention and discussion can serve to promote progress in meeting the variety of needs of persons with addictive disorders.

WHERE TO START IN GETTING THERE FROM HERE

There is the risk of complicating the issues to such an extent that it seems that you cannot get there from here when highlighting what persons with addictive disorders need. However, some perspective on the systems issues is necessary, especially when clarifying the role of managed behavioral health care in addiction treatment. The IOM (1997) clarified the dynamics of three interrelated funding and service delivery sectors, giving insight as to many of the complications and complaints surrounding managed care and addiction treatment. The three sectors are privately funded primary care, privately funded specialty care, and publicly funded care that serves as a safety net that is available to both those with public and private insurance or funding.

The recognition of these three sectors leads to other dynamics that provide an important perspective as a foundation for highlighting where to start in meeting the needs of those with addictive disorders. Much of the care for people with addictive disorders is provided in primary care settings, not in specialty programs. "Alcohol-related disorders, for example, occur in up to 26 percent of general medical clinic patients, a prevalence rate similar to those for such chronic diseases as hypertension and diabetes" ("A Guide," 1997). A Robert Wood Johnson Foundation report calculated that about 5 million users of illicit drugs and 18 million with alcohol use problems need treatment, but only one fourth receive it (Institute for Health Policy, 1993). Primary care providers have frequently not had the basic training or continuing education to improve their ability to diagnose addiction problems, intervene effectively, and coordinate the care delivered in the primary care and specialty sectors. Public services are funded and administered through a large number of categorical programs and agencies that create both duplication and gaps in service, often with different eligibility requirements.

For example, a person with co-occurring mental health and addiction problems may have difficulty receiving services as the mental health and addiction providers shunt the individual back and forth between systems. The addiction system cannot obtain payment for a psychiatric medication evaluation because there is not a primary psychiatric diagnosis or the services of a psychiatrist also may not be available. The mental health system may not accept the client until the alcohol or other drug using is under control, yet are not funded to provide addiction treatment services. Even if a program chose to provide integrated dual diagnosis care, the mental health treatment plan needs may not be funded unless the client is considered to have a major mental illness classifying him or her as severely and persistently mentally ill.

In the public care system that frequently cares for those with the most disabling conditions, there is a further dynamic that many of the service needs extend beyond health care to services and systems that encompass housing, vocational needs, education, criminal justice, and child protective and social services. When added together, the multiple dynamics serve to make managed care in addiction treatment a complex and multidimensional endeavor.

Woven together are the issues of stigma; inadequate training to diagnose, intervene, and coordinate services; multiple entry points and sectors for care (primary and specialty care and fragmented public sector agencies and systems); and the clinical realities of persons with addictive disorders (ambivalence, resistance, and readiness to change issues).

With this as a foundation, where might managed care start to realize the hopes and potential for improved addiction treatment services that offer value to those who fund care, and relief and healing for those who receive care? An IOM committee (1997) adapted the work of Donabedian to provide a framework for its study on quality improvement in behavioral health. This framework serves our purposes well here in making order out of the potential chaos of directions and dynamics involved. The framework of structure, access, process, and outcomes is useful as it orders all the main areas for attention and discussion (Table 9–3).

The issues in managed behavioral health care in general are well informed by the array of topics in Table 9–3. Those issues are addressed in even more detail within the findings and recommendations of the IOM report (1997) in 12 areas: structure and financing, accreditation, consumer involvement, cultural competence, special populations, research, workplace, wrap-around services, children and adolescents, clinical practice guidelines, primary care, and ethical concerns. However, managed care in addiction treatment has many disease-specific nuances within those issues that are worth highlighting if we are ever to move away from the stereotype and caricature of managed care as the "just say no" gatekeeper to services.

Table 9–3 Framework To Order Systems Issues in Addiction Treatment

Components	Issues and Areas Included
Structure	Types of services available
	Qualifications of practitioners
	Staffing patterns
	Adherence to building and other codes
	Public versus private service systems and financing
	Workplace systems (e.g., employee assistance programs)
	Federally supported service systems (Departments of Defense, Veterans Affairs) and distinct populations (e.g., children, seniors, and Native Americans)
Access	Utilization measures (e.g., penetration rates, use of specific services)
	Telecommunication measures (e.g., on-hold time, call abandonment rates)
	Real and perceived barriers to care (e.g., cultural differences, geographic distance, inconvenient locations and times)
	Assessment of adequacy of current access systems, procedures
Process	Measures of procedures and courses of treatment (e.g., numbers of individuals served, consumer satisfaction surveys)
	Appropriateness of care, auditing, peer review
	Practice guidelines, clinical standards
	Continuous quality improvement activities, performance monitoring
	Accreditation process, report cards and contracting
	Licensing and certification
Outcomes	Health status changes after treatment
	Consumer satisfaction with care provided
	Short-term or immediate outcomes
	Performance indicators associated with good outcomes for different patient characteristics, particular organizational and clinical treatment characteristics (types of treatment programs and managed care organizations)
	Bridging research and practice—linking outcomes data with direct input into the development of accreditation and other assessment strategies

Structural Issues in Addiction Treatment Managed Care

Managed care organizations are frequently managing a benefit designed more for the purpose of limiting cost exposure than for its clinical relevance. The types of services authorized are likely to be inadequate to meet the array of needs to be addressed for a good outcome. This is even more critical when dealing with individuals in the public sector who are socially deprived, clinically complicated, and require a greater array of services to improve outcomes. Ideally, what is needed is the ability to flex benefits (e.g., substituting or trading outpatient sessions for inpatient days); to fund services that may be outside the traditional benefit plan but make cost and clinical sense (e.g., paying taxicab fare for a client to access outpatient care instead of staying in a residential level due to lack of transportation); and broker together services from systems outside, yet supportive of the covered clinical services (e.g., accessing housing funds to join with outpatient detoxification that then prevents a residential or hospital detoxification stay).

The practitioners on the other end of a care manager's concurrent review call may have quite different qualifications from the managed care personnel. As important and valuable as the life experience of recovery may be on many different levels in care, the increasing pressure for accountability and credentialed staff has and will continue to threaten the mix and staffing patterns of addiction treatment programs that have relied on a predominance of recovering staff. Managed care companies, themselves under pressure to demonstrate clinical integrity and quality outcomes, command more control over who can and cannot be part of provider and service networks. As managed care in the public sector has increased, there have been more attempts to marry the infrastructure of private, for-profit MBHOs with the expertise and sensitivity of practitioners and programs that have served the public patient well in the past. This trend has occurred not just for its clinical sense, but for fiscal necessities as well.

With less opportunity for impressive savings through diminished inpatient care as managed care has matured in many regions, the profit margins have significantly narrowed below levels acceptable for investor-owned, publicly traded companies. A new breed of public-private partnerships and nonprofit managed care entities will likely increase to bring the principles of managed care to the public sector without the profit margins needed to be viable in the private sector. The National Council on Alcoholism and Drug Dependence (NCADD) in New Jersey is one example of a nonprofit, community-based organization contracted to provide gatekeeping assessment, referral, and care management services for welfare-to-work recipients with substance use disorder problems. Partnership of for-profit Magellan Behavioral Health with NCADD in Iowa to manage Medicaid addiction treatment is another example of this direction.

Access Issues in Addiction Treatment Managed Care

It is difficult to demonstrate good penetration rates when a great deal of addiction care is provided in primary care settings and stigma and inadequate training in diagnosis and intervention are rampant both in primary care health professionals and mental health professionals. Thus, access issues stretch way beyond relatively simple measures of education of consumers about the access toll-free telephone number, health fairs, or improved on-hold times and call abandonment rates. In addition to these are systems that recognize the nature of addiction denial, resistance, ambivalence, and stages of change. Managed care systems that do not understand the value of motivational enhancement strategies and services, that authorize services only for "motivated" clients, or that know little of how to coordinate services with referral sources who coerce or mandate care are destined to pay out excessive funds inefficiently for patients who recycle back through the revolving door of acute detoxification or mental health services and remain stuck on the high-risk, high-utilization list.

Improving access and earlier intervention through improved primary care and behavioral health practitioner education and skills may seem an almost impossible task outside of a managed care organization's capability and responsibility. This is especially true if the view is short term, and the contract is likely to turn over to another company in three years, or if the contract is a carve-out behavioral health agreement with no risk in the total health care costs of the covered lives. In managed care designed to realize the quality, cost, and societal benefits of truly managing care, improved access through earlier detection and intervention is true for all illnesses, but critical for addictive disorders still so stigmatized and inadequately detected.

Process Issues in Addiction Treatment Managed Care

Much of the wrangling that typifies unhappy relationships between practitioners and managed care companies arises from little consensus on criteria to use to determine entry and continued service in a level of care. The issues to highlight here exceed merely the measurement of numbers served, satisfaction achieved, lengths of stay, numbers of sessions utilized, or other performance measures focused on verifying delivery of services and compliance with contractual requirements. Both within the addiction treatment field and the interface with managed care, there is still too little consensus on practice guidelines, clinical standards, placement criteria, and measures of appropriateness of care.

While a major part of the interface between practitioners and managed care revolves around authorization of level of care and length of stay or number of sessions, the process issues will continue to focus on placement criteria and utilization guidelines. National efforts to reach consensus on criteria such as the ASAM criteria have attempted to: (1) define assessment dimensions that address all major aspects of an individual's addictive disorder; (2) provide a common language, definition, and description of a continuum of levels of service; (3) profile client needs and functioning through combinations of criteria and problems in a variety of dimensions that guide placement for individualized services matched to assessed needs; and (4) promote the infrastructure needed to generate outcomes data that can be compared across systems and patient populations.

Such common language and guidelines allow consumers, purchasers of a benefit, payers, and managed care organizations to know exactly how treatment programs and clinicians make decisions about client placement and ongoing care, while at the same time facilitating communication between and among all parties involved in treatment and payment decisions. Nationally accepted, consensus-developed placement criteria for assigning clients to a variety of levels of service within a continuum of care based on multidimensional severity or level of function have been available for over a decade. Yet many clients still receive one treatment model, based on diagnosis alone, as if every addiction client has an acute illness responsive to a single episode of primary treatment followed by "after-care."

With managed care's ability and power to move programs away from a fixed, traditional treatment model comes the responsibility to help find solutions to broaden the continuum of care and the range of services needed to meet the needs of persons with addictive disorders. Too often managed care denies authorization for inappropriate placement and lengths of treatment in residential or acute care settings, but it does little to help the practitioner or program to find and fund alternatives. To explain nonauthorization of care by invoking the limitations of a designed benefit, however constraining that limitation may actually be, does not advance the move to better outcomes. Care managers have the opportunity to help realize the potential for managed care not just managed cost. Managed care has the ethical imperative to use the power of its access gateway, triaging, and utilization management processes to create and promote solutions for better care management. To reap financial benefits by presiding over the management of inadequate benefits in an inadequate system of services and remain relatively inactive as the "victim" of the system raises ethical questions.

To become part of the solution for better care and outcomes, there are process issues to be addressed in the future. One important starting place is to influence benefit designers to broaden and improve the flexibility of benefits for the treatment of addictive disorders. Such flexibility would promote more efficient use of resources for a disorder that only partially fits an acute care benefit model. Although the level-of-care approach does create a framework for matching resources to client need, it simultaneously limits the practitioner's ability to choose the most appropriate combination of clinical setting, environmental structure, and overall intensity of services to meet the client's individual needs. Level-of-care criteria implicitly link the intensity of environmental supports and structure with the intensity of clinical services. For example, an individual may be ambivalent about recovery and could respond to outpatient motivational enhancement therapies. However, because he or she lives on the street, the individual most likely would be treated in a residential setting because this is the only setting that can provide supportive living needs. The predominance of available supportive living is in "recovery" homes. Such a client may need supportive living that allows for people not yet ready to embrace full recovery—a "discovery" home.

Utilization and care management guidelines or patient placement criteria, which allow for a delinking of services from settings, are yet to be fully developed. The variety of services needed to meet the client's assessed needs can be "unbundled" from the "placement" in a particular program or level. Such would provide for a broader range of both clinical and social services required by many to recover and to improve treatment outcomes (Gastfriend & McLellan, 1997; Mee-Lee, 1998; "The Role," 1995). Unless and until managed care and the treatment field address how to define, fund, and utilize a broader range of services, the benefits of managed care will remain illusive. Addictive disorders are not amenable to an acute care model of managed care and utilization review.

Managed care systems for those with addictive disorders calls for the elaboration of a coherent and more inclusive conceptual model for treatment that departs from the limiting concepts of "levels of care" and "patient placement" and extends our explicit attention to the coordinated provision of clinical and social services (McGee & Mee-Lee, 1997). A number of variables will need to be considered including a diverse set of client characteristics and needs; an array of treatment models and strategies; a participatory client service plan with specific, measurable, targeted goals; and clinicians and managed care organizations focused on a range of approaches, but committed to outcomes management. Benefit plans, funding and reimbursement of treatment, and managed care authorization of services also will need to be broader than a system that measures services in units as broad as a day or a session. Smaller units of service or other such measures of the effort, complexity, and time of a service would allow a finer accounting of the specific services needed, authorized, received, and reimbursed. Placement of the future requires further sophistication in the array of services and a comparably sophisticated way to measure and account for the services received. Measures as gross as units of a day or an outpatient session do not allow for the specificity required to tightly match a client's needs to services.

For example, a medically monitored residential program may offer physician and nursing care; subacute detoxification; psychoeducation; individual, group, and family counseling; activities therapy; and continuing care planning all bundled together in a structured, supportive residential setting where the client is safe from negative environmental influences. While a client may need some of those services, the predominant need for an inpatient setting may have arisen out of the fact of the client's homelessness or estrangement from family. Because all those clinical services are bundled together in an inpatient residential setting, the total "dose" of services—and also the cost in some cases—may greatly exceed what is specifically needed. In this example, the person could have received the intensity of clinical services needed while residing in a supportive living environment, the combined cost of which would be less expensive and less intrusive than the traditional bundled level of care. While programs and payers cannot immediately adapt to a much more flexible system than four or five fixed levels of care within a continuum, there is a need to push toward the new territory of flexible systems of care. Unless the process of moving in this direction begins, valuable resources will continue to be exhausted on administrative appeals, litigation, and ineffective fragmentation of care and repeated episodes of acute care.

Outcomes Issues in Addiction Treatment Managed Care

The bridge between research and practice remains a construction process still in its relative infancy. The performance indicators and outcome measures that can substantively meet all the talk and clamor for outcomes-driven services, funding, and accountability are still relatively rudimentary. But as the treatment and research field reaches some consensus on performance and outcomes measures and processes, care providers and care managers will increasingly be able to apply the overwhelming diversity of instruments, tools, findings, and guidelines to each aspect necessary to improve outcomes in terms of more accurate diagnosis; better inter-rater reliability and validity in the development of a multidimensional severity or level of functioning profile; more focused, pertinent problem/priority identification; better targeted strategies having proven effectiveness; and more broadly trained practitioners, skilled in a variety of methodologies, to promote greater flexibility to respond to individualized, assessed needs (Institute for Health Policy, 1993).

Managed care organizations collect and store a large volume of data, the power of which is largely lost because of a lack of coordinated efforts to utilize these data beyond the utilization and quality management functions they serve. If outcomes measurement were tied into central databanks of common assessment and client outcomes data, the field could begin to (1) refine which assessment dimensions should be discarded, added, or improved in treatment and placement criteria; (2) differentiate between two or more compared levels of care, as to whether there are intrinsic differences, or whether essential differences lie in the mix and intensity of specific strategies and services; and (3) identify which levels of care and service should be added or dropped from the continuum of care. Managed care has the opportunity for the kind of partnership with clinicians and behavioral health services that can incentivize development of systems of care more innovative and effective than what currently exists. If this potential were ever to be realized, outcomes management would need to move beyond a few measures of whether a client is readmitted within three months, whether he or she follows through on an outpatient appointment, or whether he or she feels positive and satisfied with services received. These short-term outcomes serve some purpose, but to continuously improve the system of care for persons with addictive disorders, a grander and more inclusive system of outcomes management will be necessary to develop the data that can properly inform the development of accreditation standards, clinical and practice guidelines, and bridge the gap between research and practice.

CHALLENGING DILEMMAS AND HOW MANAGED CARE COULD HELP

In the grand scheme of outcomes-driven protocols and evidence-based care and utilization management, the reality is that managed behavioral health care still has a long way to go. The incentives are overwhelming to manage cost over care and to take the short-term view of cutting sessions or days over long-term cost offsets from prevention, early intervention, and comprehensive care. If managed care is to help lead the field in the evolution to new generations of care, it must resist those overwhelming incentives and assume a stronger ethical position. This leadership position cannot be stimulated only by the increasing public restlessness with managed care, or by the threat of legislators, accreditation surveyors, or lawyers. It ideally arises from the recognition of the many opportunities to improve health care efficiently and effectively, and a commitment to better serve individuals and the community that are so negatively affected by addictive disorders. Throughout this chapter a number of challenges and hazards have been highlighted. Table 9–4 summarizes these and identifies opportunities for improvement with implications for professional development.

The attitudinal, systems, funding, and cultural challenges and hazards above often play themselves out in at least three clinical situations. These invite managed care to lead in resolving such dilemmas and to realize the potential for better outcomes through managed care. The first involves those who abuse alcohol or other drugs but who are not yet suffering from full-blown substance dependence. Related to these are adolescents who may be experimenting with alcohol or another drug, or the children, siblings, spouses, or partners of a person with an addictive disorder. In this situation, the dilemma is how to prevent initial use or further deterioration in a health care and funding system that values acute care, clear diagnostic categories, and intensive interventions over public health approaches and preventive care.

The second situation encompasses those who fall through the gaps in the addiction and mental health treatment systems—the person dealing with both a substance use and mental health problem. Third, there are the many

Table 9–4 Challenges, Opportunities, and Implications for Professional Development

Challenges	Opportunities	Implications for Professional Development
1. Limited benefit for treatment of addictive disorders	Extend parity to addictive disorders to allow flexible care and disease management to improve outcomes and eliminate wasteful "revolving-door" treatment of complications only	Educate benefit managers, employers, other payers, and health care providers about the health, cost, and social benefits of early identification and treatment of addictive disorders
2. Ambivalent attitudes of American culture that wavers between addressing addiction as a treatable disorder and focusing on interdiction and incarceration	Broaden awareness of public health approaches; harm minimization and treatment strategies that provide a greater return on investment than emphasis on supply reduction	Educate clinicians more familiar with abstinence-based treatment about harm reduction and public health approaches
3. Difficulty implementing individualized treatment because of the predominance of fixed-length, program-driven services and reimbursement mechanisms	Promote broad continua of care with funding mechanisms that encourage flexible matching of services to need; rather than placing people in programs funded by level of care, create payment for units of service that allow more flexible treatment strategies	Assist clinicians and administrators in making the paradigm shift from program-driven thinking to individualized, assessment-driven services; assist counselors in recovery to access advanced education beyond life experience and certification
4. Care management, placement criteria, and benefit design are not data driven based on analysis of outcomes	Promote the shift to outcomes management to generate data that would refine criteria and best practices; such data identify what benefit structures return what outcomes when treating which kinds of individuals with what specific problems and goals	Educate clinicians and administrators about outcomes management; assist in differentiating between performance indicators, outcomes evaluation, and the relationship to best practices and practice guidelines

continues

Table 9–4 continued

Challenges	Opportunities	Implications for Professional Development
5. Managed care process is often adversarial with mutual mistrust between care providers and care managers	Form alliances between managed care and practitioners to collaborate on efficient, effective care; create incentives for collaboration	Inform clinicians about managed care principles; improve collaborative skills of care managers; and employ those trained in addiction treatment
6. Lack of consensus on what people with addictive disorders need; different approaches toward motivation, readiness to change, and recovery process	Collaborative development of consensus statements, policies and principles (e.g., AMBHA-ASAM joint statements)	Create opportunities for direct discussion of controversial or polarized issues to develop better understanding of each other's agenda, mission, goals
7. Little acknowledgment that evidence-based, outcomes-driven systems, whether provider or managed care, have more in common than different	Move from adversarial struggles to reframe and refocus on the needs of persons with addictive disorders; collaborate on levels of care, community resources and options, and outcomes data	Develop joint approaches to best practices and criteria; practice guidelines and parameters; performance indicators; process evaluation; proximal, process, and recovery outcomes
8. Providers in isolation can be unaware of, or have difficulty accessing for clients, ambulatory detoxification, housing options, mental health services, "wrap-around" services	Managed care with a broader, cross-systems perspective can identify and broker services; such collaboration with providers promotes flexible, efficient, and focused use of resources	Help providers move to holistic, multidimensional care away from program-driven or crisis services; help managed care move to care and case management away from solely utilization review

patients who daily pass through primary care doctors' offices and health clinics, are detoxified on medical floors or treated for trauma in the emergency department, and leave that medical care with no intervention or even inquiry about their substance use and related problems. The years of stigma, inadequate training and assessment skills, missed diagnoses, and incomplete treatment interventions contributed to the focus on complications instead of on the primary causative addiction disorder. But this misguided focus cannot be laid at the feet of managed behavioral health care. Managed care did not "invent" these conditions, and it cannot resolve these dilemmas alone.

Managed care can, however, assume a position of leadership. This may be leadership in educating and raising the consciousness of benefit managers and funding agencies about the dilemma of how to authorize adequate care when contracted to manage a very limited, inadequate, or rigid benefit plan. Or, it may be leadership in coordinating and managing the many stakeholders that include, for example, the employer, the family, the probation officer, the child protective services social worker, the treatment systems, and the patient or client. By expecting proactive, meaningful discharge or transfer planning, care managers can improve coordination of care that enhances the potential for better outcomes. Leadership in the dilemmas that primary care presents may be through a variety of approaches that involve carve in of behavioral health services. This reintegration of behavioral health care back into and alongside the primary care physician, the clinic nurse, or the emergency department or trauma specialist allows managed care to literally manage the care and track the many alternative diagnoses and services that the person with addictive disorders generates. Instead of fragmented care with little follow through of treatment for an addictive disorder if even diagnosed in the first place, the promise of managed care is the promise of multidimensional care that treats a person as a whole person, instead of a fragmented set of diagnostic codes.

Leadership that exists to manage the care of persons with addictive disorders cannot espouse clinical excellence, quality, and outcomes management and be silent about what needs to be done to address the clinical dilemmas above. When a fragmented addiction and mental health system, for example, shunts a patient back and forth between detoxification and acute psychiatric crisis care, managed behavioral health care can be aware of that even as it happens. To do nothing to incentivize integration and coordination of services in the provider network is to perpetuate waste of both human and financial resources. To initiate intensive case management for high-risk patients who cycle back and forth is to truly manage the care. It marries the incentive to reduce repeated, costly, intensive treatment episodes with the improved outreach, preventive, and early intervention and treatment services that improve clinical safety and outcomes. It is the proliferation of these kinds of managed care strategies that will realize the promise of care management that does well as it does good—good clinical care, good array of services, good coordination of holistic care, and good outcomes, while doing well by cutting unnecessary spending and replacing repetitive, high-cost services with lower-cost, proactive, community-based support and wrap-around services.

In the evolution of systems of care and systems of managed care, it sometimes seems that the more things change, the more they stay the same. Despite increased recognition of the diagnostic category of substance use disorders, many persons with addictive disorders remain undiagnosed and robbed of the preventive aspects of early detection and intervention. The health, social, and family ramifications of untreated addictive disorders are so great that cold, hard dollars and cents and fiscal policy demand we manage care better for persons with addictive disorders who are present in every facet of health care. Yet so-called parity laws still overwhelmingly exclude persons with addictive disorders. The public health, social, and criminal justice benefits of harm minimization and reduction methodologies, demand reduction, and treatment are well documented. Yet the "war on drugs," mandatory incarceration, and disproportionate allocation of resources to interdiction and supply reduction continue with strong public support. It makes sound health and social policy to manage the care in every true sense of the concept. The reduction of human, financial, and social chaos makes managed behavioral health care in addiction treatment an expenditure whose return on investment is a win for everyone. The evolution to new generations of care and care management has progressed, and the hopes of ethical, effective, and innovative managed care can realistically be realized. The pace of this evolution, however, must be quickened if the generations of system failures of both care and care management are to be reversed any time soon.

REFERENCES

A guide to substance abuse services for primary care clinicians. The recommendations of a consensus panel. (1997). In *Treatment improvement protocol no. 24*. Rockville, MD: U.S. Department of Health and Human Services, Center for Substance Abuse Treatment.

American Managed Behavioral Healthcare Association and American Society of Addiction Medicine. (1997a). Effective treatment of addictive disorders. Washington, DC: AMBHA.

American Managed Behavioral Healthcare Association and American Society of Addiction Medicine. (1997b). Parity in benefit coverage. Chevy Chase, MD: ASAM.

American Managed Behavioral Healthcare Association and American Society of Addiction Medicine. (1999). Practice guidelines. Chevy Chase, MD: ASAM.

American Managed Behavioral Healthcare Association and American Society of Addiction Medicine. (2000). A guide for credentialing and privileging of clinical professionals for care of substance-related disorders. Chevy Chase, MD: ASAM.

American Managed Behavioral Healthcare Association and American Society of Addiction Medicine. (in press). Principles for outcome evaluation in the treatment of substance-related disorders. Chevy Chase, MD: ASAM.

American Managed Behavioral Healthcare Association, Committee on Quality Improvement and Clinical Services. (1998). *Performance measures for managed behavioral healthcare programs (PERMS 2.0)*. Washington, DC: AMBHA.

American Psychiatric Association, Division of Government Relations. (2000, June). *State update*. Washington, DC: American Psychiatric Association.

American Society of Addiction Medicine. (1991). *Patient placement criteria for the treatment of substance-abuse related disorders*. ASAM PPC-1. Chevy Chase, MD: The Society.

American Society of Addiction Medicine. (in press). *Patient placement criteria for the treatment of substance-abuse related disorders* (2nd ed. rev.). ASAM PPC-2R. Chevy Chase, MD: The Society.

Baum, N. (1996, September 9). How to better manage care by managing diseases. *American Medical News*, 21.

Bickel, W.K., & McLellan, A.T. (1996). Can management by outcome invigorate substance abuse treatment? *The American Journal on Addictions*, 5, 281–291.

Developing state outcomes monitoring systems for alcohol and other drug abuse treatment. The recommendations of a consensus panel. (1995). In *Treatment improvement protocol (TIP) no. 14*. DHHS publication no. (SMA) 95-3031. Rockville, MD: Center for Substance Abuse Treatment.

England, M.J., & Goff, V.V. (1993). Health reform and organized systems of care. *New Directions for Mental Health Services*, 59, 7, 5–12.

Evaluating recovery services: The California drug and alcohol treatment assessment (CALDATA) executive summary. (1994). Sacramento, CA: Department of Alcohol and Drug Programs.

Gastfriend, D.R., & McLellan, A.T. (1997). Treatment matching—Theoretic basis and practical implications. *Medical Clinics of North America, 81*(4), 945–966.

Gregoire, T.K. (1998). Factors associated with level of care assignment in substance abuse treatment. *Journal of Substance Abuse Treatment, 18*, 241–248.

Hewitt Associates. (1989). *Managing health care costs*. Lincolnshire, IL: Hewitt Associates.

Hoffmann, N.G., Halikas, J.A., & Mee-Lee, D. (1987). *The Cleveland admission, discharge, and transfer criteria: Model for chemical dependency treatment programs*.

Cleveland, OH: The Northern Ohio Chemical Dependency Treatment Directors Association.

Hoffmann, N.G., Halikas, J.A., Mee-Lee, D., & Weedman, R.D. (1991). *Patient placement criteria for the treatment of psychoactive substance use disorders.* Washington, DC: American Society of Addiction Medicine.

Iglehart, J.K. (1992). Health policy report—The American health care system—Managed care. *New England Journal of Medicine, 327,* 742–747.

Initial cost-offset findings: Cost effect study executive summary. (1996). Columbus, OH: Division of Alcohol and Drug Addiction Services.

Institute for Health Policy, Brandeis University. (1993). *Substance abuse: The nation's number one health problem: Key indicators for policy.* Princeton, NJ: The Robert Wood Johnson Foundation.

Institute of Medicine. (1990). *Broadening the base of treatment for alcohol problems.* Washington, DC: National Academy Press.

Institute of Medicine; Edmunds, M., Frank, R., Hogan, M., McCarty, D., Robinson-Beale, R., & Weisner, C. (Eds.). (1997). *Managing managed care—Quality improvement in behavioral health.* Washington, DC: National Academy Press.

Johnson, L.D., & Miller, S.D. (2000). *Session rating scale* (rev. Version 2). Chicago, IL: The Institute for the Study of Therapeutic Change.

Keller, M. (1976). The disease concept of alcoholism revisited. *Journal of Studies on Alcohol, 37*(1), 1694–1717.

McGee, M.D., & Mee-Lee, D. (1997). Rethinking patient placement: The human services matrix model for matching services to needs. *Journal of Substance Abuse Treatment, 14*(2), 141–148.

McLellan, A.T., Luborsky, L., Woody, G.E., & O'Brien, C.P. (1980). An improved evaluation instrument for substance abuse patients: The addiction severity index. *Journal of Nervous and Mental Disease, 168,* 26–33.

Mee-Lee, D. (1995). Matching in addictions treatment: How do we get there from here? *Alcoholism Treatment Quarterly, 12*(2).

Mee-Lee, D. (1998). Use of patient placement criteria in the selection of treatment. In *Principles of addiction medicine* (2nd ed., pp. 363–370). Chevy Chase, MD: American Society of Addiction Medicine Inc.

Miller, W.R., & Hester, R.K. (1986). Inpatient alcoholism treatment: Who benefits? *American Psychologist, 41*(7), 794–805.

National Committee for Quality Assurance. (1998). Health plan employer data and information set (HEDIS 3.0). Washington, DC: NCQA.

The Hay Group. (1998, November). *Substance abuse benefit cost trends 1988–1998.* Report commissioned by the American Society of Addiction Medicine. Arlington, VA: The Hay Group.

The role and current status of patient placement criteria in the treatment of substance use disorders. The recommendations of a consensus panel. (1995). In *Treatment improvement protocol no. 13.* Rockville, MD: The Center for Substance Abuse Treatment.

Tracking health care costs: Long predicted upturn appears. Issue brief no. 23. (2000, January). Washington, DC: Center for Studying Health System Change.

Weedman, R.D. (1987). *Admission, continued stay and discharge criteria for adult alcoholism and drug dependence treatment services.* Irvine, CA: National Association of Addiction Treatment Providers.

Wodak, A. (1998). Harm reduction as an approach to treatment. In *Principles of addiction medicine* (2nd ed.). Chevy Chase, MD: American Society of Addiction Medicine Inc.

CHAPTER 10

Performance, Quality, and Outcomes: Prospects for Consensus in the Behavioral Health Field

John A. Morris and Neal Adams

Purpose: This chapter states that few changes in the health care environment have so dramatically raised the awareness of quality and accountability as managed care. This chapter focuses on the challenge of useful information and data and reviews initiatives that seek field consensus on a set of performance indicators and outcome measures.

Major Topics: This chapter discusses Measuring Quality, Who Owns Quality Managed Care Concerns, Ethical Issues, and the State of Practice. The chapter also summarizes and compares the field's multiple and major measurement efforts.

INTRODUCTION

The pursuit of quality and accountability for behavioral health services predates the emergence of managed care strategies. However, few changes in the health care environment have so dramatically raised the awareness of quality concerns as the emergence of health maintenance organizations (HMOs), managed care organizations (MCOs), and their counterparts in the mental and addictive disorders, the managed behavioral health organizations (MBHOs). This chapter focuses on the challenges of data to provide useful information about quality and performance in behavioral health care that can be used by a broad spectrum of stakeholders: consumers, families, purchasers, payers, and providers. Several initiatives that seek field consensus on a set of performance indicators and outcome measures for quality management and accountability are highlighted.

MEASURING QUALITY

The much-used equation for value in the health care field is expressed as:

$$Value = Quality/Cost$$

The cost element in this equation is comparatively easy to derive, although we struggle to capture the indirect costs of both action and inattention to health concerns accurately. For the sake of comparison with the quality element in the equation, the determination of cost is the relatively easy part. Achieving a quantifiable measure for quality in order to solve the equation remains a serious challenge. One is reminded of the old joke about the naïf who is baffled by the concept of the thermos for keeping hot things hot and cold things cold: "But how does it know which to do?" And how do we know "which" to do to measure quality?

WHO OWNS QUALITY?

The simplest answer to this core question could be: the customer. But who is the customer? In a managed care environment, quality is typically what the purchaser says it is or needs to be. As is often the case, the quick and simple response is insufficient. To an increasing degree, the question is more adequately answered if the ultimate customer is understood to be the end-user, the consumer of health care/behavioral health care services. The purchaser often acts as a proxy for the primary consumer, a circumstance that is especially true for public sector populations. But even this expanded understanding excludes the role of the provider in the ownership of quality—an unfair, although common, exclusion. Yet another group of owners of quality is the national accrediting organizations, whose processes of evaluation and accreditation of providers and programs are visible and recognized signs of their commitment to quality.

MANAGED CARE CONCERNS

Although the quality movement long predates managed care approaches to the delivery of care, it is probably undeniable that public angst about managed care and a plethora of horror stories have significantly raised the ante. Increasingly, consumers are demanding guarantees that safety (at the least) be preserved in the cost savings of care management. Care management has changed the economics of service delivery. Capitation provides incentives for producing results, not generating billable fee-for-service units. In this new environment, the challenge is to find strategies that measure the results of the interventions in a way that is responsible and meaningful for all stakeholders.

In an introductory essay for a sourcebook on outcomes, Kramer (1999) succinctly outlines the reasons for the focus on performance measurement: "Purchasers are requiring more data from health plans, providers organizations, hospitals and other treatment settings; consumers are seeking more information to use when selecting health plans and specific providers; and accrediting organizations are developing report cards to address performance standards and compare the quality of care provided in various treatment settings and by third-party payers" (p. xi).

Wise purchasers and consumers have always looked for data to help in differentiating among competing products and services, as witnessed by the success of the Consumers' Union and its rating efforts. In the health sector, there have been few, if any, analogues in response to the demand for comparative data. This chapter seeks to review recent efforts to fill that void for the behavioral health care community.

ETHICAL ISSUES

There are important ethical dimensions to performance measurement. Values that drive the measurement system must be clearly identified and indicators can only be meaningfully compared in the context of these values. One such set of value statements was developed and published by the American College of Mental Health Administration (Morris, 1998). The process of identifying and elaborating these values is detailed later in this chapter.

The seven value statements, as adopted, edited, and approved by the board of the American College of Mental Health Administration (ACMHA),* are as follows:

1. Consumers and families are at the core of performance measurement.
2. Consumer/customer choice must be a driving value for all systems of care, including their design, delivery, evaluation, and accreditation.

Source: Reprinted with permission from J.A. Morris, ed., Preserving Quality and Value in the Managed Care Equation: Final Report of the 1997 Santa Fe Summit, © 1998, American College of Mental Health Administration.

3. Issues of ethnicity, race, age and developmental status, gender, language, culture, spirituality, and disability are consciously addressed in assuring access and availability of services.

4. Mental health and substance abuse delivery systems must be accountable to both internal and external stakeholders for meeting the mental health needs of the people they serve in ways that are effective and efficient, and that accountability must be based on reliable, comparable data.

5. Access to mental health and substance abuse services must be quick, easy, and convenient, and outreach and follow-up must be seen as part of the access continuum. A true public health vision of community health must drive outcomes measurement, which means that universal access and integrated primary and mental health and substance abuse care are the ultimate goal of effective systems.

6. Children who have mental health and substance abuse problems:
    • should be able to receive effective services in their home and schools without disruptive removals from either setting;
    • should be able to remain safe and out of trouble with law enforcement;
    • should remain connected to family and peers while in treatment;
    • should receive services that are family focused and health centered.

7. Adults with mental health and substance abuse problems:
    • should be able to maintain a stable, comfortable, and safe living environment;
    • should be able to engage in chosen, productive daily activity;
    • should be able to remain safe and out of trouble with law enforcement;
    • should receive treatment that is consumer-centered and which maximizes independence and self-care skills (this represents 1997 language; today we would refer to this cluster in the simpler and more powerful term: recovery);
    • should receive services designed to enhance total health and maintain social connections and improved quality of life.

While no single set of performance indicators could be expected to meet all of these ideals, ACMHA and its numerous partners continue to endorse this list of key value statements as essential to any effort toward measurement and accountability.

THE STATE OF PRACTICE

Since the early to mid-1990s, there have been numerous initiatives to address the issue of performance measurement in behavioral health. Initially these efforts gave some hope that there could be reliable report cards that would enable all stakeholders to make more informed decisions and choices in purchasing behavioral health care. These ideas spawned an exponential growth in demand for usable results. Many of the efforts focused on a particular set of stakeholder perspectives and concerns. However, the promise of reliable quality data proved more elusive than many had first hoped, as the complexities of measurement methodology and the costs associated with collecting data became clearer.

Significant among the measurement efforts has been the work of the Foundation for Accountability (FAcct), the Washington Business Group on Health, the National Committee for Quality Assurance's (NCQA) development of the Health Plan Employer Data and Information Set (HEDIS), the Mental Health Statistics Improvement Projects' (MHSIP) Consumer Oriented Report Card, the Joint Commission on Accreditation of Healthcare Organizations' (Joint Commission) ORYX™ initiative, and the National Association of State Mental Health Program Directors' (NASMHPD) framework, among others. In the public sector, the Substance Abuse and Mental Health Services Administration's (SAMHSA) Office of Managed Care, along with corollary offices with the Center for Mental Heath Services (CMHS), the Center for Substance Abuse Prevention (CSAP), and the Center for Substance Abuse Treatment (CSAT), began to devote both technical and financial assistance to state and federal purchasers.

NCQA has set the industry standard for scientific rigor in its drive for data that can legitimately be used for comparing health plans, but behavioral health measures have been difficult to include. The American Managed Behavioral Health Association (AMBHA) stepped into the breach with its own performance measurement system, PERMS, which is a set of performance indicators designed specifically for managed behavioral health care organizations and carve-outs.

The concerns of family members of persons with mental illnesses sparked the creation of the National Alliance for the Mentally Ill's (NAMI) Outcomes Roundtable, which focused especially on dangers to vulnerable populations with severe and persistent mental illnesses. These populations were seen as particularly likely to be lost in the conversion to public sector managed care strategies that were developed, in large measure, to meet the needs of employed populations, rather than persons with chronic disabilities.

In addition to these efforts and initiatives, proprietary vendors of quality surveys also began to emerge, and the national accrediting organizations began to accelerate plans to include outcomes and performance measurement as part of the accreditation process. The Joint Commission established its ORYX initiative, for example, which provided a template for providers to use in collecting, analyzing, and reporting performance information, while leaving decisions about specific methodologies to the accredited organizations. This created a new market for vendors that developed measurement systems and products to meet the Joint Commission ORYX standards, relieving providers of the need to develop their own approaches. Other examples of accrediting organizations' involvement with performance measurement are addressed later in this chapter.

The sum of these efforts has been a proliferation of indicators, measurement strategies, and reports. This has left stakeholders less certain and more confused rather than better informed and able to choose. Rather than moving toward congruence and uniformity to support comparison and evaluation of quality, there has been a divergence of measurement efforts and an increase in stakeholder frustration.

THE KUDZU PHENOMENON

Kudzu (*Pueraria thunbergiana*) is an amazing vine, introduced in the United States from Asia in 1876. In the 1930s, the federal government paid farmers $8.00 an acre to plant the vine on fallow fields to prevent erosion and to provide cheap browse for cattle—both laudable goals. Before long, however, it was discovered just how well adapted this plant was to the southern United States. In the humid, hot summer months, kudzu can grow more than a foot a day and rapidly spreads, engulfing trees, abandoned structures, and anything else in its path. The festoons of kudzu now choke fields and woodlands throughout the South and are increasingly becoming a nuisance.

In this environment, kudzu is a metaphor for the proliferation of performance and outcome measurement systems and tools in the behavioral health care field. The laudable goal of providing some form of a report card has spawned an ever-growing array of conflicting, competing instruments, some in both the public domain and in proprietary forms. The unchecked spread of these efforts has resulted in frustration and confusion on the part of all stakeholders. The proverbial canary in the mine was probably the provider community who most immediately bore the burden of satisfying an array of often duplicative or conflicting measurement requirements.

A corollary influence might be called "The Nike Phenomenon," based on the shoe company's successful ad campaign slogan, "Just do it!" Many in the field felt an enormous pressure to collect something, report something, or be left out of the game. While this is not a rational approach, it was a virtual inevitability in the volatile health care (and especially the managed behavioral health care) market of the 1990s. This haphazard approach to major policy change is not unique to the mental health and addictive disorders field, and has been described as playing "policy pinball" (Morris, 2000).

SEARCH FOR THE HOLY GRAIL

Clearly there was a need to bring some order to this pursuit of quality measures. Many began to call for the development of a core, consensus, or common set of indicators and measures—a Holy Grail for the field. A prominent and significant national effort to reach agreement on key indicators has been the work of ACMHA in collaboration with five of the leading accrediting organizations in behavioral health care.

The phrase "Preserving Quality and Value in the Managed Care Equation" was the organizing principle for ACMHA's first effort to build consensus on performance measurement and was the theme of the first Santa Fe Summit held in March 1997 (this summit was underwritten by an unrestricted educational grant from Eli Lilly and Company). The summit planning committee generated a list of individuals and organizations that were known to have an interest in performance measurement. The goal was to host a true stakeholders meeting: consumers, providers, purchasers, payers, researchers, and accreditors. The design of the summit is described in detail in an ACMHA monograph (Morris, 1998).

The premise was to present a "floor" of information about quality and measurement, and then invite the participants to work in small groups to produce recommendations to advance the field. The assembled participants settled on a modified Donabedian (1980) framework to anchor the small group work. Access, process, structure, outcomes, and prevention were selected as the five domains for the work groups. Each group was given a series of tasks that included the following: (1) to identify core values that should drive the process, (2) to define terms relevant to the topic area, (3) to specify relevant performance indicators that should be candidates for a core set, and (4) to list validated instruments that could collect data and support items 1 through 3 above. The results are detailed below.

CANDIDATE INDICATORS

The original work groups from the 1997 summit generated a number of candidate indicators in the five domains. In subsequent work (work following the summit and monograph publication were supported by a grant from the Office of Managed Care at the SAMHSA; the grant was administered by the National Technical Assistance Center for Children's Mental Health at the Georgetown University Child Development Center), only three domains retained foci: access, process, and outcomes. With regards to prevention, the ACMHA board acknowledged that its effort should defer to a work already in progress under the leadership of the National Mental Health Association; their monograph, *Preventing Mental Health and Substance Abuse Problems in Managed Health Care Settings* (Mrazek, 1998), has subsequently been endorsed by ACMHA. The structure domain, on further examination, was felt to duplicate much of what was already extant in traditional accreditation standards and further work was not seen as needed.

The indicators in the three remaining domains (access, process, and outcomes) were judged worthy of further comment and review by the field. Having made substantial progress in identifying a core set of performance indicators, a "mini-summit" was convened in March 1998—one year after the original meeting—to review the work product and present the previously cited monograph (Morris, 1998). Details of the candidate indicators are given later in the chapter.

At this meeting, a select group of leaders in the behavioral health care field participated in a roundtable discussion chaired by ACMHA Distinguished Fellow and President of the Washington Business Group on Health, Dr. Mary Jane England. Also included were representatives of three national accreditation organizations who survey behavioral health programs. Dr. England and the others invited the accreditors to join in a partnership with ACMHA and carry the effort forward. CARF, the Rehabilitation Accreditation Commission; the Joint Commission; and NCQA all agreed to accept the challenge.

MOVEMENT TOWARD CONSENSUS

The ACMHA board took seriously the offer of these three initial accrediting organizations. Invitations were then extended to The Council on Quality and Leadership in Support of Persons with Disabilities (The Council), the Council on Accreditation of Services to Children and Families (CoA), and the American Accreditation HealthCare Commission/URAC. Only the former two, The Council and CoA accepted, and a work group assembled consisting of six partners: ACMHA as convenor/facilitator, along with CARF, CoA, The Council, the Joint Commission, and NCQA. Together these organizations agreed to try and work toward further agreement on measurement. Never before had such an effort been made in behavioral health.

ACMHA then sought external funding to support the work. This effort began with the premise that if the work was to have credibility, it could not be seen as having a single underwriter and it must reflect the diversity of the behavioral health field. A consortium of funders was assembled to support a two-year work plan: the MacArthur Foundation, the Robert Wood Johnson Foundation, Eli Lilly and Company, and the SAMHSA, Office of Managed Care, agreed to fund the work; significant in-kind commitments were made by the five accreditation organizations themselves, ACMHA, and the volunteers who worked on the project.

A NEW LANGUAGE

When the ACMHA Accreditation Organization Workgroup on a Consensus Set began its deliberations, it became clear almost at once that the divergent efforts to work on performance measurement had created a contemporary Tower of Babel. Terminology could not be used interchangeably, and what one organization called a "measure" another called an "indicator," and so on through multiple examples. The first concrete task was the creation of a common taxonomy. Seemingly minor, this was an essential task. The agreed-upon elements are presented in Table 10–1.

Table 10–1 Comparison of Terms Used in Performance Measurement by the National Accrediting Organizations

Common Taxonomy	CARF Performance Indicators Version 1.1	COA	Joint Commission ORYX	NCQA HEDIS 3.0	The Council Personal Outcome Measures
Domain	Domain	Domain	Domains of performance	Domain	Factors
Concept/concern	Concern	Concern			
Indicator definition	Indicator	Outcome indicators	Performance measurement	Measure/ indicator	Performance
Measure	Measure	Measure			Measure
Specification	Data element	Data element	Data element	Data element	Data element
Benchmark					

CARF, the Rehabilitation Accreditation Commission; COA, Council on Accreditation of Services to Children and Families; Joint Commission, Joint Commission on Accreditation of Healthcare Organizations; NCQA, National Committee for Quality Assurance; The Council, The Council on Quality and Leadership in Support of Persons with Disabilities.
Courtesy of the American College of Mental Health Administrators, Pittsburgh, Pennsylvania.

The work group then turned to an exhaustive review of the candidate measures coming from ACMHA's earlier effort. This involved word-by-word dissection of the concepts, values, and candidate indicator definitions. As this process unfolded, it became necessary to construct a matrix or hierarchy of discussion; there would be momentary consensus on a concept, which would devolve into methodological dispute in the next instant. The work group adopted a framework for discussion and exacted a pledge to work systematically from top to bottom, from the conceptual to the technical. This proved a difficult commitment, as there was a natural tendency to move from concepts to data elements, from concepts and concerns to details of measurement, and so on. The framework for the discussion is presented in summary, schematic form in Figure 10–1.

Having arrived at a common taxonomy and an organizing paradigm for the work, the group then began to refine the collection of indicators coming from the 1997 summit. Initially, the group used the working principles of meaningfulness, measurability, and burden as guidelines for selecting indicator definitions to be included in a core set. Eventually it became clear that there would need to be a statement of the rationale for inclusion/exclusion of indicators. The Joint Commission, NCQA, and the American Medical Association (AMA), acting as the Performance Measures Coordinating Council (PMCC), had already developed a statement of the desirable attributes of performance measures for health care. The ACMHA Accreditation Organization Workgroup, with permission of the PMCC, modified the language of the original document and then adopted the revised set of desirable attributes as its own guiding framework. The desirable attributes statement, released in April 2000 (ACMHA, 2000), defines the desirable attributes as shown in Table 10–2.

While the accrediting organizations reached agreement on these desirable attributes, each had its own perspective and caveats as to how they should be applied to decisions about what to measure. CARF felt that it had already made substantial progress in identifying key performance indicators and associated measures for a wide array of programs. The purpose of CARF's work on indicators, which is still under development, is to provide assistance to organizations that want to gather and report uniform information to consumers and payers and to use in internal quality improvement. Because indicators may have different applications for CARF-accredited organizations, each of the attributes is important to consider, though some attributes may be more important than others.

Figure 10–1 Accrediting Organizations Work Group Organizing Schema

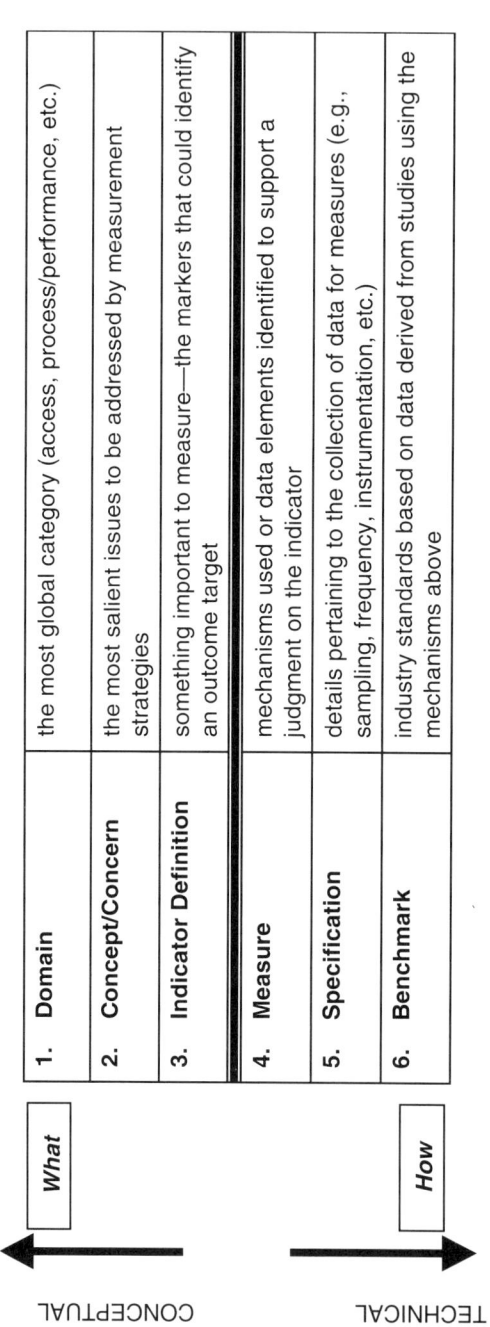

1.	**Domain**	the most global category (access, process/performance, etc.)
2.	**Concept/Concern**	the most salient issues to be addressed by measurement strategies
3.	**Indicator Definition**	something important to measure—the markers that could identify an outcome target
4.	**Measure**	mechanisms used or data elements identified to support a judgment on the indicator
5.	**Specification**	details pertaining to the collection of data for measures (e.g., sampling, frequency, instrumentation, etc.)
6.	**Benchmark**	industry standards based on data derived from studies using the mechanisms above

What → CONCEPTUAL

How → TECHNICAL

Courtesy of the American College of Mental Health Administrators, Pittsburgh, Pennsylvania.

Table 10–2 Desirable Attributes of Performance Measures in Behavioral Health

Attribute	Definition
1. Importance of topic area addressed by the measure	
1A. High priority for maximizing the health of persons or populations	The measure addresses a process or outcome that is important in maximizing the health and well-being of persons or populations. Highest priority is given to those concerns that are defined by high prevalence, incidence, mortality, morbidity, or disability.
1B. Financially important	The measure addresses an area of health or well-being that either involves high per-person burden or affects a large number of people.
1C. Demonstrated variation in care and/or potential for improvement	The measure addresses an aspect of health or functioning for which there is a reasonable expectation of wide variation in service delivery and/or potential for improvement. If the purpose of the measure is internal quality improvement and professional accountability, then wide variation in service delivery across practitioners or settings is not necessary.
1D. Strategically important	The measure addresses an area with a high level of expressed consumer and community concern.
2. Usefulness in improving individual outcomes	
2A. Based on established service or clinical recommendations	For process measures, there is good evidence that the process improves health or well-being outcomes. For outcome measures, there is good evidence that there are processes or actions that providers can take to improve the outcome.
2B. Potentially actionable by user	The measure addresses an area of health or human service that potentially is under the control of the practitioner, health care or human service organization, or system.
2C. Meaningful and interpretable to user	The results of the measure are reportable in a manner interpretable and meaningful to the intended user. For example, practitioners must be able to use the information generated by the measure to improve direct services. Health or human service organizations must find the information useful for decision-making purposes. When measures are used to compare health or human service systems, users should be able to understand the service delivery and economic significance of differences in how well systems perform on the measure.

continues

Table 10–2 continued

Attribute	Definition
3. Measure design	
3A. Well-defined specifications	The following aspects of the measure are to be well defined: numerator, denominator, sampling methodology, data sources, allowable values, methods of measurement, and method of reporting.
3B. Documented reliability	The measure will produce the same results when repeated in the same population and setting (low random error). Tests of reliability include (a) test-retest (reproducibility): test-retest reliability is evaluated by repeating administration of the measure in a short time frame and calculating agreement among the repetitions; (b) inter-rater: agreement between raters is measured and reported using the kappa statistic; (c) data accuracy: data are audited for accuracy; and (d) internal consistency for multi-item measures: analyses are performed to ensure that items are internally consistent.
3C. Documented validity	The measure has face validity—it should appear to a knowledgeable observer to measure what is intended. The measure also should correlate well with other measures or the same aspects of care (construct validity) and capture meaningful aspects of this care (content validity).

Courtesy of the American College of Mental Health Administrators, Pittsburgh, Pennsylvania.

CoA endorsed the principles and attributes as they related to CoA-accredited organizations that provide behavioral health care services to children and families. However, CoA accredits multiservice organizations that offer a diverse range of programs and services that do not fall under the exclusive domain of behavioral health care. CoA also recognized that its accredited organizations may lack the technical resources to implement performance measures at the same level of scientific rigor and sophistication reflected in the recommendations or attributes above.

The Council supported the attributes as they pertained to measures that focus on providers and emphasize specific health conditions or areas of health. However, with its publication of the Personal Outcome Measures System®, The Council remains strongly committed to measurement efforts that support a holistic approach to outcomes in behavioral health care and human services.

The Joint Commission, through the ORYX initiative, has already incorporated sets of standardized measures into its accreditation process to generate both cross-sectional comparisons and longitudinal analysis. Cross-sectional comparisons are utilized for external and internal accountability and for establishing benchmarks of excellence. Longitudinal analyses monitor and support ongoing quality improvement efforts within the individual health care organizations.

The NCQA's HEDIS is a set of standardized performance measures designed to enable purchasers and consumers to reliably compare the performance of managed care plans. Because the measures are designed to distinguish performance among managed care plans, and because the processes and outcomes of care can be affected by confounding factors over which plans may have little control, NCQA felt that some attributes might be more important than others. These measures can be used to provide valuable information that drives improvement in health care services and better informs consumer decision making.

A CONSENSUS SET OF INDICATORS

Organized according to the three domains—access, process, and outcomes—Tables 10–3 through 10–5 address the proposed indicators of the ACMHA Accrediting Organization Workgroup. These summarized lists not only reflect two years of discussion, debate, and compromise amongst the accrediting organizations, but also incorporate important consumer and other stakeholder comments and suggestions.

In March 1999, yet a third invitational meeting was held in Santa Fe to present the preliminary work of the accrediting organizations. Essentially, the following two questions were asked of the 100+ consumers, family members, purchasers, outcome system vendors, and others in attendance: From the proposed list, (1) What was the most important to measure? and (2) What was feasible? The responses yielded a few consensus ideas and concerns that further guided the workgroup. It became clear that virtually all of the indicators were important, with well-being and other outcomes perhaps at the top of the list. At the same time, there was general acknowledgment that the actual measurement of outcomes might be the most difficult task of all. In addition, consumers stressed the importance of some measure of safety to address their concerns.

Table 10–3 Access . . . Getting into Services

Topic	Concerns/Values	Things to Count	
1. **Services are available.**	Persons served perceive and experience services as available.	a.	**The rate of *persons served reporting* that they receive services they need.**
		b.	The rate of utilization of services at each available level of care expressed in treatment days per thousand of persons eligible for services.
2. **Services are convenient.**	Persons served perceive and experience services as convenient (i.e., available services are well located, offered at convenient hours, etc.).	a.	**The *rate of persons served reporting* that transportation is not a barrier to recovery.**
		b.	Geographic analysis of population-to-provider rates and travel times for behavioral health professionals.
3. **Services are timely.**	Persons served perceive and experience services as timely.	a.	**The *rate of persons reporting* timely response from first request for service to first face-to-face meeting with a mental health professional.**
		b.	**The *rate of persons served reporting* timeliness from a first appointment to a second appointment.**
		c.	The average number of days from first request for service to first face-to-face meeting with a behavioral health professional.
		d.	The average number of days from a first appointment to a second appointment.
4. **Services are provided.**	Services are available and provided to people like me.	a.	**The rate of utilization of services at each available level of care described by meaningful groupings of persons served.**

Source: A Proposed Consensus Set of Indicators for Behavioral Health. Published by the American College of Mental Health Administration in collaboration with the Accreditation Organization Workgroup. Pittsburgh, PA, 2001.

Table 10–4 Process . . . What Happens during Services

Topic	Concerns/Values	Things to Count
1. **Treatment decisions**	Persons served (and families of children and adolescents) participate meaningfully in treatment decisions.	a. **The rate at which persons served report they received useful information to make informed choices about their treatment.** b. The rate of participation in decisions regarding treatment by persons served. c. The rate of participation in decisions regarding treatment by families of children and adolescents when indicated.
2. **Responsiveness**	Services are appropriate to the clinical status of the person served.	a. **The rate of persons served who receive timely face-to-face follow-up care after leaving a 24-hour care setting.** b. The rate of persons served who receive a timely course of treatment following diagnosis of a behavioral health disorder.
3. **Non-coercive treatment**	Whenever possible, treatment should be voluntary and non-coercive.	a. **The rate of persons served who report experiencing treatment as non-coercive.** b. The rate of involuntary treatments. c. The rate of seclusion and restraint.
4. **Experience of care**	Persons served perceive and experience service providers as responsive and sensitive.	a. **The rate at which persons served report they were treated with politeness, respect, and dignity by staff.** b. **The rate at which persons served report feeling hopeful about their recovery.**

continues

Table 10–4 continued

Topic	Concerns/Values	Things to Count
		c. **The rate at which persons served report they were treated with sensitivity to their gender, age, sexual orientation, culture, religious, ethnic, and linguistic background.**
5. Co-occurring illness	Co-occurring mental illness and substance abuse are recognized and treated.	a. The rate of persons served diagnosed with co-occurring mental illness and substance abuse disorders.
6. Safe treatment	Persons served are safe in treatment.	a. **The rate at which persons served report that they feel safe in treatment.**
		b. **The rate at which persons served report that they feel safe in the community.**
		c. The rate of suicide, homicide, and unexpected deaths.

Source: A Proposed Consensus Set of Indicators for Behavioral Health. Published by the American College of Mental Health Administration in collaboration with the Accreditation Organization Workgroup. Pittsburgh, PA, 2001.

The ACMHA Accreditation Organization Workgroup was committed to remaining true to the first value statement: Consumers are at the core of performance measurement. To that end, the Office Support Agency, an Ohio-based consumer-consulting firm, was hired in spring 2000 to conduct a national survey of primary consumers about the relevance of the indicator set. A live satellite telecast initiated the review process, involving over 50 sites in 38 states, which was supported by mail surveys and a Web site for feedback. The consumer consultants also conducted a focus group with key consumer researchers.

The results of this survey process in general endorsed the work to that point, but highlighted several needed changes. The concept of recovery, while embedded in the values and product of the work group, needed more emphasis. In addition, consumer respondents wanted an indicator on transportation. These changes were made and are included in the work group's consensus set.

Table 10–5 Outcomes . . . Results of Services

Topic	Concerns/Values		Things to Count
1. Well-being	Persons served experience an improvement in health and psychological well-being as a result of treatment.	a.	**The rate of persons served who are better, worse, or unchanged at the termination of treatment compared with the initiation of treatment.**
		b.	The rate of persons served who are better, worse, or unchanged *at a standard interval following the termination of treatment* compared with the termination of treatment.
2. Work and school	Persons served are productively involved in work and school.	a.	*For adults:* The rate of employed/unemployed adults counted at the termination of treatment and at a standard interval following the termination of treatment.
		b.	*For employed adults:* The average number of days not worked counted at a standard interval following the termination of treatment.
		c.	*For children:* The average number of missed class days counted at a standard interval following the termination of treatment.
3. Safety	Treatment improves the safety of persons served.	a.	The rate of episodes of victimization reported at a standard interval following the termination of treatment.

continues

Table 10–5 continued

Topic	Concerns/Values	Things to Count
		b. *For persons served who identify victimization or vulnerability as a concern at the initiation of treatment.* The rate of perceived vulnerability measured at the termination of treatment and at a standard interval following the termination of treatment.
4. Legal Involvement	Persons served should be out of trouble with the law.	a. *For persons served who identify problems with the law as a concern at the initiation of treatment:* The rate of arrests, detentions, and/or incarcerations counted at a standard interval following the termination of treatment.
5. Housing	Housing needs are resolved.	a. The rate of domiciled/homeless persons at the termination of treatment and at a standard interval following the termination of treatment.
		b. *For adults who identify housing as a concern at the initiation of treatment:* The rate who report improvement, worsening, or no change in their satisfaction with housing at the termination of treatment and at a standard interval following the termination of treatment.
		c. *For children:* The rate of children at home at the termination of treatment and at a standard interval following the termination of treatment.

Note: For persons served with problems requiring extended treatment, evaluation should be conducted at regular intervals during the course of treatment.

Source: A Proposed Consensus Set of Indicators for Behavioral Health. Published by the American College of Mental Health Administration in collaboration with the Accreditation Organization Workgroup. Pittsburgh, PA, 2001.

The five accrediting organizations faced many tough decisions in making their final selections of indicators for inclusion in a consensus set. This process was influenced in part by the tremendous diversity of systems of care, providers, programs, settings, and populations included in accreditation by the totality of the five. Selecting indicators that were, as much as possible, broadly applicable, relevant, and meaningful across this breadth of services and consumers was a major concern.

As a result, not all concerns are addressed. Items were included by virtue of a combination of importance, broad applicability, and measurement feasibility. Having resolved issues of taxonomy, priority, and definition and considered the desirable attributes, the ACMHA Accreditation Organization Workgroup achieved internal consensus on a set of indicators. This set was intended to be a starting point in bringing congruence and uniformity in measurement efforts to the field. It was not inclusive of all concerns, and the work group acknowledged that much work remained to be done.

The included indicators are presented in a series of three tables, arranged by domain. The tables present the topic, concern, and "things to count" or indicator definition questions, as they were presented in the work group's interim report (ACMHA Accreditation Organization Workgroup, 2001). In the tables, some text appears in bold typeface. This designates items that the work group believes could be measured using a survey instrument to capture the consumer's perception of the experience of care or for which there are some established methodologies for data collection and measurement. Consumer survey–based items are highlighted with italics.

Access

The first domain is access or getting into services. This is a particularly important focus area for assessing the performance of managed care plans. Stakeholders want to be assured that cost savings are not attributable to de facto service denial by barriers to ready access.

The first three areas of concentration within access (availability, convenience, and timeliness) are straightforward. The final topic area (services are provided) is designed to understand how various subpopulations, be they diagnosis related or according to some other dimension such as race, ethnicity, language, etc., are represented in service populations. As methodological issues are raised and resolved, this information will be of great value in developing case-mix adjustment strategies.

Process

The second domain is process, or what happens in the provision of services. The topics addressed here include treatment decision making, responsiveness of service providers, non-coercive treatment, the experience of care, recognition of co-occurring disorders, and consumer safety.

Of special note here are the two items relating to non-coerciveness and safety. As the field has begun to listen to the voices of primary consumers, these issues have achieved greater importance. Seclusion and restraint concerns, along with issues related to involuntary commitment and forced medication, have special significance to psychiatric consumers, especially those served by public systems. The concepts of "sanctuary harm" and "sanctuary trauma" (psychic insults experienced in a place of perceived safety) need to be addressed in the evaluation of provider performance.

Outcomes

Outcomes, the results of care, are the ultimate arbiter of what we accomplish as a field. The well-being, employment, safety, freedom of consumers, and residence are the targets of interventions with persons who have mental and addictive disorders. These final topic areas are reflected in the items in Table 10–5.

These are some of the most critical concerns. Yet these outcome indicators pose some of the more daunting methodological challenges for the reliability and validity of the data collected.

APPLICATION OF THE CONSENSUS SET

Each of the five accrediting organizations has some expectation of data collection and analysis for quality and accountability by accredited providers. Above and beyond compliance or conformance with accreditation standards, providers are expected to measure their performance and use this information to support quality improvement and other activities.

However, each of the organizations incorporates these measurement requirements into its accreditation program differently based on different corporate cultures, stakeholder perspectives, and primary markets. NCQA, as one example, is moving to make accreditation decisions in part based on actual measures of performance. CoA, on the other hand, simply expects its accredited providers to have some ongoing data collection in place.

Regardless of what formal requirements providers face, agreement by the accrediting organizations on what is important to measure should prove to have a profound and far-reaching impact on the field over time. The challenge of reaching agreement on how to measure and collect data remains. However, it is not difficult to imagine that the outcome of this work by the accreditation organizations and ACMHA will be the de facto emergence of a core or common set of indicators for the entire field.

CRITICAL GAPS AND OTHER INITIATIVES

While the ACMHA summit and the Accreditation Organization Workgroup process have been valuable, the work has limitations that should be noted. Chief amongst them is the lack of agreement on measurement and data to operationalize each of the indicators. Because there are many possible measurement strategies, the full potential of the consensus set will not be realized without standardization in data collection and calculation. Without completion of this technical piece, broad application of the indicators, and the ability to make valid and meaningful comparisons across systems and providers, will still not be possible.

Another limitation of this consensus set is that the included indicators may not sufficiently address concerns of children, adolescents, and their families. The presence and participation of child advocates in the ACMHA process were too small to ensure adequate coverage of these concerns. The initial summit document included a special section on outcome indicators for seriously emotionally disturbed children and adolescents, and the work group has maintained contact with the SAMHSA Center for Mental Health Services' Outcomes Roundtable for Children and Families. The roundtable has provided the field with a general model for outcome-based account-ability in three steps: identification of characteristics of children and families, identification of desired outcomes, and identification of the interventions chosen to achieve those outcomes (SAMHSA, 1998). Hernandez and Hodges (2000) report on a recent effort to learn from field experience and provide a series of "lessons" learned from application efforts to measure outcomes for children and families. The first groups of lessons are clustered around planning and design, utilization, and sustainability. The second groups of lessons are grouped according to "lessons from the real world" and "lessons related to an ideal world." In addition, the work of the Health Care Reform Tracking Initiative provides useful insights into the impact of managed behavioral health care on services to children and families (Stroul, Pires, & Armstrong, 1998).

Although the ACMHA work strove to be reflective of the behavioral health field generally, stakeholders in addictive disorders treatment may find that their concerns are not adequately addressed in the consensus set. A process similar to the ACMHA Accreditation Organizations Workgroup is the Washington Circle Group, a group of substance abuse providers, researchers, and policy makers, funded by the Center for Substance Abuse Treatment. This work group has created a framework for considering performance measurement in the addictive disorders domain; it is working with the Schneider School of Health Policy and the Heller School at Brandeis University to develop a set of methodologically sound indicators and measures. The Washington Circle Group (McCory, Garnick, Bartlett, Cotter, & Chalk, 2000) proposes a linked set of four domains as essential for effective performance measurement in the substance abuse/addictive disorders area:

1. Prevention/Education. This domain covers any plan activities designed to raise awareness of substance abuse, including both broad and targeted activities.
2. Recognition. This domain captures case finding, including screening, assessment, and referral.
3. Treatment. This domain captures a broad range of services associated with an episode of care including counseling, medical services, psychiatric and psychological services, social services, and so forth.
4. Maintenance. Sustained, long-term outcomes are the focus of this domain, which includes self-management, peer supports, lifestyle changes, and other indicators (Morris & Hanley, 2000).

Adequate attention to family and children's issues, along with the concerns of substance abuse and addictive disorders treatment stakeholders, is an essential component of any truly comprehensive set of behavioral health care indicators and performance evaluation strategies.

There also have been notable efforts in public sector mental health to address the need for measurement and accountability as public care systems increasingly adopt managed care strategies. In 1997, CMHS administered the five-state feasibility study in which five states were funded to select and pilot performance indicators that would be feasible and meaningful to collect and that could be comparable across states (Ganju & Lutterman, 1998). In a nine-month time frame, five states that were different in size, organization, and geography identified 28 performance indicators to be reported comparably across states. The principal finding of this project was that although states could not report on all the selected indicators, states would be able to report performance measures if given sufficient time and resources.

A more recent effort to develop state performance indicators is the 16-state indicator pilot grant awarded from fiscal year 1998 to 2001, which is a collaborative effort between the CMHS Survey and Analysis Branch and the State Planning and Systems Development Branch (Mazade, Lutterman, & Glover, 1998). The purpose of these grants is to pilot 32 performance indicators selected from the 1997 CMHS five-state feasibility study and the 1998 NASMHPD framework of mental health performance indicators. A significant component of the grant is involvement of all key stakeholder groups in performance indicator planning, piloting, and implementation.

The performance indicators for the state indicator pilot grant address the domains of access of care, quality and appropriateness of mental health services, outcome of mental health services, and structure and plan management of services. The primary objective of the project is to pilot and implement performance indicators on a comparable basis across states and to find the best ways to report these data. Performance indicator data collection includes subgroup information on age (including children), race/ethnicity, gender, and diagnoses as well as data for hospital and community service settings. As appropriate, some indicators focus specifically on children or adults.

Another recent and related effort in the MHSIP program is the state reform grant. These grants have facilitated state efforts in the integration, synthesis, and analysis of information including reporting of performance indicators. This will hopefully help state mental health authorities to use their management information systems more appropriately in decision-making and state planning activities. Forty-five states have been funded for facilitation of these efforts, and this has resulted in increased state reporting of performance indicators for planning of mental health services. The basis of selected performance indicators was the MHSIP consumer-oriented report card in which the domains of access, quality/appropriateness, outcome, and prevention were addressed; many states have implemented the MHSIP consumer survey, as well, to obtain consumer perceptions of mental health services.

OTHER CHALLENGES TO THE FIELD

While consensus on a set of indicators for the field appears to have immediate value in addressing a wide range of stakeholder concerns, there are some particular issues that warrant special attention. These concerns are more about policy, administration, and structure rather than the immediate delivery of services; however, these domains are equally important in the pursuit of quality and accountability. One test of the value of a consensus set of indicators will be the utility and applicability of information to decision making and planning at this level.

There are four essential areas to address:

1. *Parity.* As the issue of parity in insurance coverage for persons with behavioral health disorders gains momentum in national and state policy, there are special challenges in performance measurement. Here we return to the relationship between value, cost, and quality. The critical question for policy makers and voters will be to determine the value added in return for purchasing this benefit. Hopefully competent and credible performance measurement is a source for answers.

2. *Human Resources/Professional Development.* As the behavioral health field further embraces an outcomes orientation, there is a real question as to whether or not the workforce is prepared to respond to the increasing demands for accountability and reporting. There is evidence to suggest that in fact they are not well prepared. This issue is considered in detail in a "call to action" (ACMHA, 2000), and a working paper developed by a group of academic medical centers. The gaps are especially critical in the area of children's mental health, as noted by Morris and Hanley (2000).

3. *Finances.* Given the reality that there are never enough dollars for all desired health care initiatives, who will pay for quality accountability? How are purchasers, consumers, and payers to be convinced to accept the cost burden of performance measurement? The answers to these questions are fraught with complexity. The core response is that it would be irresponsible not to make some effort to ensure that we are

buying quality and value with our health care dollars. Some expenditure on measurement must be redefined and accepted as an integral part of the cost of care. It is likely that the costs of quality accountability will be realized incrementally as initially weak or vague data yield to stronger and more compelling data. When the field is better able to achieve reliable comparative data—a true report card—then the cost-benefit balance of investing in measurement will be more visible. In the interim, all stakeholders will need to make a commitment to pursue the ultimate goal of reliable outcome data, and with this accept the costs of the inevitable false starts and blind alleys. It will probably fall to a few innovators to lead the way, but there are real incentives to take on the challenge. In the competitive managed care environment, plans that can credibly demonstrate performance and quality through data will have a valuable marketing edge.

4. *Measurement Technology.* Success in data-based quality accountability will require the widespread dissemination of sophisticated information systems and technology. The complexity of human beings makes studying the impact and value of interventions extremely difficult. The number of candidate variables in any performance measurement strategy is challenging. Technical specification of measurement strategies will create increased demands for data collection and processing, and achieving standardization presents its own special problems. If the vision of having quality information available to stakeholders is to be realized, clinical care and data management systems will need to be further developed and integrated. The potential of the Internet to address these concerns is substantial, but the needs and strategies must be well articulated.

SUMMARY

In spite of the encouraging evidence of movement toward consensus in the behavioral health community, the distance to an ultimate solution remains great. Mechanic and McAlpine (1999) offer this observation: "Quality measurement in behavioral healthcare is still relatively primitive. In the long run, the accountability of managed care will depend on our ability to develop reasonable consensus on practice standards and quality indicators." As the field pushes for this needed consensus, the enthusiasm for arriving at the goal needs to be moderated by the complexity and immensity of the task. The cautionary message issued by David Eddy (1998) is strong and bears heed: "Today's measures tend to be blunt, expensive, incomplete and distorting. And they can easily be inaccurate and misleading." As the behavioral health care field approaches an inevitable refining of measurement strategies, the challenges need to be faced with humility. Consumer benefits and concerns must come first, but interdependence of all of the stakeholders in this complex endeavor also needs to be acknowledged.

In conclusion, the insight of one of the field's leaders, Dr. Vijay Ganju (1997) is especially cogent: "In the field of behavioral health performance measurement, there has been a great deal of flapping, but *very* little flight." In the coming years, there may be no more significant challenge for the managed behavioral health care field than this: keeping aloft a meaningful and affordable set of performance indicators that genuinely speaks to quality of care for consumers of managed mental health and substance abuse services.

REFERENCES

American College of Mental Health Administration. (2000). Sounding a call to action. *Behavioral Healthcare Tomorrow*, *9*, 3, 43–44.

American College of Mental Health Administration. (2001). *Interim report 2001: A proposed set of consensus indicators for behavioral health*. Pittsburgh, PA: ACMHA.

Donabedian, A. (1980). The definition of quality and approaches to its assessment. In A. Donabedian (Ed.), *Explorations in Quality Assessment and Monitoring: Vol. I*. Ann Arbor, MI: Health Administration Press.

Eddy, D. (1998). Performance measurement: Problems and solutions. *Health Affairs, 17*(4), 7–25.

Ganju, V. (1997). A dialogue on report cards. Paper presented at the Center for Mental Health Services 46th Annual National Mental Health Statistics Meeting, Washington, DC.

Ganju, V., & Lutterman, T. (1998). State mental health agency performance measure initiatives in the public mental health system. In *Mental Health, United States, 1998* (pp. 45–51). DHSS publication no. (SMA) 99-3285. Rockville, MD: Substance Abuse and Mental Health Services Administration.

Hernandez, M., & Hodges, S. (2000). Designing, implementing and using child outcomes measurement systems: Lessons learned in the Chinsegut outcomes retreat. In *Faulkner & Gray, 2000 behavioral outcomes & guidelines sourcebook* (pp. 212–222). New York: Faulkner & Gray.

Kramer, T.L. (1999). Outcomes and guidelines agenda moves forward; but troubling policy issues remain. In *Faulkner & Gray, 1998 behavioral outcomes & guidelines sourcebook.* New York: Faulkner & Gray.

Mazade, N., Lutterman, T., & Glover, R. (1998). State mental health agency performance measure initiatives in the public mental health system. In *Mental health, United States, 1998* (pp. 52–59). DHSS publication no. (SMA) 99-3285. Rockville, MD: Substance Abuse and Mental Health Services Administration.

McCrory, F., Garnick, D.W., Bartlett, J., Cotter, F., & Chalk, M. (2000, March). *Improving performance measurement for alcohol and other drug services.* Report of the Washington Circle Group, SAMHSA, Center for Substance Abuse Treatment. Rockville, MD: TASCON, Inc.

Mechanic, D., & McAlpine, D.D. (1999). Mission unfulfilled: Potholes on the road to mental health parity. *Health Affairs, 18*(5), 7–21.

Morris, J.A. (Ed.). (1998). *Preserving quality and value in the managed care equation: Final report of the 1997 Santa Fe summit.* Pittsburgh: American College of Mental Health Administration.

Morris, J.A. (2000). Policy pinball: Making policy analysis palatable. *Administration and Policy in Mental Health, 28*(2), 131–137.

Morris, J.A., & Hanley, J.H. (2000). Human resource development: A critical gap in child mental health reform. *Administration and Policy in Mental Health, 28*(3), 219–227.

Mrazek, P.J. (1998). *Preventing mental health and substance abuse problems in managed healthcare settings.* Alexandria, VA: National Mental Health Association.

SAMHSA, Center for Mental Health Services. (1998). Building outcome accountability in child mental health and child welfare systems. In *Fitting the pieces together.* Outcomes Roundtable for Children and Families. Rockville, MD: CMHS-SAMHSA.

Stroul, B.A., Pires, S.A., Armstrong, M.I. (1998). *Health care reform tracking project: Tracking state managed care reforms as they affect children and adolescents with behavioral health disorders: 1997 impact analysis.* Tampa, FL: Research Training Center for Children's Mental Health, Department of Child and Family Studies, Division of Local Support, Louise de la Parte Florida Mental Health Institute, University of South Florida.

CHAPTER 11

Consumer Satisfaction Teams and Other Third-Party Independent Accountability Entities

E. Clarke Ross

Purpose: This chapter discusses consumers' distrust of both payers' management agents and providers, cites the professional literature documenting the relationship of consumer satisfaction to positive clinical outcomes, and offers five existing program models of independent third-party entities.

Major Topics: This chapter addresses Consumer Satisfaction Teams, Facility and Program Monitoring Teams, Ombudsman Programs, Binding and Timely Clinical Review, and Validation of Health Plan Performance.

INTRODUCTION

Consumer distrust of both payers' management agents and providers has increased with the advent of managed care. Kondracke (1998) opined, "Fueled by news accounts exposing deaths and lasting health damaged caused by HMOs [health maintenance organizations] denying access to care, even industry lobbyists admit that HMOs are barely more popular than tobacco companies" (p. 5). Blendon and associates (1998) explained the "managed care backlash" as a "negative reaction" that is inevitable on the part of persons and institutions that are affected (p. 80). Two groups founded in the 1980s—the National Association of Psychiatric Survivors and the National Association for Rights Protection and Advocacy—have long distrusted psychiatrists and other mental health providers as generally coercive, involuntary, and inhumane in their treatment of persons with mental illness (Havel, 1992). In the late 1980s, the National Mental Health Consumers Association was founded. Though not as antipsychiatry as the previously named groups, it still stresses surviving treatment and advocates consumer involvement and respect (Havel, 1992).

Rohland, Langbehn, and Rohrer (2000) documented a relationship between service satisfaction and current life satisfaction for persons with schizophrenia, affective disorder, and adjustment disorder, but not for persons with anxiety disorder. Sullivan and Spritzer (1997) established that even though community mental health centers in Mississippi serving persons with schizophrenia—a majority of whom are African American—offer similar services, there were differences in consumer satisfaction ratings by clinic, suggesting that qualities of the clinic itself may influence consumer satisfaction.

In analyzing the relationship between self-reported changes in quality of life, symptomatology, and level of functioning with consumer satisfaction, Holcomb and associates (1998) concluded that "self-reported patient satisfaction is a valid and important outcome measure that should be used in the evaluation of mental health services" (p. 934). Their study "demonstrated a significant relationship between patient satisfaction" (p. 929) and these other patient variables. Druss, Rosenheck, and Stolar (1999) reinforced the findings of Holcomb and colleagues. At the inpatient level, "satisfaction with several aspects of service delivery was associated with fewer readmissions and fewer days readmitted. Better alliance with inpatient staff was associated with higher administrative measures of rates of follow-up, promptness of follow-up, and continuity of outpatient care" (Druss, Rosenheck, & Stolar, 1999, p. 1053). The greater the satisfaction, the higher is the score on administrative measures of promptness and continuity of follow-up. Schur and Berk (1998), in an analysis from the five-state Kaiser/Commonwealth Low Income Survey (1995–1996) found that choice of health plans led to increased satisfaction regardless of which plan was chosen.

Longo and colleagues (1997) documented that the public release of consumer reports is not only useful in assisting consumers to make informed health care choices, but also facilitates improvements in the quality of hospital services offered. The more competitive the market, the more impact the release of quality public consumer reports has. This was not a mental health report; it examined obstetrical services in all Missouri hospitals.

Providers are frequently reluctant to participate in consumer satisfaction surveys. In 1998, a Minnesota project was terminated when Duluth and northeastern Minnesota clinics refused to participate in a consumer satisfaction survey that would have publicly ranked each clinic. The clinics were willing to participate only if the survey results were released in the aggregate ("Minnesota Plan," 1998).

Providers in a community mental health center outcomes-related project did not meaningfully participate in the project. The project managers concluded that the voluntary nature of the project, provider misperceptions about the project's purpose, and provider concerns about confidentiality were factors contributing to the low rate of participation (Clardy, Booth, Smith, Nordquist, & Smith, 1998).

In a study of alcohol and drug abuse treatment programs, McLellan and Hunkeler (1998) found, however, that while "more than 80 percent of patients reported being 'very satisfied' or 'delighted' with virtually all aspects of their substance abuse treatment, no significant relationships were found between the satisfaction measure and either the participation measures at any follow-up point" (p. 575).

Who conducts a consumer interview impacts the level of consumer satisfaction. While overall satisfaction with programs was high regardless of interview, Clark, Scott, Boydell, and Goering (1999) found that "clients gave a significantly greater number of extremely negative responses when they were interviewed by client interviewers" (p. 961).

Campbell (1997) observed that in the midst of all the changes in mental health services delivery, "perhaps the most far reaching is the reconceptualization of the role of the mental health services recipients" (p. 357). Campbell argues that mental health consumers are more significantly involved in service evaluation because "consumer perceptions about effectiveness, satisfaction, and quality of services determine which treatments are sought or complied with and which outcomes are valued" (p. 358). Campbell documented the "growth and acceptance" of researcher–consumer/survivor partnerships in program evaluation.

Finkel (1996) observed the following: "Managed care, if it is to work effectively, relies on an informed consumer. The majority of Americans report that they need a lot more information to help them select a specific health plan and a primary care physician" (p. 85).

The use of independent, third-party consumer and family staffed organizations is basic to health plan enrollees' public policy objective to ensure accountability by all participants in the health care arena—payers, purchasers, health plans, management agents, delivery systems, and providers (Ross, 1998–1999, 1999a, 1999b). At the moment, five types of independent third-party entities receive most of the national attention—consumer satisfaction (dissatisfaction) teams, facility and program monitoring teams, ombudsman programs, binding and timely clinical review, and independent validation of health plan performance data.

CONSUMER SATISFACTION TEAMS

The need to document consumer satisfaction is a core premise of managed care. But who does the documenting is fundamental to the meaningfulness of measures of satisfaction. And the concept itself—satisfaction—is questionable; many advocates feel that dissatisfaction and the health plan's ability to respond immediately to dissatisfaction are much more significant than satisfaction. All health care systems—not just managed care—must incorporate valid mechanisms to document and affirmatively respond to dissatisfaction.

Philadelphia's Approach

One of the very first in the nation, and probably the most advanced in terms of operational experience, is Philadelphia's Consumer Satisfaction Team, Inc. In 1990 the city of Philadelphia, which has been developing a consolidated mental health service system and today operates a citywide single managed behavioral health care system, developed a consumer satisfaction team (CST). The mission of the CST, as articulated by Ferry (1996, 1998), is to try to understand and communicate back to the funder of services what consumers like or do not like about those services. Recognizing that it often takes a long time to build trust with a person with serious and persistent mental illness, the CST in Philadelphia conducts multiple interviews with the same consumer over the course of a year.

CSTs provide written documentation of each consumer visit and hold regular meetings with the payer. With Philadelphia's development of a managed care program in 1996, the CST expanded its responsibility to include consumer outreach and education. Also in 1996, the scope of the CST was broadened to include people with addictive disorders as well as those with serious mental illness.

Most managed care organizations (MCOs) use their own internal marketing or, hopefully, quality assurance teams to determine consumer satisfaction. Whether marketing or quality improvement staff perform the function, they are internal employees of the organization. Marketing staff tend to focus on overall satisfaction, and they assume that when overall rates of satisfaction are high everything is okay. Quality improvement staff tend to focus on areas of operation requiring improvement. This is helpful, but still is skewed by the situation of internal staffing. Some MCOs use outside agencies, most frequently university departments or professional surveying organizations. This practice avoids the internal staffing bias; however, consultants may not fully understand the situations of consumers and family members directly affected by mental illness.

Valerie Byrd of Philadelphia's CST (Ross, 1999b) emphasized that Philadelphia's CST focuses on the value of listening to the consumer while recognizing the importance of the treating professional. Byrd made it clear that, "We do not blame anyone. We point out consumer dissatisfaction. The first visit to a provider is announced. All subsequent visits are unannounced. We want to see the program in its natural environment" (p. 13). This CST is funded directly by the city and county of Philadelphia, and it issues its reports not to the provider, but to the payer, which is the city and county administrating agency. The purchasing agency must ensure provider accountability and responsiveness. Philadelphia's CST assumes that consumers and families will share things with their peers that they will not share with providers or professional reviewers.

Philadelphia's CST uses two-member teams. The two-member teams include one family member and one consumer. Interviewed consumers and providers are not asked to fill out a standardized questionnaire. Instead, CST staff ask questions in a conversational format. Questions can range from patients' treatment goals and how they are being met to whether the MCO has helped them change providers. This approach can prove more enlightening than questions asking consumers to rank services on a scale of 1 to 5.

"It's more about what people want to tell us, rather than what we want to know," says Loretta Ferry, CST's executive director. "I call us reporters rather than evaluators" (Rudd, 1999a, p. 2). To keep the conversational atmosphere with consumers and providers, CST staff do not take notes during an interview. Instead, team members record their findings after leaving a site. Written questionnaires do come into play when CST staff visit partial hospitalization programs, however. But even the simple four-question survey, with questions such as, "What's the best thing about being here?" requires conversational follow-up with consumers to ensure they have understood what was being asked.

Team members are not always allowed to express their opinions to consumers or providers, and CST's hiring works to ensure people do not join looking to settle grudges. "If we do that," Ferry says, "we'll be doing what I always accuse the system of doing: judging for us" (Rudd, 1999a, p. 2). The bottom-line assumption is that satisfied clients are probably using services more cost effectively. Payers and providers better tailor services in response to direct consumer experiences.

Georgia's Approach

With Philadelphia as a model, similar, but different, versions of CSTs have begun in other states—Georgia, Massachusetts, Alabama, and Ohio. The Georgia Evaluation and Satisfaction Team (GEST) is a consumer- and family-staffed independent agency that positions itself as the provider's guest. GEST currently contracts with two of Georgia's regions and directly with provider agencies. With no guaranteed source of income, GEST customizes its services according to the payer's requests. Regional boards in Georgia are responsible for services not only for mental illness and addictive disorders, but also for persons with mental retardation. One GEST contract is for monitoring community care for 80 persons with mental retardation who most recently resided in a 24-hour institutional facility. This contract requires a clinical component, so the monitoring team also employs clinical staff.

In another region of the state, GEST consumer and family staff sit down with providers after their interviews with consumers and families to give them immediate feedback. All interviews are one-on-one encounters. The first provider visit is announced, but subsequent visits are not. Statistical reports are provided to the regional authorities.

Survey instruments are tailored to satisfy GEST's regional board contractors. Consumers and providers are not subjected to a written question sheet calling for simple answers. "We really like to use open-ended questions," explains Ginny Riley, GEST's administrator. "That way, we get what is uppermost in the consumer's mind regarding their quality of life, without presupposing what we think they want to tell us" (Rudd, 1999a, p. 3).

GEST evaluators usually ask consumers 8 to 10 questions along the lines of "What do you like most about the services you receive?" GEST evaluators also talk with program staff to get their take on how services are being delivered.

Evaluation team members are part-time GEST employees. The size of GEST's evaluation teams varies depending on the site. A day-service program with 30 people usually calls for a team of three GEST staff members, while a residential program with only one to four consumers may require only one or two evaluators. Reports from GEST site visits go to the regional board and the site's director.

GEST also handles more involved service monitoring contracts. Those contracts call for GEST to combine site visits with an evaluation of program capabilities. That function includes a checklist approach to gauge performance in such issues as safety, appropriateness, staff training, and record keeping. A GEST leader conducts that portion of the review with program administrators. Under service monitoring contracts, GEST meets with individual consumers face-to-face once a month, with a second mandated contract with a consumer's family members or providers.

Massachusetts' Approach

Rudd (1999a) described the Massachusetts CST within a Medicaid managed mental health program: "Massachusetts mental health officials like the consumer satisfaction team approach so much, they wrote the creation of teams into their contract with the Medicaid carve-out organization Massachusetts Behavioral Health Partnership. With plenty of push from consumer advocacy groups, the Bay State made consumer satisfaction teams part of their performance standard for 1999, with a $400,000 bonus if the Partnership begins the program" (p. 3).

"It's a way to get very valuable input on the services consumers are receiving, both negative and positive," says Laurie Ansorge-Ball, director of the state's mental health and substance abuse program. "The feedback will be very useful to providers and the Partnership in their quality improvement efforts" (Rudd, 1999a, p. 3). Evaluation teams will report to providers and the partnership, which will use the information in its provider network management.

Alabama's Approach

The Alabama Department of Mental Health (DMH), wishing to promote greater accountability through its community mental health centers (CMHCs), developed FACTS—Family and Consumer Team Satisfaction. Operating with a grant from DMH, FACTS has only one full-time staff member, its executive director. Alabama has 24 CMHCs, with a variety of satellite centers, serving the state's 60 counties. The state requires CMHCs to contract with FACTS for review. Each FACTS team consists of a consumer and a family member who are from the location where the interviews are done. All consumer clients are asked the same five questions, and results are reported using a scale of responses. Open-ended questions also are asked, and unsolicited ideas are recorded. The state DMH provides all data analysis and reports to the CMHCs (National Alliance for the Mentally Ill, 1999a).

Ohio's Approach

Ohio operates a program that is more complex and multidimensional than the other states. The Ohio Department of Mental Health directly finances the Consumer Quality Review Team (CQRT), which runs three projects covering 26 Ohio counties. The program is a result of a DMH planning and advisory panel developed for this purpose. Two of the projects cover adults with severe mental illness, while the third covers children's services in metro Cincinnati.

CQRT does not perform consumer satisfaction per se, but instead studies service delivery. CQRT teams, composed equally of consumers, families, and providers, evaluate availability, accessibility, acceptability, and appropriateness of service delivery. Much of the evaluation is performed using focus groups. CQRT maintains evaluation findings on satisfaction, cultural competence, consumer knowledge, service utilization, family inclusion, staffing, referrals, and housing. As reported by Rudd (1999b), the state-funded teams include consumers and family members, who pair up to conduct face-to-face interviews with consumers. Team members pose questions on four quality-related areas: accessibility, availability, appropriateness, and acceptability. Teams also interview mental health providers and family members.

Queries are split evenly between closed- and open-ended questions. The state hired a researcher to help team members analyze and quantify answers from open-ended questions. The researcher and team members have developed methods for codifying answers and translating them into workable information.

The teams submit reports to the local mental health boards, which manage local services. Team members meet with the boards to explain the finding via Microsoft PowerPoint presentations and discuss possible system improvements. "Consumers are not only identifying problems, but identifying solutions," Townsend says (Rudd, 1999b, p. 4). Reports also go to the National Alliance for the Mentally Ill (NAMI) of Ohio, which combines reports from the three consumer quality evaluation team programs into a single report for the state. The key finding of the April 1999 report (Rudd, 1999c) was that while consumers were very satisfied overall with the public mental health system, the quality of their treatment was problematic. Consumers also were poorly informed about the availability of services and the treatment options available.

Other Efforts

The U.S. Department of Health and Human Services Office of Inspector General (2000) recommended that Medicaid managed mental health programs "establish independent, third party mental health systems for conducting beneficiary satisfaction survey" (p. 2). Notably, efforts also are under way in South Carolina, Michigan, and California.

FACILITY AND PROGRAM MONITORING TEAMS

At least four states (NAMI, 1999b) have developed independent, third-party consumer and family groups that monitor state psychiatric hospitals. All four of these groups are operated by chapters of the NAMI. These states are Delaware, New Hampshire, Oklahoma, and Pennsylvania. Efforts also have been made in Massachusetts and New Jersey.

The U.S. General Accounting Office (1999) concluded: "Advocates and state administrators we interviewed often expressed the view that the most effective monitoring system involves a combination of internal and external oversight" (p. 21). The General Accounting Office further observed:

External monitors complement internal quality control systems by providing an independent perspective. In addition to accreditation or state licensing surveyors and P&As [Protection and Advocacy agencies], some states allow trained lay monitors to visit mental health facilities unannounced and assess environmental conditions. In Delaware, for example, if a monitor reports a concern about conditions in the state psychiatric hospital, the facility must respond within 10 days. Because staff at the facilities know the reports are reviewed and acted on by management, they sometimes inform monitors about concerns that affect patient care, such as low staffing. In some cases, courts have appointed independent monitors to ensure compliance with specific requirements and safeguarding of basic patients rights in facilities that have had serious problems. (p. 21)

Each monitoring team negotiates a voluntary agreement with the state mental health authority (SMHA). Consequently, the operational details for each state differ. None of the monitors are allowed to see patient records. While monitors may come any hour of any day, in Delaware and Oklahoma hospital staff escorts must accompany monitors. In Delaware and Oklahoma, monitors are assigned to specific units or wards for fixed periods of time. While all states have monitor training programs, Delaware and Oklahoma have mandatory four-hour training programs that must cover a fixed set of issues.

While three of the states prohibit payment of volunteer monitors, Pennsylvania pays each volunteer for his or her time. While all four states have consumer and family teams administered by the state NAMI chapter, Pennsylvania also funds an independent exclusive primary consumer monitoring team.

While three of the states allow monitors to work freely and independently, Oklahoma monitors work in teams of two. While Delaware prohibits monitors from discussing personal questions or personal situations with facility residents, Oklahoma requires that all facility residents be interviewed a minimum of three separate times by facility monitors. While three states do not permit monitors to be involved with overseeing treatment, in Pennsylvania monitors actually meet with treatment teams. While most require monitors to wear hospital identification badges, Delaware monitors wear a special NAMI identification badge. While three of the states allow monitors to go anywhere in the hospital, Delaware prohibits monitors from entering security areas.

While the Protection and Advocacy (P&A) Agency (a federally financed legal rights agency in all 50 states) in New Hampshire routinely sees hospital monitoring reports, in Delaware the P&A has to file a Freedom of Information Act request to see the reports. New Hampshire reports are made to the hospital; the monitors meet monthly with the SMHA and quarterly with hospital administration. In Delaware, all monitor reports are posted in the ward/unit being monitored. In Pennsylvania, hospital monitoring teams receive monthly reports on each unit and each ward of such incidents as restraint and seclusion use. Delaware monitors see medication profiles in the aggregate for the hospital.

OMBUDSMAN PROGRAMS*

Ombudsman programs, particularly those in managed care, have two purposes: (1) help consumers navigate administrative processes and (2) help consumers resolve grievances (Gately, 1999). Gately outlines five key responsibilities:

1. Educate prospective enrollees about their options.
2. Educate current enrollees on their rights and responsibilities.
3. Provide assistance to consumers who have problems navigating the health or mental health system.
4. Collect and analyze comprehensive information regarding the true scope of consumers' problems with access to quality services, as well as the health plan's strengths and weaknesses in addressing the problems.
5. Work with all components of the health care system.

Following these potential responsibilities Gately concludes: "Few exist to date, and those that are currently operating are considered experiments, are under-funded, are under-staffed, and have not yet established a track record" (p. 1).

The U.S. Congress established a federally financed long-term care ombudsman program in every state of the nation that is primarily focused on nursing homes. In 1995 these programs investigated 218,000 com-

---

*Portions of this text are reprinted with permission from J. Gatley, *Mental Health Ombudsman Programs: Working to Improve Mental Health Delivery Systems for Consumers*, © 1999, National Mental Health Association.

plaints made by 162,000 individuals residing in nursing homes and board and care homes (Gately, 1999).

Eighteen states, through their DMH, operate mental health ombudsman programs. These states are Alabama, Arizona, Arkansas, Colorado, Connecticut, Indiana, Louisiana, Massachusetts, Maine, Michigan, Minnesota, Montana, New Jersey, Ohio, Oklahoma, Rhode Island, Tennessee, and Washington (Gately, 1999). Five states have general ombudsman programs that include mental health—California, Florida, Oregon, Utah, and Wisconsin—but three of these (California, Florida, and Wisconsin) are just operative in some counties (Gately, 1999).

Gately outlines 11 ingredients for success. They are as follows:

1. A clear definition of the population to be served
2. A clear understanding of the services to be provided
3. Adequate funding
4. Independence from overseeing bodies and health plans (Indiana and Tennessee Mental Health Associations hold contracts to provide ombudsman services)
5. Staff and volunteers who are well trained and have a grounding in advocacy
6. Up-to-date technology to track and analyze complaints
7. Effective coordination with health plans, purchasers, regulators, and other consumer assistance programs
8. Systematic sharing of strategies with other ombudsman programs
9. Access to legal and mental health expertise
10. Regular consumer satisfaction surveys
11. Formal evaluations

The National Mental Health Association (Gately, 1999) recommends four existing ombudsman programs as the most effective ones—Colorado (created by the State Mental Health Planning Council), Indiana (created by legislation to serve persons discharged from state institutions), Tennessee, and Washington State.

Ombudsman programs are clearly needed. In October 1998, NAMI tabulated the results of its second annual survey of member views about experiences with managed care. The number one finding was that 55% of survey respondents did not know how to file an appeal. Obviously, consumer education has been grossly inadequate, and all parties in health care must develop more concentrated programs to educate health plan enrollees about their opportunities and rights to file grievances and appeals (Ross, 1999a).

BINDING AND TIMELY CLINICAL REVIEW

Another technique to protect the interests of health plan enrollees is the use of third-party independent entities to decide clinical conflicts between health plan utilization reviewers and treating clinicians. As of June 29, 1999, 29 states mandated such entities (National Conference, 1999).

In July 1999, the National Association of Insurance Commissioners (NAIC) recommended the following components to external review legislation:

- Reviews should be binding
- For emergencies, decisions should be made within 72 hours
- Decisions should be based on:
  - patient's medical records
  - physician's recommendation
  - consulting reports from health care professionals
  - health plan's terms of coverage
  - practice guidelines
  - plan's clinical review guidelines
- If patients are required to pay review fees, the fee should not exceed $25.00; it should be waived for those who cannot afford it

The Georgetown University Law Center (1999) identified the following kinds of external reviewers mandated by state laws:

- Regulatory agency is the reviewer or selects the reviewer: Five states
- Independent review organizations (IROs) are selected by the state— health plan or consumer chooses (in Rhode Island the consumer selects the reviewer from this state-approved IRO list): Five states
- Plans contract directly with the IRO: One state
- IROs are accredited by a state-recognized nonprofit organization, health plan chooses: One state

The U.S. Congress is considering national managed care patient protection legislation. Both the Senate and the House of Representatives have passed such legislation. The Senate legislation, though less protective than most consumer groups desire, is viewed as stronger than the House legislation. The Senate-passed provision (1999) reads as follows:

> Enrollee shall have access to an independent external review with respect to an adverse coverage determination (denial of coverage or reimbursement) if such service exceeds a significant financial threshold or if there is a significant risk of placing the life or health of the enrollee in jeopardy. The enrollee must exhaust the internal appeals process. Within 5 working days the plan must select an external appeals entity and provide notice to the enrollee. Information shall be forwarded to the external review within 5 days. The health plan shall select the external review entity (recognized by the state, under contract with the federal government, recognized by the federal government, or accredited as such an entity). The reviewer shall be identified within 30 days, the review performed within 72 hours after identification, and the review completed within 30 days after identification. The determination shall be binding. Process may be speeded up given "the medical exigencies of the case" and in emergencies must be completed within the 72 hours. Decisions must be based on the health plan's definition of medical necessity. (Section 121[e])

INDEPENDENT VALIDATION OF HEALTH PLAN PERFORMANCE DATA

In 2000, the National Committee for Quality Assurance (NCQA) required that health plans submitting Health Plan Employer Data and Information Set (HEDIS) performance information data have such data independently validated to ensure credibility with the public.

CONCLUSION

The mechanisms discussed in this chapter—consumer satisfaction/ dissatisfaction teams, facility and program monitoring teams, ombudsman programs, independent clinical review, and validation of performance data—all use independent third parties to overcome the distrust of health plans and their management agents. They are all mechanisms intended to restore confidence in managed care entities.

REFERENCES

Blendon, R.J., Brodie, M., Benson, J.M., Altman, D.E., Levitt, L., Hoff, T., & Hugick, L. (1998, July–August). Understanding the managed care backlash. *Health Affairs, 17*(4), 80–94.

Campbell, J. (1997, June). How consumers/survivors are evaluating the quality of psychiatric care. *Evaluation Review, 21*(3), 357–363.

Clardy, J.A., Booth, B.M., Smith, L.G., Nordquist, C.R., & Smith, G.R. (1998, February). Implementing a statewide outcomes management system for consumers of public mental health services. *Psychiatric Services, 49*(2), 191–195.

Clark, C.C., Scott, E.A., Boydell, K.M., & Goering, P. (1999, July). Effects of client interviewers on client-reported satisfaction with mental health services. *Psychiatric Services, 50*(7), 961–963.

Druss, B.G., Rosenheck, R.A., & Stolar, M. (1999, August). Patient satisfaction and administrative measures as indicators of the quality of mental health care. *Psychiatric Services, 50*(8), 1053–1058.

Ferry, L. (1996, November/December). Ensuring consumer satisfaction. *Behavioral Health Management*, 15–17.

Ferry, L. (1998, March/April). Involving consumers and families in managed care. *Behavioral Health Management*, 34–37.

Finkel, M.L. (1996). *Health care cost management: A basic guide*. Brookfield, WI: International Foundation of Employee Benefit Plans.

Gately, J. (1999, June). *Mental health ombudsman programs: Working to improve mental health delivery systems for consumers*. Alexandria, VA: National Mental Health Association.

Georgetown University Law Center, Institute for Health Care Research. (1999, November). *External review of health plan decisions: An overview*. Washington, DC: IHCR.

Havel, J.T. (1992, September). Associations and public interest groups as advocates. *Administration and Policy in Mental Health*, 27–44.

Holcomb, W.R., Parker, J.C., Leong, G.B., Thiele, J., & Higdon, J. (1998, July). Consumer satisfaction and self-reported treatment outcomes among psychiatric inpatients. *Psychiatric Services, 49*(7), 929–934.

Kondracke, M. (1998, April 20). Congress is likely to avoid both bad and good on HMOs. *Roll Call*, 5.

Longo, D.R., Land, G., Schramm, W., Fraas, J., Hoskins, B., & Howell, V. (1997, November). Consumer reports in health care: Do they make a difference in patient care? *Journal of the American Medical Association, 278*(19), 1579–1584.

McLellan, A.T, & Hunkeler, E. (1998, May). Patient satisfaction and outcomes in alcohol and drug abuse treatment. *Psychiatric Services, 49*(5), 573–575.

Minnesota plan to measure consumer satisfaction at clinic level fails to get providers' support. (1998, May). *State Health Watch, 2.*

National Alliance for the Mentally Ill. (1999a, September 21). Consumer satisfaction teams. Briefing of U.S. Health Care Financing Administration headquarters staff, HCFA headquarters, Baltimore, MD.

National Alliance for the Mentally Ill. (1999b, September 28). Facility monitoring teams. Briefing of U.S. Health Care Financing Administration headquarters staff, HCFA headquarters, Baltimore, MD.

National Association of Insurance Commissioners. (1999, July 15). *Independent external clinical review, working group recommendations.* Kansas City, MO: NAIC.

National Committee for Quality Assurance. (1999). *HEDIS 2000.* Washington, DC: NCQA.

National Conference of State Legislatures. (1999, June 29). 29 States mandate external appeals [Press Release]. Washington, DC: NCSL.

Rohland, B.M., Langbehn, D.R., & Roher, J.E. (2000, February). Relationship between service effectiveness and satisfaction among persons receiving Medicaid mental health services. *Psychiatric Services, 51*(2), 248–250.

Ross, E.C. (1998–1999, December–January). Consumer staffed monitoring teams in managed care assessment. *NAMI Advocate,* 10.

Ross, E.C. (1999a, March 11). Using independent entities to ensure accountability in managed behavioral health care. *Managed Behavioral Health News,* 6–7.

Ross, E.C. (1999b, August–September). Consumer satisfaction teams ensure accountability. *NAMI Advocate,* 12–13.

Rudd, T. (1999a, March 25). Consumer satisfaction teams take off; payers boost quality management. *Managed Behavioral Health News,* 1–4.

Rudd, T. (1999b, April 22). Consumer survey teams help performance monitoring. *Managed Behavioral Health News,* 2–5.

Rudd, T. (1999c, April 29). Follow seven steps to form consumer evaluation teams. *Managed Behavioral Health News,* 5.

Schur, C.L., & Berk, M.L. (1998, Fall). Choice of health plan: Implications for access and satisfaction. *Health Care Financing Review, 20*(1), 29–43.

Sullivan, G., & Spritzer, K.L. (1997). Consumer satisfaction with CMHC services. *Community Mental Health Journal, 33,* 123–131.

U.S. Department of Health and Human Services, Office of Inspector General. (2000, January). *Mandatory managed care: Changes in Medicaid mental health services.* OEI-04-97-00340. Washington, DC: U.S. Department of Health and Human Services, Office of Inspector General.

U.S. General Accounting Office. (1999, September). *Mental health: Improper restraint or seclusion use places people at risk.* GAO-HEHS-99–176. Washington, DC: GAO.

U.S. Senate. (1999, July 15). Patients' Bill of Rights Plus Act. S. 1344.

CHAPTER 12

Can Provider-Sponsored Organizations Successfully Manage Care?

Allen S. Daniels and Charles G. Ray

Purpose: This chapter examines the experiences of provider-sponsored systems of care in managing care.

Major Topics: This chapter discusses the evolution of provider-sponsored organizations including Provider Participation, Financial Mechanisms, Benefit Options, Controls, and Sponsors. It reviews the stages of development and the structures of management (Network Development, Delivery Systems, Credentialing, Member Services, Access and Triage, Utilization Management, Information Management, Quality Improvement, Claims Adjudication, Finance and Contract Management, and Marketing and Business Development). The chapter also presents survey results from provider-sponsored organizations. The authors conclude that provider-sponsored organizations are successful in their efforts to manage care.

INTRODUCTION

In recent years, there have been myriad evolving organizations responsible for the management of behavioral health care. These organizations have developed throughout the spectrum of stakeholders including both providers and payers. Based on the experiences of these organizations and the rapidly changing health care marketplace, a fundamental question arises: Can providers of care successfully manage care? The evaluation of this issue must be expanded to include provider-sponsored systems of care, and their ability in both the public and private sector to manage care.

313

Managed care in its most basic definition represents an approach that superimposed organizational structure, control, measurement, and accountability on the health care system to effect a balance in the utilization of health care resources, cost containment, and quality or value. The rationalizing of the balance between access to care, the cost elements of care, and quality parameters have been traditionally controlled in the commercial sector through the three-legged stool of finance, benefit design, and the resulting delivery system components. The rapid movement of public payers into managed care methodologies in the mid-1990s introduced a fourth element, public policy interests. An additional fifth component is in the emerging stage; it is characterized by recent legislative health care reform initiatives that foster increased consumer rights in managed health care.

The traditional fee-for-service environment generated clinical practices, administrative structures, and financial mechanisms that were 180° out of alignment with the concepts of managed and organized care. Providers in the acute, intermediate, and long-term segments of health care were incentivized to produce billable encounters or "clinical widgets" in order to maximize revenue. Providers were not paid based on "outcomes" but on treatment encounters. The financial systems required in such an environment were retrospective audit and accountability systems that yielded little applicability toward proactive clinical or administrative management. Quality assurance mechanisms tended to be retrospective, audit-based approaches that utilized focused studies, clinical tripwires, and other post hoc indicators. Provider organizations were production driven, reactive, and tightly constricted as to where, how, and under what circumstances services could be provided. The introduction of prospective payment and the assumption of financial risk have introduced dramatic new challenges and opportunities for community-based providers. As noted above, the concepts of managed care attempt to superimpose a structure of standards measurement and accountability over the formerly fragmented fee-for-service system with an additional element of increasing financial and clinical risk for providers.

The current and anticipated health care environment, both public and commercial, is driven by the following trends:

- Intensifying pressures for both managed care organizations and provider-based organizations to achieve economies of scale and risk-bearing capability through mergers, consolidations, and acquisitions

- Growing focus on the integration of behavioral health care and primary health care
- Adapting and adopting of managed health care concepts by public sector payers
- Increasing numbers of uninsured individuals and families placing additional burdens on already underfunded public systems and fostering cost-shifting in the commercial arena

THE EVOLUTION OF PROVIDER-SPONSORED ORGANIZATIONS

The factors outlined above have altered the roles of providers in managed care. Some of these elements have contributed to the evolving roles that providers have adopted to meet these changes. One result is the development of provider-sponsored organizations (PSOs) for the management of behavioral health care. These organizations have developed along a parallel track with carve-out managed behavioral health care organizations (MBHOs). The principal feature that distinguishes an MBHO from a PSO is the role and direction of providers in the ownership and management of the entity. In both the public and private sector, providers have assumed the functions and roles for the management of care and the financial risk for the delivery of services.

The factors that have shaped the evolution of health care and its management in behavioral health care provide a framework to examine the evolution of PSOs and their structural requirements. These factors are significant for their impact on the systems that manage care and the providers that deliver the services. These factors include provider participation in managed care plans, financial mechanisms for the reimbursement and management of care, the structure and evolution of benefit plans, controls on the practice of behavioral health care, and the sponsors or purchasers of care.

Provider Participation

Provider access to organized systems of care has been an issue throughout the evolution of managed care programs. The development of credentialing and accreditation standards, the creation of select panels by managed care organizations, and the establishment of discounted reimbursement systems have significantly impacted the role of providers in managed care. This influence has been seen in both commercial and public systems of care. The trend toward selective contracting, delegated care management, and the assignment of risk or preferential referral patterns to designated core providers has led to new roles for providers.

Financial Mechanisms

In recent years, the various reimbursement models have been powerful drivers of health care delivery systems. Discounts and financial and clinical risk coupled with control of access are critical and essential elements in the design of managed care programs. Early generations of managed care were based on aggressive discounts off usual and customary rates, negotiated per diems for facilities, and capitation arrangements for large-volume contracts of covered lives. Successive market changes have seen the introduction of per-episode or per-case rates and subcapitation, generally between larger health organizations and smaller specialty providers. The allocation of a percentage of premium dollars for specialty care also has been introduced. Each of these financial models carries a risk to providers. These risks include discounting and under-costing services; overutilization, given higher acuity or adverse selection of risk-covered populations; or discounts that are coupled to withhold models that result in the inability to control cash flow and predictability of revenues.

Structure and Evolution of Benefit Plans

The evolution of the definition of covered benefits, medical necessity criteria, structures of copayment, and exclusions and lifetime limits is among the most profound components in the contemporary health care environment. These features are uniquely important in both the public and private sectors. For the public mental health systems, dealing with chronically and persistently, physically and behaviorally ill individuals creates a need for a comprehensive benefit that incorporates medical and social requirements. These services are built on a legal entitlement to "all Medicaid necessary care." As a result, profound and complex design management issues have occurred in many public systems. In commercial health plans the behavioral health benefit options are often limited and exclude parity with other health benefits. The design of benefits is a vital issue for providers.

Controls

Controls have generally evolved as utilization management and review techniques. The spectrum of these controls includes preauthorization, second opinion, and concurrent reviews to a complex array of inpatient, outpatient, and referral authorizations. Treatment protocols, case management, claims review, provider privileging, and selected credentialing criteria also have been used as control mechanisms. Regrettably, in some managed care programs providers are hampered by an overlay of control mechanisms, standards, and accountabilities that add an extended burden of responsibility with a decline in reimbursements. As provider groups assume greater management responsibility, this presents a problem for the management of care and the promotion of provider efficiency.

Sponsors or Purchasers of Care

The role of sponsors or purchasers of health care also has evolved over successive generations in managed care. During the early 1980s employers and purchasers primarily used the traditional models of indemnity plans, small emerging health maintenance organizations (HMOs), and the service providers themselves. Community-based systems in strong "home rule" states were largely funded and managed through county-based programs. In the recent past there has been a proliferation of models that have included HMOs, preferred provider organizations (PPOs), and other managed plans.

Future Directions

The current and future environment projects an extraordinarily hybridized mix of organizations that performs functions commonly associated with health insuring organizations. These include behavioral health carve-out organizations, horizontally and vertically integrated health care delivery systems, and regional networks of providers. These organizations can be risk-bearing entities, which will contract and deliver health care either through subsidiaries, networks, or other alliances. Public sector designs have embraced partnerships between government and commercial organizations with various risk-sharing arrangements.

THE SUCCESS OF PROVIDER-SPONSORED ORGANIZATIONS

As noted above, the success or failure of organized health systems is predicated on a precarious balance between access, cost, and quality. The interplay of capital resources, the benefit designs, medical necessity criteria, and the restructuring of the service delivery system to both bear risk and meet accountability standards is critical to successful outcomes. The restructuring of publicly supported systems is complicated by the traditional tensions between federal, state, and county governments and public interests.

The future for provider-based organizations (both profit and nonprofit) is not necessarily bleak provided they have adequate capital resources and can develop programs and services appropriate to their market. Provider organizations have generally developed the attributes necessary to accept delegated responsibilities for the management of care over time. Generally, these organizations demonstrate better coordination with other elements of the health care and community-based systems, and they are attentive to consumer needs.

Additional strengths for provider-sponsored organizations include their ability to build multidisciplinary staffs, teams, or networks. A true biopsychosocial approach may enhance their ability to integrate with primary, other specialty, and mainstream health care systems. This is due in part to providers having a primary role in the organization and their commitment to the growth and evolution of the organization.

STAGES OF DEVELOPMENT FROM SERVICE DELIVERY (PROVIDERS) TO MANAGED BEHAVIORAL HEALTH CARE ORGANIZATIONS (PSOs)

There are common steps that many PSOs follow in the development of care management attributes and organizational sophistication. These stages are discussed in the paragraphs that follow.

MBHOs have been developed in both the public and private sectors. Both payer and provider systems have developed these organizations. In either case the fundamental components are generally similar (Zieman, 1998). It also is possible to chart the common stages of development for provider-sponsored managed care systems. This is the process of moving from isolated provider systems to a structured MBHO. This process of development can be divided into six stages. While these steps are generally similar for most organizations, the timeline for the progression through these steps can be different due to opportunity and process.

The initial level involves the integration of delivery system resources (i.e., the provider or service delivery systems that will embark on the course to develop managed care capabilities). Most service delivery systems are designed to accommodate the access of patients and consumers into the necessary care. The availability of various levels of care will be dependent on the complexity of the service delivery system. At the early stages of evolution, this care may be provided in isolated sites with little system integration. The provider system is designed to provide its own level of care, and the organizational structures are designed to support this as well as the billing and collection for these services.

At the second level of development the service providers move from independent practitioners to become an organized system of care. It includes the development of the organizational structures that are capable of facilitating the integration of levels of care and operations. This can be in community-based systems or networks of providers or facilities. In either case a central organizing entity begins to emerge that facilitates this integration. The development of integration may include quality improvement programs, centralized information systems, or clinical programs. As these integrated systems develop they will frequently establish relationships with payers and purchasers of care. These may include insurance companies, behavioral carve-out systems, and community or state and federal programs.

Based on the establishment of these relationships with purchasers of care the newly integrated delivery system is now capable of accepting an enhanced level of responsibility for the process of care management. In this third stage, the organization is now able to perform selected functions that might include utilization management or quality improvement. Initially, these services may be limited to the internal programs of the delivery system. As the organization evolves it gains the capacity to increase the level of operation and assume broader responsibility across delivery systems.

As evolving service delivery systems gain the capacity to perform core managed care functions, then movement to the next level of development is possible. In the fourth stage the organization is able to accept delegated responsibility for certain functions. This contractual agreement transfers the responsibility for designated functions to be performed by the integrated system. A common course of development is for these to begin with the delegation of utilization management or quality improvement and expand over a course of successful performance.

The fifth level of development involves the integrated provider system becoming an MBHO. It is now able to accept more comprehensive levels of contracting. The organization is now able to assume the management of predefined populations, and it is able to accept financial risk for the treatment needs of the population. The ability to assume risk may be comprehensive or targeted to case performance or designated levels of care. A comprehensive review of the core functions necessary to achieve this level of operation also will help to provide a road map for this organizational development.

The final level of development is achieved when the organization receives accreditation or certification as an MBHO. This external validation of the comprehensive spectrum of resources certifies that the program is able to meet its contractual requirements in a consistent and measurable fashion. For commercial programs this accreditation may be by the National Committee for Quality Assurance, the Joint Commission on Accreditation of Healthcare Organizations, or other accrediting bodies.

The course of development from a service provider to an organized delivery system and eventually to an MBHO follows a generally consistent course. However, it will always have unique features including the starting point of the delivery system and local market conditions. This course also will vary due to the market influences of existing managed care programs, competition, the populations served, and state and federal laws.

There are certain core functions that are necessary for an MBHO to sustain comprehensive operations. The following review provides a framework to assess the capacity of provider systems to manage care and assume comprehensive risk for pre-defined populations.

THE STRUCTURE OF MANAGED BEHAVIORAL HEALTH CARE ORGANIZATIONS

The development and operation of MBHOs involve ten strategic components. These key elements are sometimes combined within operational units, but must be present to provide the framework for the process of managing care for defined populations (Daniels, Zieman, Kramer, & Furgal, 1997).They include network development and delivery system, credentialing, member services, access and triage, utilization management, information systems, quality improvement, claims adjudication, finance and contract management, and marketing and business development. An examination of these central components provides a framework to evaluate the structure and operation of provider-sponsored MBHOs. Within the review of each of these structural components the challenges for PSOs are examined.

Network Development and Delivery System

In order to be able to provide care for a defined population, an MBHO requires a well-developed provider network and delivery system. It can take a number of forms, and various models have been used. Two of the more common approaches are the staff and network models. In a staff model the members of the defined population are cared for in organized systems of care, which are run by the organization. The staff in these programs constitute the delivery system. In a network model, an organized panel of providers and facilities provides care. In many cases the delivery system may be a mix of these two models.

Challenges for PSOs: A comprehensive delivery system must include all levels of care and be geographically accessible. This continuum includes outpatient, partial, and inpatient levels of care for mental health and chemical dependency. For provider-sponsored organizations the difficulty arises when clinical resources are needed beyond the scope of the founding organization. For community-based programs, there also are social system needs that must be developed.

Credentialing

The cornerstone of a well-developed network is the credentialing process for all providers. NCQA has established standards for credentialing providers in managed care networks (NCQA, 1998). This review customarily includes the primary source verification of graduate training, professional licensure, malpractice coverage, any history of claims against a provider, and site reviews. This review certifies that the location of practice is accessible to all people and that certain safety standards including fire detection and prevention are met. A review of medical records also can be a part of the initial process, and it is required for recertification.

Challenges for PSOs: For these organizations, an established credentialing committee is established and customarily reviews and grants provider status. The development of a network can be an expensive undertaking for a PSO. The cost of credentialing applications and primary source verification for an individual provider is between $50 and $100 per two-year cycle. In addition, a site visit for each provider including medical record review can cost between $50 and $150 per provider. Therefore, an established network can require significant capital investment.

Member Services

In order to meet the needs of a defined population it is imperative to have a system of member services. This component is responsible for the day-to-day questions and service issues that arise among the constituent members. Generally, this is a telephone-based service. However, some MBHOs are exploring Internet-based customer services. Some MBHOs also have incorporated customer services into their clinical access components.

Challenges for PSOs: There are significant differences between the level of customer service for provider groups and managed care organizations. This level of service requires additional information resources to support benefits information, review claims payment, and provide other member assistance. In some PSOs, enhanced scheduling also is available.

Access and Triage

The principal responsibility of any organization that is managing care is to provide rapid access to those individuals who need care. This is a 24-hour per day, 7-day a week commitment of service. Established standards for access include urgent, emergent, and routine care. In order for a provider group or MBHO to manage care there must be a commitment to this level of service. Some provider organizations accomplish this through facility-based emergency departments. Other programs utilize rapid access assessment teams who are able to evaluate and triage patients to the correct service disposition.

Challenges for PSOs: The triage and referral for services are essential aspects of managed care systems. For PSOs the challenge is to develop the availability of these services to support evaluation and referral to comprehensive levels of care. The access and triage system can be linked to the utilization management program, which is usually a new program for PSOs.

Utilization Management

The management of care requires an established set of criteria for determining the level and scope of care to be provided. The utilization management (UM) program provides this resource. UM decisions must be available 24 hours a day, and they are frequently linked to the access and triage systems. In most managed care programs, clinicians at any level can issue authorizations and approvals. However, in order for a denial of care to be made, a physician must make that determination.

There are several steps in the development of a UM program. First, it is necessary to identify a set of level-of-care guidelines. These can be a commercially purchased set or internally developed. In either case they should be based on commonly agreed-upon criteria, and they should be broadly available to all providers of care in the system. In addition, there should be a mechanism in place to determine that all UM decisions are consistently made among the staff.

Challenges for PSOs: The principal challenges for PSOs center around their ability to provide self-oversight. The development of UM systems requires clinicians to develop mechanisms to examine the work of their peers and authorize or deny the proposed course of treatment. There is a tendency to avoid difficult or contentious clinical reviews among colleagues. This can result in inconsistencies in the clinical review process.

Information Systems

There are data tracking requirements that are present in any managed behavioral health care organization. These are different from the elements frequently found in provider systems. For managing care, there is the necessity to track the enrollment of the covered population. In order to track episodes of care, information systems also must have the capacity to generate referrals and monitor authorizations. These are tied to the scope of covered benefits and track the network provider who is authorized to provide the care. This process also is linked to the UM decision and may be the source to record these decisions. Once a referral is authorized and care is provided, the information system also must be capable of adjudicating a claim. In this process the information system matches a claim for payment with an authorized provider and an approved level of care. The final component of the information system is the generation of reports. These are generally linked to both financial management and the quality improvement program.

Challenges for PSOs: The purchase or development of an information system capable of managing care can be an expensive proposition for a provider system or an MBHO. This represents a major capital expense of both hardware and software. This can be a prohibitive investment for some organizations. In addition, since each program is different, there are customizations needed for each system.

Quality Improvement

Quality improvement (QI) has become a fundamental component of managed care programs. A number of accreditation programs have developed within the managed health care field. A comprehensive program will have an organizational structure with a QI plan and target activity for the program.

Challenges for PSOs: The development of a comprehensive program requires a high level of organizational commitment. This includes the dedication of the necessary resources to evaluate, propose improvements to the program, and assess the impact of the changes on the program. This can be an expensive commitment of resources for an organization to bear. In addition, an accreditation evaluation can be extremely costly.

Claims Adjudication

While delivery systems are accustomed to providing care and billing for these services, the adjudication of claims can be a different process. For an organization that is assuming risk for the services provided by an established network, it will be necessary to develop the capacity to adjudicate and pay claims. This can either be done internally or contracted through a third-party administrator.

Challenges for PSOs: An important issue that faces the development of the claims payment process is the determination of the fee schedule by which providers are paid. Many MBHOs will pay network providers on a fee schedule that is linked to their professional credentials. Since providers with doctoral degrees are generally paid more than those with a master's degree, this can pose a problem for PSOs with multidisciplinary owners. For staff model programs, providers are generally reimbursed on a salary basis, and the adjudication of claims is a tracking system of effort and work. The cost for the development of a claims process can be a substantial investment for the development of a managed care organization.

Finance and Contract Management

The management of care requires a substantial commitment to business services. This includes the tracking of payments to providers and the monitoring of the financial stability of the risk contract. In addition, there are all of the business requirements commensurate with the size of the organization. The combination of these factors can result in a need for a more comprehensive business operation than is commonly seen in provider organizations.

Challenges for PSOs: The management of care requires a broad spectrum of contracts. These include the payer contracts and the agreements with providers and facilities. All of these require a monitoring and compliance process that is often provided by business operations in consultation with legal services. Other financial and management services include human resources and general operating structures.

Marketing and Business Development

Successful managed care organizations have a range of contracts and multiple business relationships between payers and providers. A marketing program can effectively provide the necessary linkage for these. This also can be important in the development of new business and the management of existing business.

Challenges for PSOs: For provider organizations these complex relationships are different from those commonly seen in clinical practice. In addition, the marketing and business development issues will vary widely between commercial and publicly funded contracts. For public systems there are unique state and federal requirements for the bidding and contracting for services.

AN EXAMINATION OF PROVIDER-SPONSORED ORGANIZATIONS

One of the more interesting evolutions in the behavioral health care industry that has taken place in the past several years involves the rapid growth of organizations created to organize and oversee the delivery of services by diverse provider panels. These PSOs are generally consistent with MBHOs. Both commercial and public purchasers of behavioral health care have encouraged the growth of these organizations. Commercial purchasers, such as self-funded plan administrators or third-party administrators, have wanted vertically aligned providers who have financial incentives for improved access and cost efficiencies. Public programs administered by the Health Care Financing Administration (e.g., Medicaid and Medicare) have recognized and regulated ways for providers to organize and share risk in care delivery. Community-based behavioral health providers have responded to these demands and incentives by purchasers and created a range of organizational structures. Dyer and Barkey (1998) initiated a survey to explore some of the features of PSOs. A review of their study illustrates how providers have been able to respond to the evolving challenges and develop organizations designed for managing and providing care.

The Survey

Noting the scarcity of data and information involving behavioral health PSOs, Dyer and Barkey undertook the design of a survey that would begin the process of categorizing and examining these new structures. Their project was hampered by the lack of a national trade association or clearinghouse for such entities. The researchers approached the National Council for Community Behavioral Healthcare (NCCBH), a national trade association for community behavioral health providers, state associations, funding authorities, and integrated delivery systems. NCCBH agreed to sponsor the effort. It proved difficult to identify such entities, since no trade association existed, no formal part of any annual conference was dedicated to these entities, and no mailing lists existed. The first task was to determine how to obtain a sample.

The Sample

The target population for the study was limited to ventures between two or more provider entities in which a separate entity was formed and employed its own staff. While survey responses were received from representatives of some ventures that no longer existed, the principal goal was to identify and catalog current existing ventures. Preliminary research yielded 60 potential PSOs in 24 states. Designed as an ongoing sampling process, subsequent responses were received from 35 entities in 15 states. (Results were skewed by incomplete responses yielding some questions with less than 35 entity responses.)

The Findings

Exhibit 12–1 data illustrates that PSOs have been developed with substantial numbers of participants in the venture. These are established organizations with longevity and evolving histories. In addition, these are public, private, and not-for-profit ventures.

The scope and purpose of these PSOs also are varied. Exhibit 12–2 indicates the development and mission of these organizations. There is a range of reasons why these organizations have been developed; the primary purpose is to support business operations. The findings of this study support the notion that these organizations have been created to provide publicly funded contracts. This is in part due to the sampling population of the study and the NCCBH partnership.

Additional Findings

The median Medicaid venture was administering over $25 million in annual benefits, while the median commercial or participant administra-

Exhibit 12–1 Number of Participants, Ages, and Types of PSO

Number of Participants of Venture	
10%	Two Partners
45%	Less than 10 participating organizations
42%	Between 10 and 40 participating organizations
3%	Over 40 participants
Age of Venture	
12%	Less than one year old
32%	One to two years old
32%	Three to four years old
24%	More than four years old
Type of Entity	
54%	Not-for-profit
19%	Public/private partnerships
15%	Public entities (authorities)
12%	Private ventures

Source: Reprinted with permission from R. Dyer, *NC News*, May, © 1999, National Council for Community Behavioral Healthcare.

tive services venture was generating less than $1 million to support the venture. Eighty-five percent of the dollars administered on average were being utilized for purchasing clinical services. The majority of ventures over five years old were financially self-sustaining.

Respondents were asked to identify those elements they believed critical for venture success. Findings included the following: adequate capital, a strong chief executive officer (CEO) for the venture, task-appropriate management information system, CEO or senior staff with managed care competence and experience, strong financial management/oversight/presence, protocols for managing risks, and resources. Some of the positions/functional areas cited in the study included the following: CEO/president, chief operating officer, chief medical officer, provider relations, access services, claims administration, marketing, account management, member services, quality improvement, and management information systems. These are consistent with the core areas described earlier. Services that are typically outsourced included the following: financial oversight (often stated as transitional until entity is self-sustaining), provider source verification (for credentialing), claims administration, and actuarial (rate-setting) services.

Exhibit 12–2 Purpose, Capitalization, and Products and Services of PSOs

Purpose of Venture	
42%	Customer mandated (Medicaid)
24%	Decrease administrative costs
20%	Seek new revenues and/or customers
14%	Create new internal services or products
Capitalization	
6%	Less than $100,000
18%	$100,000–$500,000
6%	$500,000–$1 million
60%	$1 million–$2 million
6%	Over $2 million
Products and Services Sold	
54%	Medicaid behavioral health benefits management
28%	Insurance/behavioral health benefits management
20%	Management information system for behavioral health providers (participants)
16%	Government program operations or oversight (e.g., Head Start or corrections)
12%	Claims administration
12%	Employee assistance programs
8%	Credentialing
8%	Human resources
8%	Hospital inpatient management

Source: Reprinted with permission from R. Dyer, *NC News*, May, © 1999, National Council for Community Behavioral Healthcare.

Respondents identified the following items as most likely to threaten success of the venture: inadequate capital, distrust between participants (do not trust your partners), poor communication between participants, inadequate business skill (or inadequate business focus) particularly regarding managed care–related resource management, and inadequate market analysis/sales effort or product packaging.

All but two respondents were enthusiastic about the benefits of the venture to the participating provider organizations. Positioning, potential consolidation, and evolving improved managed care skills and focus were the most commonly mentioned positives of participation despite lack of overall financial benefits. Helping to cut costs, protecting current business, and developing new revenues that were previously unavailable also are cited as important features.

Respondents were asked what advice they would give others contemplating a provider-sponsored venture. Their responses included the following: organize and implement venture to rigorous business standards; have a market-based business plan; determine and execute a methodology for quick, clear decision making; assure that incentives exist for a healthy entrepreneurial culture; assure adequate capital for the sustained period of dependency; keep participants focused on the venture accomplishing its strategic purpose; spend the time to clarify values and commitments; revisit and reinforce commitments and steps to success of strategic purpose; and actively promote efforts to reduce distrust among participants.

The findings of this study suggest that PSOs have been successful in the development and management of care. They have effectively entered both commercial and public markets, and they have withstood the tests of start-up and development.

CONCLUSIONS: CAN PROVIDER-SPONSORED ORGANIZATIONS SUCCESSFULLY MANAGE CARE?

Private Sector

The evidence is clear that PSOs are currently managing care successfully. This is supported by the evolution of behavioral health systems presented in this chapter, illustrated in the evolution of core competencies for MBHOs, and documented in the study results presented. Two corollary questions for the commercial managed behavioral health care market are raised by this presentation: (1) What do provider-sponsored managed care programs offer that is unique to their organization? and (2) Can PSOs survive in the changing health care environment?

In the commercial marketplace, provider-sponsored managed care organizations provide a distinct set of favorable attributes over their insurance-based competitors. Provider organizations generally serve a local or regional market. Their strength is in their ability to achieve integration with the broader health care systems. In addition, these types of systems are generally more committed to consumers because their future is linked to their local success. As evidenced by the study described above, these types of organizations achieve a measure of horizontal integration that is based on core values and common goals.

MBHOs that are not provider sponsored often have a core tension between the providers of care and those who manage it. There is an inherent mistrust that cost and control are the driving values of the management of care. Consumers are often caught in the middle of this contentious relationship. Bureaucratic systems that make access, care authorization, and continued care difficult to obtain frustrate both consumers and providers. When providers also sponsor the management of care, there is a shift to a more central commitment to effective and efficient care.

The principal question that remains is: Will PSOs be able to continue to survive in the evolving health care systems? It is clear that managed care has successfully reduced the cost of health care. This has had a significant impact on behavioral health care, with declining amounts of the benefit dollars being allocated to behavioral health (The Hay Group, 1998). This trend, combined with increasing capital requirements for the establishment and maintenance of PSOs, makes the future picture less certain.

Nationally, there has been a consolidation of both commercial health insurers and MBHOs. This trend has increasingly challenged the survival of PSOs. This combination of the decline of premiums allocated for behavioral health and the consolidation of payers has fostered a shift to the lowest-cost approach to provider contracting. As the future unfolds, it is unlikely that PSOs will be able to survive in a lowest-cost model. For these organizations to prosper, there must be a commitment to both effective and efficient care delivery systems. In this environment, PSOs do provide the best potential resource.

Public Sector

Board-governed, community-based organizations as well as consumers often have difficulty in understanding the changing market and in translating their traditional advocacy issues to the more complex and interlocked resource-based care debates. Regrettably, in some communities they may have encountered negative public images typically associated with traditional public providers regarding both quality and clinical effectiveness. These organizations also have had limited experience in marketing to private pay segments and in accumulating the management competencies associated with effective and contemporary business practices.

Consumer and customer sensitivity will require that providers must continually demonstrate that their services are functionally effective, beneficial, and contribute to creating and maintaining healthy and safe communities. Consumer involvement will continue to affect both payers and providers, particularly in view of this current anti–managed care mood. Consumers in both public-sponsored and private systems will continue to influence what, where, and how behavioral health care services are provided.

A review of salient information presented would lead to the conclusion that, yes, providers can indeed manage care. However, the issue of whether or not providers can manage care well can balance the inherent ethical and operational tensions between being both a risk-based management organization and a clinical and delivery service.

Despite the theoretical long-term benefit that PSOs might bring to health care, the current and anticipated environments show that the development of such enterprises carries extremely high risk. The survey presented in this chapter (Dyer & Barkey, 1998) and "Survey of Behavioral Health Organizations," a NCCBH survey conducted by the Gallup Organization (1999), indicate some of the commonly experienced barriers to success, particularly in public sector restructuring. The three chief barriers may be loosely described as follows: (1) inexperience in developing and managing complex business structures including managing conflicts of interest, business modeling and planning, and conflict management skills; (2) lack of access to capital, specialized business knowledge and systems, and the steep learning curve associated with beginning a new enterprise; and (3) the public politics of Medicaid.

The ultimate outcome of any managed behavioral health care system must support the needs of consumers and the principal role of care providers. These types of organizations must support effective and efficient care. There must be sufficient levels of capital to support the start-up and evolution of either public or private organizations, and there must be a commitment to continuous quality improvement.

REFERENCES

Daniels, A., Zieman, G., Kramer, T., & Furgal, C. (1997). *The behavioral healthcare quality and accountability toolkit.* Tiburon, CA: CentraLink Publications.

Dyer, R., & Barkey, M. (1998). Behavioral Health PSOs. Rockville, MD: National Council of Community Behavioral Health.

National Committee for Quality Assurance. (1998). *Behavioral health accreditation standards*. Washington, DC: NCQA.

National Council for Community Behavioral Healthcare. (1999, September). Survey of Behavioral Organizations (www.nccbh.org/gallup.htm).

The Hay Group. (1998, May). *Health care plan design and cost trends—1988 through 1997*. Prepared for National Association of Psychiatric Health Systems, Association of Behavioral Group Practices, and National Alliance for the Mentally Ill. Washington, DC: The Hay Group.

Zieman, G.L. (1998). *The handbook of managed behavioral healthcare: A complete and up-to-date guide for students and practitioners*. San Francisco: Jossey-Bass.

CHAPTER 13

Interest Group Competition and the Regulation of Managed Behavioral Health Care

E. Clarke Ross

Purpose: This chapter summarizes the competition between structural interests over access to and control of behavioral health services and reviews major federal and state regulations of managed care.

Major Topics: This chapter discusses Interest Groups, Market-Related Policy Approaches, Regulation, President's Advisory Commission on Consumer Protection and Quality in the Health Care Industry.

Plaintiffs' economic complaint boils down to distress that the defendants reimburse their membership at lower rates than plaintiffs were accustomed to charging or would like to charge. . . . Plaintiffs merely wish to protest the buying power of managed care organizations. . . . For the reasons stated . . . I dismissed the complaint in its entirety with prejudice. . . . I denied plaintiffs' request for leave to amend their complaint. (*Stephens et al.*, 1998, p. 3)

In *Stephens et al.* (1998) mental health providers attempted to argue that consumers of mental health services were illegally harmed by managed

Source: Adapted with permission from E.C. Ross, Regulating Managed Care: Interest Group Competition for Control and Behavioral Health Care, *Journal of Health, Politics, Policy and Law*, Vol. 24, No. 3, © 1999, Duke University Press.

behavioral health care organizations accepting capitated payments from purchasers, using provider networks that were not open to every behavioral health care professional, and requiring provider contracts using quality performance and discounted fees. Plaintiffs argued that these provisions were the result of antitrust actions by the managed care organizations. The case was dismissed with prejudice; there were no reasonable grounds for complaint and, as such, provider plaintiffs were refused permission to re-plead their case.

The Stephens case is a typical vignette of the power dynamics involved between managed behavioral health care organizations and organized interests of behavioral health care providers. Managed care is a massive paradigm shift in the organization, payment, and delivery of mental health services. Organized professional guilds of mental health providers have launched judicial, legislative, and public relations initiatives to reclaim the autonomy and financial rewards of pre–managed care days. Provider litigation success is very questionable, but legislative success, which is likely in some degree, will depend on public relations success.

This chapter describes, from both the professional literature and personal experience, the tension between interest groups in advocating professional, regulatory, and market-based approaches to accountability; explains the competition to control the purse strings; differentiates between concepts of consumer protections and provider privileges; and explains why some for-profit managed behavioral health care executives, and their national trade association, operate as policy outliers in relation to historic and expected patterns of public policy behavior. The chapter concludes with an identification of major current regulatory issues confronting managed behavioral health care.

COMPETITION AMONG INTEREST GROUPS

As Alford (1975) observed two decades ago, the struggle among interest groups in a democratic society is inevitable. When systemic changes occur, such as we are now experiencing with the advent of managed care and intensifying congressional debate about its regulation, competition among core structural interests is certain to accelerate. By conceptually outlining three different types of structural interests in the health care field, all of which remain relevant to contemporary health care politics, Alford's work provides a framework for exploring and understanding the organizational dynamics currently at play.

The first category of organizations includes those representing "dominant structural interests," such as organized professional guilds. They seek to protect and reinforce the logic and principle of professional monopoly over the production and distribution of health services. These groups are in competition with "challenging structural interests," bureaucratic organizations such as hospitals and public health agencies, that must tailor professional services to meet the objectives of not only improved health, but also broader social needs within the resource constraints of society. Managed care organizations (MCOs), the management agents of health care purchasers, emerged as a new breed of challenging structural interests. Some observers would argue that MCOs have now become the dominant interest, with the previously dominant professional guilds, as the new challengers, striving to restore their lost status. Finally, in Alford's schema there are "repressed structural interests." They are the family, patient, and consumer groups that wish to maximize the responsiveness of health professionals and bureaucratic organizations to their needs, including access to high-quality medical care.

Past analyses of health care organizational dynamics and politics have demonstrated the utility, either directly or indirectly, of Alford's classification of interests. In previous work, for example, Ross (1992a, 1992b), Havel (1992), and Rickhards (1992), this approach has been used to examine national mental health interests. Starr, in *The Social Transformation of American Medicine* (1982), wrote the definitive social history of organized medicine, the core dominant structural interests in American health care politics. Feldstein (1980), employing economic analysis, also investigated this "struggle for control." Thinking of organizations' interests in these terms allows considerable leverage in explaining the nature of group positions and politics in the debate over managed care.

Bauer (1994) and Samuels (1996) discussed how professional guilds, particularly physician groups, have strongly defended maintenance of the status quo. They define the status quo as the fee-for-service approach that relies on "consuming" services. In this paradigm, systems and resources are not mobilized for individuals until they become "patients." Samuels (1996) observed that initial managed care approaches relied on "a series of procedural hoops to discourage consumption" to offset "the protection of the status quo" by "a powerful self-interest in this country" (pp. 7, 11–12).

In this scheme, MCOs can be viewed as either "dominant" or "challenging structural interests." They are challenging the historic dominance of solo practice fee for service. They are dominating by insisting on integrated delivery, documented clinical performance, and discounted fees.

Alford's (1975) three categories of health interest groups tend to be associated with three societal approaches to accountability.

DOMAINS OF ACCOUNTABILITY

Darby (1998), Emanuel and Emanuel (1997), Levin (1980), and Zelman (1996) each described domains for promoting accountability in health services. Interestingly, Alford's structural interests are associated with these domains of accountability. The "professional" approach is the historic reliance of the professional guilds on state licensing and board certification and purchasers' reliance on third-party professional accreditation. The "market-driven" or "economic" approach is the purchaser of health care's use of the contract authority and performance data to demonstrate performance compliance. Competitive requests for proposals (RFPs) are used in this approach. The role of profit in health care is a major issue of controversy. The "public policy" approach uses the regulatory authority of government to alter behavior and conditions. Absent such regulation, behavior and conditions would most likely be different.

In the professional model, physicians establish the standards of accountability and hold each other accountable through professional organizations. Physicians are certified by the profession and its specialty boards and are expected to adhere to professional standards. It is assumed that the professional is dedicated to the patient's well-being.

In the ideal economic model of accountability, consumer-patients shop for the best combination of price and quality to satisfy their preferences. Switching between competing health plans and providers is a fundamental premise of this approach. Competition and choice are expected to deliver appropriate services. As Daniels and Sabin (1998) observed, market accountability requires plans to inform purchasers and consumers about performance and options. When consumers make informed choices among plans, they give "informed consent" to the limits the plan imposes.

Emanuel and Emanuel (1997) expanded the "public policy model" with what they termed the "political model." In it, the community's representatives determine how to pursue patient well-being. The voice of the citizens and the community's good are stressed. The community, however, does not need to be a formal governmental unit; it may be other organizations, such as unions, professional associations, community health centers, and patient cooperative health maintenance organizations (HMOs). This complexity of community interests is recognized, but not addressed in this chapter. The "political" and "public policy" approaches are treated as different formulations of using the regulatory authority of government to alter behaviors and the nature of interactions among individuals and health care organizations. This chapter focuses on how behavioral health care interests compete for influence over the national government. (Purchasers, both private and governmental, currently use the term "behavioral health." Many national associations also use the term "behavioral health" in their titles, reflecting the predominant use by purchasers. But the term is controversial within the behavioral health field. Behavior implies willful control and choice by the individual. Many organizations prefer and use terms such as "brain disorders," "serious and persistent mental illness," "addictive diseases," "addictive disorders," and "chemical dependency" to emphasize the biological nature of these conditions. Such organizations also tend not to use the terms "mental health" or "substance abuse.")

The three categories of structural interest have each typically supported the approach to accountability that is ideologically consistent with its projected interests and sources of strength. Professional guilds, for example, have largely preferred the "professional" approach (APA, 1997), which grants considerable advantage to those who can lay claim to what Starr (1982) called "cultural authority" based on scientific expertise. Purchasers of health care coverage and services, on the other hand, have tended to favor the "market" approach, where their control of the flow of dollars can give them the most leverage. Lacking either of these resources, the "repressed" family and patient groups have relied more extensively on the "regulatory" approach, counting on the power of representative government to reflect and protect their interests.

FOCI OF CONFLICT

Zelman (1996) argues that interest group struggles for control have largely focused on two goals—"access to and control over the premium dollar," and the "proper positioning to lead, be essential to, or function productively in the emerging breed of organized delivery systems" (p. 75).

While the issue of control over the premium dollar and delivery of care is the area of fundamental conflict, Wilkerson, Devers, and Given (1997) wrote: "The impetus for market-based reform and price-competitive managed care comes largely from the demand side of the health care market—that is, from large purchasers of health benefits. A key element of price-competitive managed care is the enhancement and use of bargaining power by large purchasers" (p. 55). MCOs may be viewed as management agents of the purchaser. Human attitudes tend to be most negative when "agents" of those in power are active. Agents include tax collectors, estate managers, overseers, bounty hunters, and MCOs.

This view of who the purchaser is and what role the management agent has is being challenged. Consumer groups argue that ultimately the purchaser is the consumer—the employee, the insured beneficiary, and the tax-paying citizen. Advocates of medical savings accounts, vouchers, defined contributions, and equalizing income tax treatment of health expenditures, which are frequently "think tanks" and not nationally organized consumer organizations, all begin from the common philosophical premise of the consumer as purchaser. Interestingly, professional guilds also are major advocates of medical savings accounts, vouchers, and equalizing tax treatment. To professionals, once they have obtained a license to practice from the state they should be free to bill any source of payment connected to their patient. The health payment relationship should, in their view, be entirely a two-party concern—the provider of professional services and the consumer patient who is the purchaser. Access to, and control over, the premium dollar is a major battleground. Consumers desire control in order to have choice. Professionals want the autonomy to practice as they have been trained. Neither has been sensitive to costs.

Managed care, at its core, integrates financing and delivery of care. This is the second major battleground. O'Neil and Finnocchio (1997) observed that market pressures—the large purchasers—are increasingly emphasizing primary care, prevention, population-based practice, interdisciplinary teamwork, clinical effectiveness research, and integrated clinical delivery. Specialists, who largely operate as autonomous practitioners, particularly in the area of behavioral health, will be required to function within coordinated, comprehensive, and continuous care delivery settings. Zelman (1996) argued that the professional guilds are competing to control, be recognized as essential to, and function properly in these newly organized delivery systems. To emphasize this point, Cummings, Pallak, and Cummings (1996) published a book, *Surviving the Demise of Solo Practice.*

Blackwell (1998) argues that as long as Americans, encouraged by the professions, rely on open networks, point-of-service plans, and extensive use of subspecialists, health care will never be integrated. The current regulatory public policy agenda of the professional guilds is to mandate any willing provider (AWP) laws, mandatory point of service, and mandatory reliance on specialty care. They desire to use the regulatory authority of the government to mandate their control over both the premium dollar and the delivery site.

MARKET-RELATED POLICY OPTIONS

While the current dominant model for health care organization and financing relies on market forces, Zelman (1996) outlines four policy options to respond to instances where the market is failing. These options are:

1. Encourage or foster activities that seem fully compatible with market trends, but might not occur without some policy action. An example would be enactment of insurance reforms that increase the probability that insurers will compete on quality.
2. Accept a market trend but recognize the need to contain or protect against some negative fallout from that trend. An example would be that capitation incentives might reduce utilization too far under some circumstances.
3. Reject a market trend and prohibit it. An example would be APW mandates aimed at prohibiting managed care's reliance on networks that are focused on quality, accountability, and contract obligations. Zelman (1996) observed that the American Medical Association and other professional guilds have done a marvelous public relations job in getting the public and legislators to refer to these APW initiatives as "patient protections." It reminds this writer of the marvelous public relations effort of this nation's Founding Fathers—nationalists, who referred to themselves as "federalists," thus forcing the true federalists to be branded in the public image as "anti-federalists," a portrayal that remains to this day.

4. Do nothing. Zelman (1996) observed: "Of course, there is always a fourth option. And today, it is often the most popular—do nothing" (p. 11). It appears legislators have rejected this do-nothing option.

NATIONAL AND STATE LEGISLATIVE CLAMOR TO REGULATE THE MARKET EXCESSES OF MANAGED CARE

Kondracke (1998) opined, "Fueled by news accounts exposing deaths and lasting health damage caused by HMOs denying access to care, even industry lobbyists admit that HMOs are barely more popular than tobacco companies" (p. 5). Kondracke's remark is merely typical of the many media and political commentary offered on negative attitudes about managed care. Blendon and associates (1998) give an excellent analysis of the managed care backlash. Given that managed care is a "forceful revolution," they argue that "a negative reaction is inevitable on the part of persons and institutions that are affected" (p. 80). This chapter identifies multiple factors that have contributed to this backlash.

Consistent with the theme of this chapter regarding the competition between professional guilds and managed care interests, Blendon and colleagues (1998) observed that physicians "regret the demise of fee-for-service indemnity insurance . . . fear loss of income . . . and have suffered a loss of autonomy and authority."Meanwhile, they argued that HMOs "at times seem to be their own worst enemies" by being "insensitive and unresponsive to consumers and have treated employers instead as their primary customer. . . . Some plans have resisted market-improving legislation, in part because they may benefit from market imperfections," and "many health plans have antagonized physicians rather then finding ways to win their cooperation." They explain that over the past decade, millions of "consumers have been converted—often involuntarily" from fee-for-service indemnity coverage to managed care, "often without much explanation of the relationship between the limitations and cost containment." While overall consumer satisfaction with health plans is quite high, chronically ill and hospitalized patients report problems with their plans.

Numerous legislative proposals have been introduced in the U.S. Congress. A comparative analysis of these proposals is beyond the scope of this chapter. The U.S. House of Representatives passed legislation on October

7, 1999, while the U.S. Senate earlier passed a bill on July 15, 1999. This chapter summarizes the major regulatory issues while attempting to differentiate concepts of "consumer protections" and "provider privileges."

INTEREST GROUP APPROACHES

On the issue of the national regulation of managed care, in many ways structural interest groups line up on the issue in expected and traditional ways. For example, the Health Benefits Coalition for Affordable Choice and Quality is opposed to any national regulation and proposes a series of voluntary market-based improvements. This coalition is composed of major business interests, such as the National Federation of Independent Business, National Association of Manufacturers, and U.S. Chamber of Commerce; major insurers, such as the Blue Cross–Blue Shield Association and Health Insurance Association of America; and the major trade association representing managed care organizations, the American Association of Health Plans. This coalition's argument is straightforward: Every government mandate increases the cost of health care. It cites studies by the U.S. Congressional Budget Office (CBO) that a 10% increase in premiums results in 3.5% of currently insured persons voluntarily giving up insurance. Another CBO estimate is that a 1% increase in premiums nationwide causes 200,000 people to voluntarily drop insurance coverage (Patient Access to Responsible Care Alliance).

Consumer, patient, and advocate groups, such as Families USA, the American Association for Retired Persons (AARP), the National Mental Health Association, and the National Alliance for the Mentally Ill, endorse the strongest possible national regulation of health plans and their management operations. For every documented abuse by a health plan, advocates tend to want a regulatory protection.

The approaches of the business and advocate communities rely almost exclusively on one ideological view—market versus regulation. These views are completely consistent with Alford's (1975) concept. And each community uses dueling actuaries to make their public policy arguments. Affordability and cost impact are important decision factors. While the approaches of the professional guilds are ideologically consistent, they are more complex. Several MCOs have demonstrated an ability to cross ideological boundaries and advocate a more mixed approach.

MANAGED BEHAVIORAL HEALTH CARE ORGANIZATIONS—A UNIQUE FLEXIBILITY

In September 1997 three managed care plans—Kaiser Permanente, Group Health Cooperative of Puget Sound, and HIP Health Insurance Plans—joined with Families USA and AARP in advocating 18 principles to govern the national regulation of managed care. This was a unique partnership and an important model to managed behavioral health care organizations.

The American Managed Behavioral Healthcare Association (AMBHA), a trade association created in 1999 and representing 13 managed behavioral health care organizations that serve over 112 million health plan enrollees, advocated utilizing all three domains of accountability—professional, market, and public policy approaches.

The purchaser is a major participant, and health plans must be accountable for meeting contract requirements. The use of voluntary national performance reporting, through such entities as the National Committee for Quality Assurance (NCQA) Health Plan Employer Data and Information Set (HEDIS), and accreditation activities is a significant way of documenting accountability. In addition, AMBHA supported national standards targeted to health plan consumers, enrollees, and patients in an effort to restore consumer confidence in the credibility of managed health plans. AMBHA also defended the ability of health plans to manage health benefits effectively while holding providers accountable for the services they deliver.

AMBHA has joined a coalition for consumer protections that includes the National Alliance for the Mentally Ill, National Mental Health Association, and Bazelon Center for Mental Health Law. This coalition advocates protections that go beyond those proposed by the Advisory Commission on Consumer Protection and Quality in the Health Care Industry (1997).

The AMBHA public policy agenda is unique and significantly strays from Alford's (1975) formulations and expected ideological predispositions. Why is this the case? AMBHA members, though for-profit MCOs, are almost exclusively dedicated to the management of health benefits for the treatment of mental illness and addictive disorders. This so-called "carved-out" managed care industry is unique in American health care organizations and financing.

Unlike any other category of health disease, since colonial times America has operated a state-owned and -operated public mental health system. Of the nation's 1997 direct mental illness and addictive disorders treatment expenditures of $82.2 billion, only $34.3 billion, or 42%, is derived from the private sector (Coffey et al., 2000). Thus government—national, state, county, and municipal—expended $47.9 billion in the direct treatment of mental illness and addictive disorders.

Another topic for another day is the interface, or lack thereof, between the public mental health system and the private insurance sector and between "full service" health plans and carved-out specialty health plans. The importance to this discussion is that many of the AMBHA members' senior executives and chief clinical officers have their roots in the public mental health system, either as public mental health executives or clinicians working in public sector programs. Public sector executives and clinicians are salaried employees working in programs attempting to integrate and coordinate systems of care. Responsibility is to the public mental health authority, an entity of government and community. Solo practice, fee-for-service payment, and responsibility only to the professional guild are not components of public sector employment. AMBHA's executive director, for ten years the deputy executive director of the National Association of State Mental Health Directors, was hired by the AMBHA president, the current chief executive officer of the nation's largest managed behavioral health care organization (MBHO), who had previously served as the state of Maryland mental health director. Concepts of the public interest and public sector values are important to these for-profit managed care executives and clinical officers. It should be noted that several large MBHOs are not members of AMBHA; one reason given is that AMBHA's current leadership has too great a focus on the public interest and public sector values. Other MBHOs have expressed no marketplace advantage to belonging to such a national association. (The concept of "the public interest and public sector values" is a complex one. Here, three proposals are used. In 1995 six national groups [Mental Health Policy Resource Center et al., 1995] outlined ten suggested interests and values: to provide leadership that involves citizens and consumers in planning and public policy, in partnership with other parts of the health care and human service system; to promote access of vulnerable populations to community-based, integrated systems of care; to collect, manage, and analyze mental health– and health-related information for the purpose of prospective decision making; to define and evaluate performance, outcome, effectiveness, and costs of mental health–related services and systems; to ensure that savings are treated as a return on public investment;

to improve the health status of communities, families, and individuals; to promote safe communities; to provide a safety net for individuals unable to access needed services elsewhere; to promote innovation and best practices in services and systems; and to provide disaster-related mental health services at times of local, regional or statewide emergencies. In 1997 four national associations [AMBHA et al.] published a white paper that declared two major purposes of public behavioral health services: to improve the health states of individuals and to create and maintain healthy and safe communities. These then are among the public interest and public sector values. A 1995 Eleventh Annual Rosalynn Carter Symposium on Mental Health Policy work group "defined the public interest as a dynamic constellation of values that fosters the achievement of the highest level of health and well-being for all citizens and safeguards the needs and values of the most vulnerable" ["Managing Care," 1995, p. 610].)

Given this uniqueness of AMBHA, the organization operates as a policy outlier. For-profit MBHOs recognize the advantages of market-driven reform and defend the ability of health plans to manage health benefits effectively while holding providers accountable for the services they deliver. Thus AMBHA opposes the agenda of the professional guilds to return to providers autonomy and fee-for-service approaches. But AMBHA's members also see the crisis in consumer confidence, recognize the dysfunctional aspects of the current system, and are comfortable with appropriate regulation to protect and promote the public interest, consistent with the philosophies and notions of collective responsibilities as identified above. Some, particularly the leaders of AMBHA, but clearly not all executives of for-profit MBHOs, continue to advocate private sector social contract responsibilities to the larger society. Being comfortable with reasonable regulation in times of crisis, AMBHA is not part of the larger business-purchasers health plan community.

Perhaps Elazer's (1998) description of the public interest best represents the thinking of the leadership of AMBHA. Elazer described the "public interest" as a halfway position between the classical notions of "virtue" and "interest." "Republican virtues" were a core premise for proper political behavior. With the adoption of the U.S. Constitution and acceptance of Madison's notion of ambition countering ambition, "interests" were recognized as the basis of individual motivation. There are private economic interests, and there are common or community interests. The public interest at any point in time is the balance between the efficiency of the private market and the fairness of a common distribution of resources.

AMBHA's leadership not only is a strong advocate of the efficiency of the market but also recognizes social responsibilities to the common good.

AMBHA's strategic relationships also are unique, in comparison with, for example, the American Association of Health Plans (AAHP), the major association representing managed care organizations. AAHP is aligned with the business and purchaser communities. AMBHA has published joint papers and statements and works legislatively with the major mental health consumer and advocacy organizations—the National Alliance for the Mentally Ill, the National Mental Health Association, and the Bazelon Center for Mental Health Law. There is a tenseness to this collaboration as well. The advocacy groups are highly critical of many aspects of managed care and instinctively turn to more national government regulation as a response to perceived problems. But the advocacy groups also believe in organized and integrated delivery systems, accountability by all participants including providers, and in not wanting to return to the previous unmanaged fee-for-service provider autonomy arrangements, goals shared with AMBHA.

AMBHA has published joint papers and statements with the major public sector administrators—the National Association of State Mental Health Directors, the National Association of State Alcohol and Drug Abuse Directors, and the National Association of County Behavioral Health Directors. There is tenseness to this collaboration, too. Many public administrators resent for-profit managed care organizations coming into their jurisdictions to take over much of the health benefit and clinical management functions. Yet the public administrators recognize the reality of managed care, the management and information strengths that MBHOs bring with them, and the historic public values many MBHO executives bring. Both public administrators and MBHOs recognize the need to improve the public procurement process.

AMBHA also has engaged in strategic partnering with national provider organizations supportive of organized and integrated delivery systems—the National Council for Community Behavioral Healthcare, the National Association of Psychiatric Health Systems, and the Council for Behavioral Group Practices. There is always tenseness to this collaboration as well. Organized provider groups ultimately see no need for a third-party management agent of the purchaser, particularly when this third party is a for-profit entity that, at the purchaser's direction, is reducing provider payments. Yet these providers also are creating unique joint ventures with MBHOs as purchasers continue to insist on organized and integrated delivery; many MBHOs have experience and expertise unmatched by provider groups.

The area where AMBHA has little strategic partnering is with the professional guilds, of which there are many in the area of behavioral health. There are over 600,000 individual behavioral health care professionals in the United States. The leading mental health professional societies have declared "war" on "the scourage of managed care" and have declared their goal to be the return to the "Golden Age" of mental health when there was fee-for-service payment and professional autonomy (Dixon, 1997; Eist, 1997; Ross, 1997).

But even with the professional guilds there is partnering, which also usually includes the advocate groups. Here the larger public interest of behavioral health is at work. AMBHA was a founding member of the Coalition for Fairness in Mental Illness Coverage and the Coalition for Nondiscriminatory Coverage of Addiction Treatment, coalitions devoted exclusively to the attainment of parity for mental illness and addictive disorders in health benefit design. AMBHA also is a member of the major behavioral field national coalitions, the Mental Health Liaison Group and the National Coalition on Alcohol and Other Drug Issues.

While insurers, business representatives, most health plans, and consumer/advocate groups have remained consistent with Alford's (1975) concept, some managed behavioral health care organizations have developed unique, largely unexpected, and flexible approaches to public policy. The jolt of managed care has driven professional guilds to increasingly advocate national regulatory approaches.

PROPOSED LEGISLATIVE CONSUMER PROTECTIONS

The Advisory Commission on Consumer Protection and Quality in the Health Care Industry (1997) recommendations are generally conceded to be "consumer protections." They include the following:

- *Information disclosure*. Consumers and enrollees have the right to receive accurate information about the health plan's benefits and operations.
- *Provider network adequacy*. Each health plan must have sufficient numbers and types of providers.

- *Access to specialists.* Enrollees with specialty needs can directly access specialist providers.
- *Continuity of care (transition, outside network).* Newly enrolled consumers who are undergoing treatment for chronic conditions can continue to be treated by their previous non-network provider.
- *Access to emergency care (prudent layperson standard).* Persons with symptoms and pain, such as a prudent layperson would reasonably expect, can immediately access emergency care.
- *Timelines for authorization for reimbursement of care.* Health plan decisions will be made within standardized time frames.
- *Prohibition on "gag clauses."* Health plans may not prohibit or influence a provider giving consumers advice about treatment options.
- *Enrollee right to appeal denials through an external and independent peer review entity.* The Consumers Union (Bureau of National Affairs, 1998) argues that "an impartial external grievance and appeals system is the linchpin for all other consumer protections aimed at providing the delivery of quality care" (p. 445).
- *Mandatory choice of health plans (wherever feasible).* Choice should be a goal.

REGULATING MANAGED CARE

An outline of the fundamental provisions of the patients bill of rights legislation passed by the House and Senate (Borzi & Rosenbaum, 2000) identifies the core issues. These core issues, which include both patient protections and provider privileges, are as follows:

- Point-of-service (POS) requirement
- Choice of medical provider
- Access to emergency care
- Access to specialty care
- Access to obstetrical and gynecological care
- Access to pediatric care
- Continuity of care
- Access to prescription drugs

- Access to clinical trials
- Disclosure of treatment options required
- Access to information
- Information about providers
- Interference with medical communications ("gag clauses")
- Discrimination against providers based on licensure
- Physician incentive plans
- Prompt payment of claims
- Protection for patient advocacy ("whistleblower provisions")
- Access to behavioral health services
- Minimum hospital stays for mastectomies
- Genetic information

Notably, the first ten are recognized as fundamental patient protections by Families U.S.A. (2000).

Benefit claims and appeals procedures are as follows:

- Utilization review
- Internal plan appeals
- Independent external review
- Grievances

Employee Retirement Income Security Act (ERISA) preemption and plan liability provisions include the following:

- Applicability of state law regarding patient protections
- Plan liability (ERISA preemption of state remedies)

States continue to enact managed care regulations. The Bureau of National Affairs (2000e, 2000f), citing the National Conference of State Legislatures, reported the information summarized in Table 13–1.

Health plan medical liability is an issue that the U.S. Congress has avoided. However, six states have granted managed care plan enrollees the right to sue the MCO for negligent care (AMBHA, 1999; "Arizona To Become," 2000; Bureau of National Affairs, 2000a, 2000b). The six states are Arizona, Georgia, Louisiana, Oklahoma, Texas, and Washington. Both consumers and providers strongly support such legislation.

Table 13–1 State-Managed Care Laws/Regulations

Issue	No. of States with Laws/Regulations
Bans on gag clauses	48
Inpatient care after childbirth	42
Direct access to OB/GYN services or OB/GYN as primary care physician	40
Emergency care service mandate	39
Prudent layperson standard	39
Prompt payment to providers	38
Independent appeals	37
Disclosure of restrictive drug formularies	31
Written notification of contract termination between provider and plan	28
Bans on use of financial incentives	27
Continuity of care	27
Standing referrals	26
Hold harmless	25
Report cards	24
Licensing of medical directors	23
Freedom of choice	22
Definition of medical necessity	22
Any willing provider	21
Procedures for covering nonformulary drugs	20
Inpatient care after mastectomy	19
Point of service	19
Provider due process	17
Independent ombudsman programs	10
Insurer liability	7
Collective provider negotiations	1

Courtesy of the National Conference on State Legislators, Washington, D.C.

Texas, in 1997, was the first state to enact law. MCOs are liable for "adverse health care treatment decisions" when "ordinary care" is not exercised. Georgia and Louisiana enacted laws in 1999. In Georgia, plans must "exercise ordinary care in a timely and appropriate manner," while in Louisiana medical necessity may not be "rendered in bad faith," and the MCO may not be involved in "negligence" or "intentional misrepresentation." Enacted in 2000, Washington health plan enrollees may sue for damages if they were "harmed through negligence." In Arizona, enrollees may sue "for damages caused by the delay or denial of medically necessary services or claims" if there was no reasonable basis for the delay or denial. The most recent state to enact law is Oklahoma (enacted April, effective

July 1, 2000). It allows MCOs to be sued "for harm caused by medical treatment decisions."

In December 1999, the Institute of Medicine (IOM) issued a report stating that as many as 98,000 people die annually from hospital medical errors. The IOM report provided national visibility to a problem discussed for years within health care quality circles. President Clinton and members of Congress discussed the creation of a new National Center for Patient Safety. Legislation was proposed to require reporting to and maintenance of a national database of error reports. Disagreements between supporters revolve around whether identified best practices could then be required of hospitals by the U.S. Department of Health and Human Services (Bureau of National Affairs, 2000d). Professionals and providers generally oppose such legislation while consumers generally favor it.

The IOM medical errors report also stimulated national and state legislators to propose consumer and citizen access to the National Practitioner Data Bank (Borzo, 2000; Bureau of National Affairs, 2000h, 2000i). While the databank was established in 1986 as a clearinghouse for information relating to the disciplinary and malpractice records of physicians, consumers still have no access to it. Current law permits only hospitals, licensing boards, and other health care institutions to access it. New York State is about to join Massachusetts as the only state to allow consumer Internet on-line public disclosure of malpractice settlements and judgments.

Consumers support all these efforts to allow consumer access to information; professionals, led by the American Medical Association, oppose such access. Professionals are strongly advocating physician bargaining laws (Bureau of National Affairs, 2000c, 2000g). Texas is the first state in the nation to allow physicians to negotiate fees and other contract matters jointly with health plans under immunity from antitrust laws. On June 30, 2000, the U.S. House of Representatives passed legislation (H.R. 1304) that would allow competing health care professionals—such as independent physicians, dentists, and pharmacists—to bargain collectively with health plans.

A PUBLIC UTILITY MODEL FOR REFORM

The ongoing competition between structural interest groups will never stop. Should we accept that public policy and the public interest are merely the temporary accommodations that public decision makers make with structural interests? The fundamental goal of the professions remains consistent with Alford's (1975) concept—autonomy. What is new is the profession's endorsement of national regulation to mandate (and restore) autonomy. The fundamental goal of patient groups is access to care that is affordable.

An alternative, which accepts structural interest group competition within a framework, is to adopt a national public utility model as proposed by Etheredge (1997) and Senators Jeffords and Lieberman (S. 1712, 1998). This model would apply the Securities and Exchange Commission model to health care organization and financing. This model accepts the fundamental operation of a market approach. But the model declares there is a primary public interest and a national governmental body must oversee the market to prevent harm (externalities). The model uses government in a less heavy-handed way than direct operational regulation.

The Securities and Exchange Commission (SEC) uses full-time commissioners and staggered five-year terms; ensures adequate and accurate disclosure of information through registration; and has investigative authority and sanctions. A Financial Accounting Standards Board develops standards for financial accounting mandated by the SEC and uses seven full-time members serving five-year terms and an expert advisory committee. Etheredge proposed a National Health Care Market Commission, which would establish and enforce standards in information disclosure and consumer protection and contract with accrediting and regulatory agencies for certification.

Senators Jeffords and Lieberman envision government as an arbiter and clearinghouse for information. Their legislation, S. 1712, would establish a health quality council to advise Congress and the president and develop population-based benchmarks. The council and the Agency for Healthcare Research and Quality, formerly the Agency for Health Care Policy Research (AHCPR), would develop measures for comparing plans, developing standardized reporting forms, and distributing such information to the public.

A public utility model has appeal to many interests. It recognizes the effectiveness and efficiency of marketplace operations. It recognizes the public interest to correct market failures. It recognizes the primacy of consumer knowledge and information to make informed choices. It combines all three domains of accountability into a unified governmental market strategy. It also recognizes that interest group competition will continue.

CONCLUSION

Wilkerson, Devers, and Given (1997) declared: "Society must ultimately decide how it will balance competing values. In case of market-based health care reform, the ultimate question concerns how much efficiency Americans are willing to give up in order to promote a more equitable distribution of health care or how much inequality they are willing to accept in order to promote a more efficient health care system" (pp. 26–27).

Emanuel and Emanuel (1997) advocate a "stratified model" of accountability where "different types of accountability govern different interactions." Given their professional ties to the American Medical Association, they advocate that the physician-patient relationship be entirely governed by the professional model. They argue that the political model should govern the other aspects of accountability.

AMBHA, in actual political practice, is advocating a mixed model using all different types of accountability. AMBHA's emphasis is on the market model, but when the market fails, the political arena must be resorted to. Restoring consumer confidence in health plans at this moment in time requires a political response. But the political response, like all responses, has inherent weaknesses. Emanuel and Emanuel (1997) recognize these weaknesses with the political model—inefficiency, domination by extremists or experts, paralysis, fragmentation dealing with diversity, and stigmatization of minorities.

The current focus is on more traditional regulatory responses. But, "the issue still has time to fizzle. Some polls suggest that the more voters learn about managed care reform, the less they like it. When polls link patient protections with higher costs, support for new HMO regulations goes way down" (Carney, 1998, p. 1558).

Stalemate, even in 2000, an election year, is possible. As Moore (1998) opined: "Make no mistake, this is a battle between two heavyweights, despite the media's refrain that managed care opponents are underdogs taking on the system. When it comes to campaign contributions, the nonphysician providers are outspending the managed care companies" (p. 1518). Spending is more balanced when employer and business spending is added with physician provider spending. But as Center for Responsive Politics research associate Jennifer Shecter observed (in Moore, 1998), "This fight is not David against Goliath" (p. 33). Weissenstein (1998) reported: "With about six months remaining until the November 3 midterm elections, groups that support regulation are spending $2.4 million vs. opponents' expenditures of $1.8 million" (p. 33). Shector (in Bresnahan, 1998) further observed: "A lot of members of PARCA [Patient Access to Responsible Care Act] have been around forever . . . and have always been generous givers. The HMOs are new at this" (p. 10).

Ultimately, Emanuel and Emanuel (1997) are correct: "The choice about which domains of accountability should be made primarily is a value judgment. . . . It is a choice about how to value health care, whether it is a commodity or a nonmarket good, a matter of justice or a community service" (p. 172). A major influence complicating and compromising these judgments will be Alford's (1975) interest group competition dynamics. And last, as Blendon and associates (1998) observed: "Americans must reconcile their demands for lower costs with their demand for unlimited care."

REFERENCES

Advisory Commission on Consumer Protection and Quality in the Health Care Industry. (1997, November). *Consumer bill of rights and responsibilities: Report to the president of the United States*. Washington, DC: Office of the President.

Alford, R. (1975). *Health care politics: Ideological and interest group barriers to reform*. Chicago: The University of Chicago Press.

American Managed Behavioral Healthcare Association. (1999, June 24). *Health plan medical liability—State legislative tracking*. AMBHA's executive director's report 99-55. Washington, DC: AMBHA.

American Managed Behavioral Healthcare Association, National Association of County Behavioral Healthcare Directors, National Association of State Mental Health Directors, and National Community Mental Healthcare Council. (1997, February). Improving public/private partnerships in managed behavioral healthcare. *Behavioral Healthcare Tomorrow, 6*(1), 67–75.

American Psychiatric Association. (1997, September). *General principles for the operation of managed mental health and substance abuse organizations*. Washington, DC: APA.

Arizona to become fifth state with right to sue managed care plans. (2000, April 3). *Managed Care Week*, 1.

Bauer, J.C. (1994). *Not what the doctor ordered: Reinventing medical care in America*. Chicago, IL: Probus.

Blackwell, B. (1998, April 30). "Barriers to the Integration of Behavioral Health Care." Presented at CNR Managed Care Conference, Milwaukee, WI.

Blendon, R.J., Brodie, M., Benson, J.M., Altman, D.E., Levitt, L., Hoff, T., & Hugick, L. (1998, July–August). Understanding the managed care backlash. *Health Affairs, 17*(4), 80–94.

Borzi, P.C., & Rosenbaum, S. (2000, March). *Pending patient protection legislation: A comparative analysis of key provisions of the House and Senate versions of H.R. 2990*.

Washington, DC: George Washington University, Center for Health Services Research and Policy.

Borzo, G. (2000, September). New York poised to post physician profiles: Plan resembles Massachusetts system. *Clinical Psychiatry News*, 35.

Bresnahan, J. (1998, July 13). Healthy donations flow from HMOs and PARCA. *Roll Call*, 10.

Bureau of National Affairs. (1998, March 16). Advisory panel approves final report, hedges on remedies for injured patients. *Health Care Policy Report*, 445–446.

Bureau of National Affairs. (2000a, March 20). Washington governor signs patients rights bill with health plan liability provision. *Health Care Policy Report*, 445.

Bureau of National Affairs. (2000b, May 8). Oklahoma Governor Keating signs bill allowing patients to sue HMOs for medical harm. *Health Care Policy Report*, 735.

Bureau of National Affairs. (2000c, May 22). Texas attorney general issues final rules allowing joint physician bargaining. *Health Care Policy Report*, 834.

Bureau of National Affairs. (2000d, June 21). Senators Jeffords, Frist unveil bill to create safety center, urge reporting. *Health Plan and Provider Report*, 725.

Bureau of National Affairs. (2000e, June 28). Despite deadlock in Congress, states moving forward on key managed care issues. *Health Care Policy Report*, 758–759.

Bureau of National Affairs. (2000f, June 28). Despite deadlock in Congress, states moving forward on key managed care issues. *Health Plan and Provider Report*, 758–759.

Bureau of National Affairs. (2000g, August 5). Health provider bargaining bill passes House by 2-to-1 margin. *Health Plan and Provider Report*, 792–793.

Bureau of National Affairs. (2000h, August 14). Most doctors disciplined for serious offenses not required to stop practicing temporarily. *Health Care Policy Report*, 1395–1396.

Bureau of National Affairs. (2000i, August 28). Commerce chairman plans bill to make physician records public. *Health Care Policy Report*, 1434–1435.

Carney, E.N. (1998, July 4). Bitter medicine. *National Journal*, 1554–1558.

Coffey, R., Mark, T., King, E., Harwood, H., McKusick, D., Genuardi, J., Dilonardo, J., & Buck, J. (2000, July). *National estimates of expenditures for mental health and substance abuse treatment, 1997*. Rockville, MD: Substance Abuse and Mental Health Services Administration.

Cummings, N.A., Pallak, M.S., & Cummings, J.L. (1996). *Surviving the demise of solo practice: Mental health practitioners prospering in the era of managed care*. Madison, CT: Psychosocial Press.

Daniels, N., & Sabin, J. (1998, September–October). The ethics of accountability in managed care reform. *Health Affairs*, 50–64.

Darby, M. (1998, February). *Health care quality: From data to accountability*. Washington, DC: George Washington University, National Health Policy Forum.

Dixon, K. (1998, February). Enough already! Myths and realities of managed behavioral healthcare. *Behavioral Healthcare Tomorrow*, 7(1), 37–41.

Eist, H. (1997, Spring). The scourge of managed care. *Paradigm Magazine*, pp. 10–11.

Elazer, D. (1998). *Covenant and constitutionalism: The great frontier and the matrix of federal democracy.* New Brunswick, NJ: Transaction Publishers.

Emanuel, E.J., & Emanuel, L.L. (1997, February). Preserving community in health care. *Journal of Health Politics, Policy, and Law*, 147–184.

Etheredge, L. (1997, November–December). Promarket regulation: An SEC-FASB model. *Health Affairs, 16*(6), 22–25.

Families U.S.A. (2000, February). *The 106th Congress: How federal managed care legislation affects you.* Washington, DC: Families U.S.A.

Feldstein, P.J. (1980). The political environment of regulation. In A. Levin (Ed.), *Regulating health care: The struggle for control* (pp. 6–20). New York, NY: The Academy of Political Science.

Havel, J.T. (1992). Association and public interest groups as advocates. *Administration and Policy in Mental Health, 20*(1), 27–44.

Institute of Medicine. (1999, December). *To err is human: Building a safer health system.* Washington, DC: IOM.

Kondracke, M. (1998, April 20). Congress is likely to avoid both bad and good on HMOs. *Roll Call*, 5.

Levin, A. (1980). The search for new forms of control. In A. Levin (Ed.), *Regulating health care: The struggle for control* (pp. 1–5). New York, NY: The Academy of Political Science.

Managing care in the public interest. (1995, November 15–16). Paper presented at the Eleventh Annual Rosalynn Carter Symposium on Mental Health, Atlanta, GA.

Mental Health Policy Resource Center, National Association of State Mental Health Program Directors, National Association of Countries, National Association of County Behavioral Health Directors, National Community Mental Healthcare Council, & Technical Assistance Collaborative. (1995). *The public interest: The role of public mental health authorities in the emerging healthcare system.* Alexandria, VA: NASMHPD.

Moore, W.J. (1998, June 27). Playing footsie with health care. *National Journal, 30*(26), 1518.

O'Neil, E., & Finnocchio, L. (1997). The future of the health professions under managed care. In J.D. Wilkerson, K.S. Devers, & R.S. Given (Eds.), *Competitive managed care: The emerging health care system* (pp. 113–135). San Francisco, CA: Jossey-Bass.

Patient Access to Responsible Care Alliance. (1998, February). *Premium impact analysis: H.R. 1415.* Washington, DC: U.S. Congress Budget Office.

Rickards, L.D. (1992). Professional and organized provider associations. *Administration and Policy in Mental Health, 20*(1), 11–26.

Ross, E.C. (1992a). Guest editor's introduction—the role of advocacy groups in mental health. *Administration and Policy in Mental Health, 20*(1), 5–10.

Ross, E.C. (1992b). Success and failure of advocacy groups: a legislative perspective. *Administration and Policy in Mental Health, 20*(1), 57 66.

Ross, E.C. (1997, Fall). Managed behavioral healthcare objectives: Accountability within integrated and coordinated care. *Paradigm Magazine*, 10–11.

S. 1712, 105th Cong., 2d Sess. (1998).

Samuels, D.I. (1996). *Capitation: New opportunities in healthcare delivery*. New York: McGraw-Hill.

Starr, P. (1982). *The social transformation of American medicine: The rise of a sovereign profession and the making of a vast industry*. New York: Basic Books.

Stephens et al. vs. CMG Health et al. (U.S. District Court for the Southern District of New York, 96 Civ 7798) (April 30, 1998 Judge Kimba Wood decision and July 21, 1997 Magistrate Judge Naomi Buchwald Report and Recommendation).

Weissenstein, E. (1998, July 13). Donations heating up: Managed care debate has healthcare organizations opening up their wallets. *Modern Healthcare, 28*(28), 33.

Wilkerson, J.D., Devers, K.S., & Given, R.S. (Eds.). (1997). *Competitive managed care: The emerging health care system*. San Francisco, CA: Jossey-Bass.

Zelman, W.A. (1996). *The changing healthcare marketplace: Private ventures, public interests*. San Francisco, CA: Jossey-Bass.

CHAPTER 14

Concluding Observations

E. Clarke Ross

Purpose: This chapter provides a summary of the major topics covered in this book.

Major Topics: This chapter discusses some of the successes and failures of managed care and describes some of the challenges that face the managed behavioral health care field.

MAJOR ISSUES

The major goals of managed care are to control costs, reduce unnecessary or inappropriate utilization, increase access to preventive care, and maintain or improve quality of care (Edmunds, Frank, Hogan, McCarty, Robinson-Beale, & Weisner, 1997). These are, of course, also the goals of managed behavioral health care, and the chapters in this book have been written to identify the extent to which these goals have been met and to describe the challenges that remain before they can be fully achieved.

Ultimately, in order for managed care, including managed behavioral health care, to work to the full benefit of persons in need, our society must create a seamless system of care. We have to get away from the notion that a person, when privately insured, is entitled to one type of health care but can be reduced, upon the exhaustion of insurance benefits, to a kind of second-class citizen, able to access only a sharply curtailed set of services through a government-sponsored public sector safety net program. We have to move away from the status quo model shown in Figure 14–1 and toward an alternative model of the kind indicated in Figure 14–2.

359

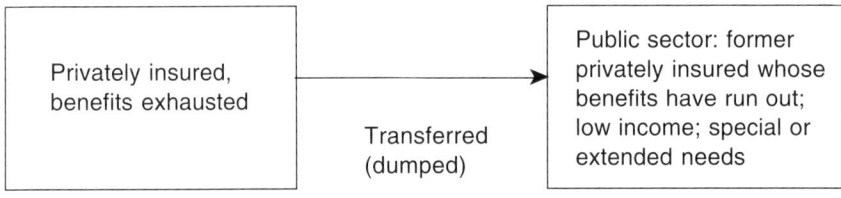

Figure 14–1 Predominant (Status Quo) Private-Public Model. *Source:* From T.R. Watkins and J.W. Callicutt, eds., *Mental Health Policy and Practice Today,* pp. 541–575, © 1996 by Sage Publications, Inc. Reprinted by permission of Sage Publications, Inc.

A single-payer system may not be necessary, but universal insurance coverage based on the use of a single network of providers is clearly in order. The recommendation to bring about such coverage, however, is so controversial that it is not likely to be implemented by this generation of Americans.

ACCOMPLISHMENTS AND CHALLENGES

The managed behavioral health care industry can be justly proud of some of its accomplishments, chief of which is perhaps cost containment. In 1998, one of the managed behavioral health care industry's founders published an article on the "Spectacular Accomplishments and Disappointing Mistakes" of the industry (Cummings, 1998). He cited cost containment, industry growth, saving the mental health benefit, account-

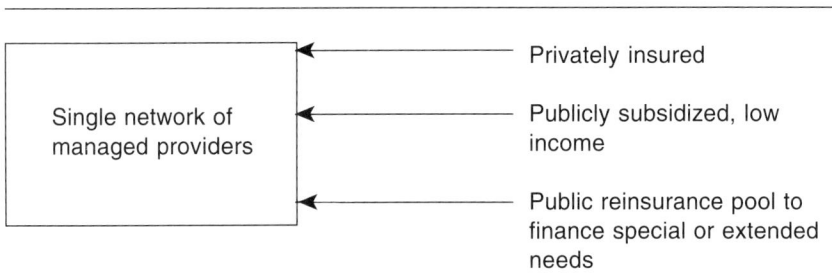

Figure 14–2 Alternative Model. *Source:* From T.R. Watkins and J.W. Callicutt, eds., *Mental Health Policy and Practice Today,* pp. 541–575, © 1996 by Sage Publications, Inc. Reprinted by permission of Sage Publications, Inc.

ability, continuum of care, and self-regulation as the accomplishments. Cummings identified the disappointments as loss of clinical focus, price merger mania, the public relations disaster, competitive paranoia, and integration with primary care. However, as Mechanic and McAlpine (1999) conclude, the "mission" is unfulfilled. Although more persons with mental illness now receive more care and at a uniform level of treatment, the very standardization achieved has undermined care for persons with the most serious forms of mental illness. And whereas some managed care plans have reduced hospitalization and increased alternative services, many other plans have merely reduced hospitalization and increased their profits.

The challenges that remain to be tackled include the following. First, as noted in Chapter 3, the concept of medical necessity, which is central to attempts by managed care organizations to restrict the provision of services and prevent waste of resources, needs to be clarified. Second, the causes of treatment variability (e.g., differences in belief systems and in educational background) need to be understood and addressed so that the care provided to persons with behavioral disorders will be based on evidence and not on accidents of training or location of practice.

Behavioral health care and general health care (primary care) are insufficiently integrated. We remain far from the seamless system of care mentioned above. One of the obstacles to greater integration is the tendency of people to resist giving up traditional ways of doing things, for full integration will entail significant role changes for providers and health plan agents. One of the worst consequences of the lack of integration is that many mental disorders are undetected and undiagnosed. Chapter 4 offers strategies for increasing the integration of care. One of the most important is to increase communication, not only among health professionals but also between health plans and consumers, so that the latter fully understand the benefits to which they are entitled. Other strategies include making health screening more effective, increasing the accountability of behavioral health care providers, modifying payment arrangements to reward improvements in care, making treatment guidelines consistent across managed care organizations, establishing best practices, developing "virtual" systems of care, and improving the education and training of practitioners.

One of the thorniest challenges facing the managed care industry is how to regulate the industry (if at all) and what types of regulation to establish. The latter topic is the focus of Chapter 5, which looks carefully at issues associated with patients' rights. Among the rights that patients arguably possess are the right to appeal an adverse coverage decision, the right to obtain an external review of a coverage decision, the right to obtain an external review of treatment, and the right to a judicial review of coverage decisions or treatment. If these are indeed rights worthy of being respected, regulations will need to be instituted to ensure that they are not infringed upon. As for how to regulate the managed care industry, Chapter 13 recommends looking at a public utility model of regulation. Following this model, the federal government would create an oversight organization resembling the Securities and Exchange Commission to supervise the industry and ensure, through the development of standardized performance measures and reporting forms, that the public will be provided with valid comparisons between health plans and between individual providers. The appeal of this model is that it allows for the efficiency of marketplace operations while recognizing the benefits to be gained by giving consumers the information they need to make informed choices.

If consumers of health care (i.e., enrollees in health plans) want to make informed choices, so do purchasers of health care (the companies and government agencies that contract with health plans for coverage of their employees). One of the difficulties purchasers face is the lack of meaningful outcomes-based quality indicators to help them choose effective health plans with which to contract. As noted in Chapter 6, companies are now trying to fashion their own indicators to make up for this lack. Another frustration companies have is related to the rapid increase in prescription drug costs. Yet, at the same time that they want to control health care costs, they also want to know the value, in terms of health outcomes, of prescription drug use. That is, they recognize that increased use of pharmaceuticals, while it pushes up their health care spending, might actually decrease their total costs by vastly reducing productivity losses (e.g., losses due to employee depression). Public purchasers of health care are also interested in suppressing costs and improving quality, but in addition they look to managed care as a means of enhancing the management and delivery of mental health and substance abuse services, expanding the range of such services, and easing the burden on them of administering public health systems.

As mentioned above, one of the most obvious failings of the managed behavioral health care industry is its poor performance in serving persons with severe mental disorders. Whereas the employed population is generally healthy, the population covered by Medicaid is not, or at least it is much less healthy. Further, the capitation rates that are adequate for covering a basically healthy population will be inadequate for a population with a high proportion of serious illnesses, including severe mental disorders. Managed care organizations thus have an incentive to disenroll such patients or give them insufficient care. Chapter 8 identifies four areas in which public managed care systems have done poorly, especially in regard to treating the seriously ill. Recommended strategies for improvement include increasing the integration of care delivery, ensuring that capitation payments are adequate to cover the needs of the severely ill, increasing provider accountability for treatment outcomes, and fostering meaningful consumer and family participation in operations and decision making.

Another population at special risk consists of persons with addictive disorders. As Chapter 9 states, one challenge facing the managed behavioral health care industry is to increase the provision of clinical, outcomes-driven treatment for this population (replacing older types of treatment, such as complications-driven treatment, which wastes resources by repeatedly treating complications rather than resolving the root problem). To do this, the industry must work toward generating more extensive treatment-outcomes data to provide the basis for true data-driven care. Other challenges include ensuring that authorized services are adequate to meet the needs of the socially deprived (who are at special risk for addictive disorders); that the benefits are suitably flexible (e.g., allow substitution of outpatient session for inpatient days); that care providers understand the nature of addiction denial, resistance, and ambivalence and the value of motivation enhancement; that managed care organizations and providers reach a consensus on practice guidelines, clinical standards, placement criteria, and the like; and that the measurement data collected are used, among other ways, to assess the effectiveness of treatments and determine which should be dropped from the continuum of care.

One of the major changes brought about by the transition to managed care is the increased focus placed on health plan and provider accountability. If a workable set of outcomes measures could be devised and applied, plans and providers could be held accountable for the treatment outcomes they were able to achieve. Further, they could be compared with each other, allowing purchasers and consumers of health care to choose plans and providers with the best track records. As Chapter 10 notes, one of the main obstacles to comparing plans and providers is the proliferation of inconsistent performance measurement systems. As a consequence, leaders in the behavioral health care field have tried to develop a core set of accepted measures. Not surprisingly, the "consensus set" arrived at has some limitations, and in particular it may not adequately address concerns regarding children and persons with addictive disorders.

Even if an adequate set of measures was fashioned, other impediments to implementing full accountability would remain, including the lack of needed performance measurement training among the health care work force, the lack of funds to support performance measurement, and the added technical burden that demands for accountability will place on information management systems. On the other hand, one already existing method of enhancing accountability is to use consumer satisfaction teams to discover what consumers like and dislike about the care they have been given. Chapter 11 presents case studies that illustrate the use of such teams, and it also describes other types of third-party entities, such as facility- and program-monitoring teams and ombudsman programs, that can be employed to increase the accountability of health plans and providers.

An important question is whether provider-sponsored organizations are able to successfully manage care. The question arises because providers in the past, during the fee-for-service era, had an incentive to increase the number of billable encounters and were seemingly responsible for the overutilization of health care resources. Nonetheless, the results of a survey of behavioral health provider-sponsored organizations indicate that such organizations can indeed manage care successfully. This claim is further defended in the conclusion of Chapter 12, which cites certain characteristics of provider-sponsored organizations that give these organizations an advantage over other managed care organizations when it comes to the efficient provision of health services.

SUMMARY

As shown above, managed care, including managed behavioral care, faces a range of challenges. In some areas, it has not been as successful as some proponents had hoped; in other areas, it has not been as disastrous as some critics had feared. In any case, managed care is here to stay, at least for the foreseeable future.

As medical ethicists Philip Boyle and Daniel Callahan (1995) remark, "Our contention is that managed care is inevitable, but this need be no more morally troubling than the present fee-for-service mental health system. If anything, attempts to manage care are or could be less morally doubtful" (p. 11). Later, in the same article, they claim, "To the extent that managed mental health care is making, and continues to make, good-faith attempts to curb abuses, rectify ethical problems, and address treatment effectiveness issues, it should prove superior in the whole to fee-for-service medicine" (p. 20).

REFERENCES

Boyle, P., & Callahan, D. (1995, Fall). Managed care and mental health: The ethical issues. *Health Affairs, 14*(3), 7–22.

Cummings, N. (1998, August). Spectacular accomplishments and disappointing mistakes: The first decade of managed behavioral health care. In *Behavioral Healthcare Tomorrow.* (pp. 61–63). Tiburon, CA: CentraLink.

Edmunds, M., Frank, F., Hogan, M., McCarty, D., Robinson-Beale, R., & Weisner, C. (Eds.). (1997). *Managing managed care: Quality improvement in behavioral health.* Washington, DC: National Academy Press.

Mechanic, D., & McAlpine, D.D. (1999, September–October). Mission unfulfilled: Potholes on the road to mental health parity. *Health Affairs, 18*(5), 7–21.

INDEX

A

Access to care
  addictive disorders, 253
  quality measurement, 282, 288
Accountability
  domains in health services, 338–339
  as managed care issue, 16–19
  See also Health interest groups; Third-party accountability
Actuarial cost models, 34–38
  data sources for development of, 36–38
  examples of, 40–41
  general rules, 35–36
  patient data requirements, 35
Addictive disorders
  access to care, 253
  Alcoholics Anonymous, 242
  American Society of Addiction Medicine (ASAM) diagnostic criteria, 233, 243, 248, 254
  assessment dimensions, 243
  attitudes about addicted persons, 230
  benchmark development, 78
  case management, 244, 246–247
  clinically-driven treatment, 232–235
  complications, treatment of, 227–229
  disease management, 239–241
  dual diagnosis, 247, 249–250
  improvement of service, basis of, 244–246, 258–262
  outcomes-driven treatment, 235–239
  outcomes issues in treatment, 257–258

performance measures, 237–239
  and primary care detection, 77
  process issues in treatment, 253–256
  program-driven treatment, 229–232
  service delivery sectors, 249–250
  structural issues, 250–251
  treatment failure, 226–229
Administrative performance, 187
  levels for improvement, 188
Administrative services, 43–44
Administrative services organizations (ASOs), function of, 3
Advisory Commission on Consumer Protection and Quality
  consumer bill of rights, 111, 122–123
  consumer protection, areas of, 348–349
Agency for Healthcare Research and Quality, 107, 353
Alcoholics Anonymous (AA), 242
ALERT system, outcome management, 88–89
Allies and Adversaries: The Impact of Managed Care on Mental Health Services (Schreter, Sharfstein, and Schreter), 20
American College of Mental Health Administration (ACMHA), 17
  development of quality measures, 273–277, 281, 284–285, 290
  value statements of, 269–270
American Managed Behavioral Healthcare Association (AMBHA), 17, 202–204
  on attributes of managed behavioral health care, 202–203

367

About the Editor

E. Clarke Ross, DPA, is the chief executive officer for Children and Adults with Attention-Deficit/Hyperactivity Disorder, Inc. (CHADD). Dr. Ross previously served as deputy executive director for public policy for the National Alliance for the Mentally Ill; executive director, American Managed Behavioral Healthcare Association; deputy executive director, National Association of State Mental Health Program Directors; and director, Government Activities Office, United Cerebral Palsy Associations. For two years, Dr. Ross served as assistant professor of public administration, Troy State University—European Region, Weisbaden, Germany. He holds adjunct faculty rank at the University of Maryland and Central Michigan University. His doctorate in public administration is from The George Washington University.

ABOUT THE CONTRIBUTORS

Neal Adams, MD, MPH, currently serves as director for Santa Cruz County Mental Health and Substance Abuse Services. Previously he was medical director for the New Mexico Division of Mental Health. In these roles, Dr. Adams functions as a clinical administrator involved in program and policy development as well as quality management and daily operations. He has taught treatment planning at CARF, the Rehabilitation Accreditation Commission's annual international meetings for the behavioral health division as well as provided training to a wide range of clinical organizations, including adult and child mental health and substance abuse treatment settings. In addition to his current administrative duties, Dr. Adams serves on numerous committees and boards. He serves as an accreditation surveyor for CARF, a utilization review physician for a national behavioral managed care company, and is a member of the Mental Health Statistics Improvement Project (MHSIP) Policy Group. Dr. Adams is president-elect of the American College of Mental Health Administration and is chair of its Workgroup on Quality Measurement. In addition, he has been part of the National Association of State Mental Health Program Directors (NASMHPD) President's Task Force on Performance and Outcome Measures Technical Workgroup and serves on CARF's Advisory Council on Performance Measurement.

Dr. Adams received his MD from Northwestern University in 1978; he also received his MPH from Harvard University that same year. Following completion of his residency in psychiatry at Stanford University, he participated in the Robert Wood Johnson Clinical Scholar Program.

Christy L. Beaudin, PhD, LCSW, CPHQ, is the corporate director of quality improvement at PacifiCare Behavioral Health. Dr. Beaudin earned her doctorate in health services research from the UCLA School of Public Health and master's of social work from San Diego State University. She has served at the vice-president level with other behavioral health care organizations and has worked extensively as a consultant, health services researcher, and program administrator. In addition to evaluation research projects, Dr. Beaudin has completed needs assessments for nonprofit organizations, health care systems, and state Medicaid programs. She is widely published and serves as a reviewer for five peer-reviewed publications.

Martin D. Cohen, MSW, is the founding president/chief executive officer of the MetroWest Community Health Care Foundation, an independent philanthropy serving the unmet health care needs of a 25-town area west of Boston. Prior to joining the foundation Mr. Cohen served as the executive director and senior consultant of the Technical Assistance Collaborative, Inc. (TAC), a national health and human services consulting firm. While at TAC, Mr. Cohen focused much of his work on issues of governance in state and local mental health authorities and the use of managed care in behavioral health services. Mr. Cohen previously served as a deputy director and program director with the Robert Wood Johnson Foundation and was a deputy assistant secretary in the Massachusetts Executive Office of Human Services. He is on the faculty of the Harvard Medical School Department of Psychiatry.

Allen S. Daniels, EdD, LISW, is the chief executive officer for Alliance Behavioral Care, a regional managed behavioral health care organization. He also is the executive director for University Psychiatric Services, a multidisciplinary behavioral group practice. Both of these organizations are affiliated with the department of psychiatry at the University of Cincinnati. Dr. Daniels is a graduate of The University of Chicago School of Social Services Administration and the University of Cincinnati. Dr. Daniels is a professor of clinical psychiatry at the University of Cincinnati, College of Medicine. As the chief executive officer of Alliance Behavioral Care, Dr. Daniels has established one of the largest and most successful academically based managed care programs. His leadership in the managed care community has been recognized by his election as chair of the American Managed Behavioral Healthcare Association. This is the trade association for the managed behavioral health care industry, and its member companies serve over 100 million lives. As the executive director of University Psychiatric Services, Dr. Daniels has established a successful, academically based behavioral group practice. His leadership in group practice operations has been recognized by his appointment as the chair of the Council of Behavioral Group Practices and his appointment to the board of the Association of Behavioral Group Practices. In 1995, Dr. Daniels received the Annual Commitment to Excellence award from the Council of Behavioral Group Practices. This award recognized the development of a national outcomes assessment program for group practices and managed care organizations. Dr. Daniels has extensively published in the area of managed care and group practice operations, quality improvement and clinical outcomes, and academic health care. He has consulted both nationally and internationally on these subjects.

Stephen L. Day, MSW, is co-founder and executive director of the Technical Assistance Collaborative, Inc. He has provided consulting services to over 30 state and local mental health and human service agencies on a variety of issues from organizational change to managed behavioral health care. He has assisted mental health authorities in Georgia, North Carolina, South Carolina, Pennsylvania, Washington, Ohio, Oklahoma, Iowa, Texas, Connecticut, and Michigan in their preparation for managed care initiatives. Mr. Day has assisted these and other public and nonprofit organizations in developing and implementing organizational, service system, and financing innovations in support of state-of-the-art community services for people with serious mental illness and other disabilities. He specializes in organizational development and management, strategic planning, and consumer-based outcome and performance measurement. Mr. Day previously served as deputy commissioner of mental health and as assistant secretary for the executive office of elder affairs health for the Commonwealth of Massachusetts.

Veronica V. Goff, MS, is a principal with the Business Health Network. Previously she was vice president for the Washington Business Group on Health (WBGH), a nonprofit health policy organization representing the nation's largest employers. Ms. Goff oversaw all facets of administration and day-to-day operations for WBGH. She also led the Health and Productivity Management Initiative and Depression Awareness, Recognition, and Treatment (D/ART) National Worksite Program, a cooperative initiative of

WBGH and the National Institute of Mental Health to identify workplace and health system practices that reduce the costly impact of depression. Before joining WBGH in 1989, Ms. Goff was a research associate at the University of Virginia Health Sciences Center. She worked for AT&T, supervising a Chicago-based corporate health promotion facility and was marketing director for a shared-use corporate health promotion facility in Richmond, Virginia. Ms. Goff holds a master of science degree and a bachelor of science degree in education from Southern Illinois University.

Daniel Lieberman, MD, is the northeast regional medical director for ValueOptions, Inc., a major national behavioral health care organization. He has been a senior medical director with the two largest behavioral health care companies in the country over the past decade. He is currently involved in program development and innovative clinical delivery initiatives for behavioral health care for ValueOptions. Dr. Lieberman is a board-certified child/adolescent and adult psychiatrist. He is a formally trained short-term dynamic psychotherapist for the New York Institute for Short-Term Dynamic Psychotherapy. Dr. Lieberman has been a surveyor for the National Committee for Quality Assurance since 1994, where he also served on the scoring Task Force for Behavioral Healthcare.

David Mee-Lee, MD, is involved in full-time training and consulting focused on developing and promoting innovative behavioral health treatment that values clinical integrity, quality, and cost-consciousness. He is a board-certified psychiatrist with added qualifications in addiction psychiatry and addiction medicine. Dr. Mee-Lee is an assistant clinical professor, University of California at Davis, School of Medicine, Department of Psychiatry. He is chair of the Criteria Committee (and Standards and Economics of Care Section) of the American Society of Addiction Medicine (ASAM). Dr. Mee-Lee's clients include both provider and practitioner groups, as well as managed care organizations. (He is a consultant to managed care companies, where he assists in shaping and teaching corporate policy on addictions treatment.) Dr. Mee-Lee was a consultant in the first major managed care Medicaid project for substance abuse in Massachusetts, as well as public sector managed substance abuse care in Iowa.

Stephen P. Melek, FSA, MAAA, is a principal and consulting actuary with the Denver office of Milliman & Robertson, Inc. His areas of expertise include health care product development, management, and financial analysis. He has experience with plan design, pricing, capitation and risk analysis, reimbursement analysis and strategies, health care revenue distribution, and utilization management analysis. He has worked extensively in the behavioral health care specialty field. He has advised hospitals, physician groups, physician-hospital organizations, health maintenance organizations, preferred provider organizations, managed care organizations, behavioral health care firms and associations, insurance companies, employers, and state insurance departments. He is a graduate of the Illinois Institute of Technology, a fellow of the Society of Actuaries, a member of the American Academy of Actuaries, and a master fellow of the Life Office Management Association.

John A. Morris, MSW, CHE, has devoted his professional career to public mental health. Beginning as a ward attendant at the South Carolina State Hospital, he has served in a number of capacities in two state systems, finally serving a 20-month interim appointment as state director of mental health for South Carolina. Since 1997, he has been teaching and doing research at the USC School of Medicine as Professor of Neuropsychiatry and Behavioral Science. In early 2000, he was named the first director of the South Carolina Center for Innovation in Public Mental Health. At the time of this writing, he is serving a two-year term as president of the American College of Mental Health Administration. He serves as an advisor on behavioral health performance indicators to CARF, the Rehabilitation Accreditation Commission and to the National Committee for Quality Assurance (NCQA). He is a member of the National Advisory Councils for the Technical Assistance Center for Children's Mental Health at Georgetown University and for the Kentucky Center for Mental Health Studies.

Charles G. Ray, MEd, is currently the president and chief executive officer of the National Council for Community Behavioral Healthcare (formerly the National Community Mental Healthcare Council), based in Rockville, Maryland. He is known nationally for his ability to inspire and motivate audiences while explaining intricate health care concepts. He is particularly adept at facilitating complex negotiations among groups with overlapping (and sometimes competing) visions and missions, at strategic planning and positioning, at political strategizing, and at design of health care delivery systems. Known for his articulate speeches, he also is a superb executive coach and systems consultant. His role as national council president and chief executive officer involves him with federal, regional, state, and local organizations regarding provision of behavioral health services, strategic planning, public policy, and program development.

Sara Rosenbaum, JD, is the Harold and Jane Hirsh Professor of Health Law and Policy at the School of Public Health and Health Services, The George Washington University. Ms. Rosenbaum also directs the Center for Health Services Research and Policy and the Hirsh Health Law and Policy Program at The George Washington University. From 1993 to 1994, Ms. Rosenbaum served as a consultant to the White House Domestic Policy Council and directed the drafting of the Health Security Act. Prior to joining the faculty at The George Washington University in 1992, Ms. Rosenbaum was a legal services attorney and later worked for the Children's Defense Fund, where she directed its health work and later its department of programs and policies. She has authored numerous studies, reports, and journal articles in the areas of maternal and child health, health care financing, civil rights, health care for the medically underserved, health insurance, and managed care. She is co-author of *Law and the American Health Care System*, published by Foundation Press.

Ian A. Shaffer, MD, MMM, is the executive vice president and chief operating officer of University Alliance for Behavioral Care, Inc. in Reno, Nevada. Previously he was the executive vice president for quality and outcome strategies at ValueOptions and chief medical officer responsible for clinical services. He is a child and adolescent psychiatrist, board certified in psychiatry, addiction medicine, and utilization review and quality assurance. Trained at the University of Manitoba in Canada and the University of Southern California, he spent 18 years in private practice before becoming the chief medical officer for American PsychManagement, a predecessor company to ValueOptions. He is a member of the National Advisory Committee for the Center for Mental Health Services and the National Committee for Quality Assurance subcommittee on managed behavioral health. He was the chairman of the American Managed Behavioral Healthcare Association (AMBHA).

Joel B. Teitelbaum, JD, LLM, is an assistant research professor of health services management and policy at the School of Public Health and Health Services, The George Washington University. Mr. Teitelbaum is also the associate director of the Hirsh Health Law and Policy Program, specializing in legal and policy issues in the areas of managed care, Medicaid, behavioral health, and civil rights. Prior to joining The George Washington University in 1997, Mr. Teitelbaum worked for a private law firm and the Children with Special Health Needs Law Project, both in Milwaukee, Wisconsin.

Jerome V. Vaccaro, MD, is president and chief executive officer of PacifiCare Behavioral Health, Inc. He is a board-certified psychiatrist and associate clinical professor of psychiatry at UCLA's School of Medicine. He was the chairman of the American Managed Behavioral Healthcare Association (AMBHA) in 1999, and he is the author of *Practicing Psychiatry in the Community,* published by American Psychiatric Press, Inc. This textbook, hailed as the definitive text in community psychiatry, has been translated into three languages. He has published articles in leading mental health publications including the *American Journal of Psychiatry, Community Mental Health Journal, Journal of Addictive Diseases, Discharge Planning and Psychiatry, Hospital and Community Psychiatry, Handbook of Psychiatric Rehabilitation, Alcoholism Treatment Quarterly, New Directions in Mental Health,* and *Behavioral Healthcare Tomorrow.* Dr. Vaccaro has been named in several editions of *Who's Who,* was honored as one of its "750 Best Physicians in America," and was named by *Los Angeles Magazine* as one of Los Angeles's best physicians.